PRAISE FOR
*NATURE, OUR MEDICINE*

"No surprise that Dr Dimity Williams brings her nurturing nature as a compassionate GP, a wonderful mother and nature lover to this honest, heartfelt and healing book. Through her scientific expertise, life experience and common sense, she doesn't sugar coat the challenges but also leaves the reader hopeful with practical solutions from making space in our lives for nature, inspiring the next generation, and even writing nature prescriptions for her patients. Immerse yourself in its pages like one of the beautiful forest baths Dr Williams describes."

Dr Grant Blashki, Lead Clinical Adviser, Beyond Blue
Associate Professor in Global Health University of Melbourne

"With an engaging and unique blend of medical knowledge and passion for the natural world, Dr Williams reminds us we are not above nature, but that our health is intimately connected to that of the planet and all living things...and that we ignore this at our peril."

Associate Professor Marion Carey, Public Health Physician

"A comprehensively researched, powerful book that will leave no reader in doubt of the inextricable link between our health, our wellbeing and humanity's life support system – Earth. A planet of once thriving ecosystems that now urgently needs each and every one of us to care for, nurture, and protect. Our health depends on it, as Dr Williams convincingly argues through her book whilst reminding us all: 'If not us then who? If not now, then when?'"

Dr Eugenie Kayak, anaesthetist
Enterprise Professor in Sustainable Healthcare University of Melbourne

"Incredibly timely. This impactful book should be required reading. Dr Dimity Williams articulates everything that has been needed to be said and has been ignored for too long. We have bought into a way of living that has deteriorated our humanity which has resulted in a major health crisis. May everyone read this, leave their screens and start re-engaging with nature. Your health will thank you for it!"

Julie Postance, author of *Breaking the Sound Barriers*

"This book is riveting, essential reading in these times. We've lost our way in this world and lost our connection to the earth. This book is a signpost back. It highlights how imperative nature is for health, wellbeing, and healing. Humanity has spent generations moving out of nature and into technology. It's time we returned."

Suze Male, writer and yoga teacher

# DR DIMITY WILLIAMS

Dr Dimity Williams is a mother, nature lover, and family doctor. Following her medical degree, she completed further training to become a fellow of the Royal Australian College of General Practitioners. She has worked as a Family Physician for 25 years in inner Melbourne on Wurundjeri Country, and enjoys looking after the whole person from pre-conception to old age. Dimity has completed additional training in obstetrics, paediatrics and mental health, particularly mindfulness meditation.

She has worked in environmental advocacy with multiple organisations from grassroots community groups to large associations. Dimity is an alumna of the Centre for Sustainability Leadership, a co-founder of the Kids In Nature Network, and founder of Doctors for the Environment Australia's Biodiversity Special Interest Group. Passionate about integrating nature into healthcare, she has written and spoken about the 'nature: health interface' in various forums and delights in issuing nature prescriptions. A wish for all children to have every opportunity to experience, love and look after nature guides her.

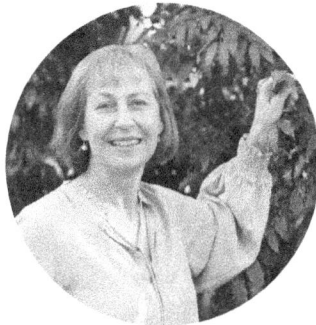

# NATURE,
*Our*
# MEDICINE

Published in Australia by
Currawong Books
Level 1, 12-14 Glenferrie Road, Malvern. Victoria. 3144
Email: info@natureourmedicine.com
Website: www.natureourmedicine.com

First published in Australia 2023
Copyright © Dimity Williams 2023

National Library of Australia Cataloguing in Publication entry

A catalogue record for this book is available from the National Library of Australia

ISBN: 978-0-6455092-0-5 (paperback)
ISBN: 978-0-6455092-1-2 (hardback)
ISBN: 978-0-6455092-2-9 (epub)

Cover layout and design by John Bryll Pulido
Photos by Shutterstock and Andrew Edwards
Interior layout and design by Sophie White
Printed by Ingram Spark

Although every effort has been made to ensure that the contents of this book are accurate, it must not be treated as a substitute for qualified medical advice. Always consult a qualified medical practitioner. Neither the author nor the publisher can be held responsible for any loss or claim arising out of the use, or misuse, of the suggestions made or the failure to take advice.

All contact details given in this book were current at the time of publication, but are subject to change.

**Currawong Books acknowledges the Traditional Custodians of the country on which we work, the Wurundjeri Woi-wurrung people of the Kulin Nation and recognises their continuing connection to the land, waters and culture. We pay our respects to their Elders past, present and emerging.**

# NATURE,

## *Our*

# MEDICINE

*How the natural world sustains us*

DR DIMITY WILLIAMS

*To all who love and look after nature,*

*especially those on the front lines.*

# AUTHOR'S NOTE

*This book touches on grief and suicide and contains historical references which include racist slurs. Please read it with self-care and if any of the content raises issues for you, seek support from friends or trained professionals.*

*The name of a deceased First Nations person is used, and I wish to thank Amos and Eban Roach for providing permission for their father's name and work to be referred to at this sad time.*

*For authenticity and voice this book uses Australian English grammar and conventions.*

*Dimity*

# CONTENTS

# FOREWORD

*Nature, Our Medicine* takes me back to my first rafting trip down Tasmania's Franklin River in 1976. I was a General Practitioner in Launceston and had been struck by how many of my patients' maladies like hypertension, skin rashes and insomnia were fuelled by anxiety. Valium had become the drug of choice. I found in the Franklin's waterfalls, sea eagles, platypuses, ferny side-canyons and, at night, glowworms, starry skies and ringtail possums whistling in the riverside forest, a spiritual uplift that no drug could emulate. So why drown it all behind a dam to make more electricity to power more tranquilliser factories? In the following years, I left direct medical practice to concentrate on environmental activism – that is, preventative medicine. Keeping what is left of nature is keeping the best storehouse for human mental and physical wellbeing that was or ever will be.

Dr Dimity Williams brings science and experience to the simple proposition that nature is humanity's best restorative. She explains why taking nature out of our lives is at the expense of health and happiness and how putting it back is cost-free and easy.

This birthright was stolen by capitalism, which perceives nature as best used by its conversion into share market dividends. However, our re-immersion in nature offers personal dividends that are not available in any stock exchange.

Every child has the right to time and space to play in nature, as children had for millions of years before our industrialisation. Modern urban society with its ear buds, screens, artificial noise and light, manufactured smells and endless concrete has robbed children of nature.

Dr Williams quotes educator David Sobel: "let us allow them to love the Earth before we ask them to save it". She has a simple recipe: "Bush kinders, kitchen gardens and outdoor learning and adventure for young people accessible throughout their lives".

She calls for a nature-fuelled revolution and lays out how easily everyone can be part of it – from installing a window box to regular visits to the local park or bushland, to spending days in a wilderness like Tasmania's Tarkine Rainforest.

But why be bothered? Because the personal health benefits are real and your happiness quotient, in the only life you'll ever live, will go up and stay up if you are 'bathed in nature'. Just as clean air, chemical-free food and pure water are guarantees of a healthier body, so regular time amongst trees or the waves ensures a healthier, happier mind.

In what Dr Williams calls the 'tsunami of anxiety', nature is better and cheaper for us than reaching for another beer, cigarette or chocolate.

Sigmund Freud's Industrial Age dictum that "nature is externally remote. She destroys us – coldly, cruelly and relentlessly" is being turned on its head as medicine returns to the reality that nature cures because it is essential to our being. 'She' breathes life into us – offering warmth and happiness, without limit. As Dr Williams puts it, "nature is an intrinsic part of human wellbeing rather than separate from it".

Williams compares and contrasts the closed-off 'windscreen view of your suburb' with the First Nations connection to country. This book is not about us reverting to live in the wilds but it expounds the common sense that we have a great deal to gain from more time spent in natural settings.

Here is a U-turn in modern medicine on the delivery of human health and wellbeing. While prescription medicines can be life savers, none has the benefits of nature.

A free walk in the local woods or dunes or by the riverside has no debilitating side-effects, is in tune with our instincts, and reconnects with the world which evolved our minds and bodies.

*Nature, Our Medicine* is a life-changing proposition. It takes us through the rapids of our high-stress world to the calming balm of nature – just like rafting the Franklin.

Bob Brown

# PREFACE

After we've unpacked the car, I walk down to the beach. My footsteps are quiet as I pad through the ancient, gnarled trees sheltering behind the dunes. The breeze carries the ocean's brine and the scent of gumtrees and saltbush. It flows warm and gentle across my face. I breathe deeply. Tilting forward, I make my way under the twisted trunks and along the sandy track winding through the grove and over the sand dune. Before reaching the beach there's a gully filled with the thin, sparse branches of tea trees. The ground is a carpet of their tiny green leaves. It is still here. Quiet. The sound of the sea diminished to a gentle rumble. I pause and notice little brown birds flitting amongst the foliage, seemingly oblivious to my presence. Their tinkling chirrups make me smile.

I push on, keen to get to the water, and emerge into the fading sunlight behind the last sand ridge. Shucking off my shoes, the sand is cool and fine between my toes and the view is breathtaking. Creamy dunes are studded with grasses, delicate silvery plants and yellow flowers. Their undulating forms flow into the distance as far as I can see up and down the beach. Looking south, the ocean swells denim blue to the horizon while along the shoreline wavelets are frilled as if with lace. The sun slowly drops to the water and as it does the sky turns golden, fringing clouds iridescent. A mist hangs low, shimmering like a veil. Seagulls swoop and dive, seizing their dinner.

The dark shape moving along the water's edge, catching waves, seems like a surfer at first. It's a seal, riding wave after wave, its body twisting and turning in the current. The creature moves along the shoreline slowly getting farther and farther away, until eventually it's out of sight. I nestle into the dune. Here, protected from the wind, the sand is still warm from the day. I lie back, sighing as my head sinks to the ground. My mind clears and my breathing and heart rate slow as my body shifts into its relaxed state. If nature is medicine, this is a bolus dose infused into my bloodstream. I feel at home, held by Earth, lulled by her rhythms and profoundly connected to the life around me.

# INTRODUCTION

It may seem strange for a scientifically trained medical doctor to regard nature as medicine. Yet many years of work and study as a doctor and in advocacy for environmental protection and community change have brought me to this view. Experiences like the encounter with a surfing seal have allowed me to feel for myself the profound sense of rejuvenation that comes from being deeply immersed in nature.

This book brings together all I have learnt about the natural world and how it provides the wellspring of healing desperately needed right now. It also outlines the precarious and fragile state of Earth's biome, the complex layer of life we live in. Pulling together information from scientific and medical journals, public health and other experts and translating it into a more digestible format, I hope to pique your curiosity and encourage you to deepen your relationship with nature into one of reciprocity and care. To begin, I'd like to share a little of my own journey, from white coats and stethoscopes to forest bathing and nature prescriptions.

As a university student in the 1990s I was taught what, at the time, was a progressive view of human health. For rather than just focussing on the body and its systems, we were encouraged to think of the psychological and social determinants of health—how our thoughts, emotions, social situation and living conditions affect our physical body. Factors like poverty, home life, and access to education and employment were all understood to influence if and how illness arose in individuals and communities. So, along with enquiring about physical and psychological symptoms, we were instructed to ask patients about their home and work life and social practises. This helped us formulate a clear picture of why a person was seeking our help and how we may best alleviate their suffering.

During this time the AIDS epidemic was sweeping the globe and famine was devastating Africa. These events shaped our understanding of how human behaviour and social shifts on a grand scale affected the health of individuals. We learnt that the human immunodeficiency virus (HIV) had arisen as a zoonosis—an infection which jumps from another species into humans. The virus had crossed from primates to people living in Central Africa and then throughout the world, infecting and killing millions. It is thought human exposure to blood and other secretions from the hunting of apes for food facilitated the virus' transmission. Bushmeat hunting had been a longstanding practice in pockets of rural sub-Saharan Africa. However, with the rise of industrial logging, remote areas of forest became accessible for the first time and the extraction of timber and bushmeat amplified habitat destruction for these apes. While social and economic forces were key, ultimately it was the disruption of the natural separation between populations of people and primates which was responsible for the generation of this new zoonosis. The loss of the protective environmental buffer provided by the rainforest allowed these different species to come together in a new and profoundly unhealthy way.

Elsewhere in Africa, severe drought and crop failures, together with prolonged armed conflict and poverty, provided the perfect storm for the Ethiopian famine. Once again, the combination of eroded natural ecosystems and the human tendencies toward greed and conflict led to catastrophic outcomes for health. To simply provide emergency aid and medical treatments, without also investigating and addressing the underlying social and environmental factors would see the cycle repeat, both within Africa and throughout the world.

Even though some academics at the time were highlighting the life support systems provided by nature to humans, describing them as ecosystem services, this knowledge was not imparted to us aspiring doctors. Learning about human health without considering these broader factors made our medical education seem incomplete. I left university having been taught that health and the natural environment were separate domains but deep down I knew this to be untrue. I had always felt my wellbeing was inextricably linked to, and dependent upon, nature.

Over the ensuing decades, having worked in hospitals and the community, I have come to think about health through a much wider lens. Many years in general practice, where entire families are known and cared for throughout life's phases, has shaped my perspective. I've also learnt to zoom out from the 'street view' of the individual sitting in front of me to take in the 'Earth view'. To see the vast environmental forces which shape human wellbeing. During this time, alongside my parenting journey, the spectres of climate change and ecological destruction have arisen, disrupting everything.

Having children unearthed memories of my own childhood. This prompted me to notice troubling changes in seasonal weather patterns. My sons were young during the millennial drought. So, they had no experience of the seemingly endless, drenching rains of a Melbourne winter that had contextualised my childhood. Instead, they grew up with a bucket in the shower to catch water for the garden as this precious resource was carefully rationed. Trees, which had blossomed in the springtime of my 1970s' primary school years were now flowering weeks earlier, in late winter. The changes I was observing in the natural environment were compelling, and I sought to understand them by reading the work of climate and ecological scientists. What I learnt about global warming, the threat it posed to all life on Earth and how it could compromise my children's future was deeply distressing. But the most shocking thing of all was the ignorance and passivity of our leaders, and of their possible corruption.

I was not alone with my concerns; other parents were also noticing the changing climate and worried about the future for their children and the natural places they loved. Naively, I thought once our politicians understood the science of climate change and how it threatened every aspect of our lives, especially our health, they would act. Along with other parents, I formed a community climate action group to raise awareness and impress upon our local member of parliament the need for urgent action. Over the following years we held many meetings, colourful public events and direct actions in parks and out the front of parliamentarian's offices. I even loaned our political representative Tim Flannery's book explaining climate science and the solutions needed to stop the unfolding climate catastrophe. The Federal Treasurer returned the book with a polite note of thanks but no positive action followed. Perversely, when publicly challenged on his government's poor climate policies he said, "in 2030, we'll all be dead anyway".

Despite the frustration of political intransigence in the face of looming climate catastrophe and the psychological toll of this activism, there was great strength to be found in standing side by side with others in peaceful protest. There were also times of levity and bemusement at the absurd over-reaction from authorities to a small group of suburban mothers and their children disrupting the peace. The wry smile of one of the five federal police officers called to monitor our presence outside our local member's office will stay with me for a long time. And walking through the city streets with tens of thousands of other concerned citizens singing and chanting and sometimes silent in peaceful collectivism can be uplifting. These moments sustain those of us who push for change against a system beholden to the extractive industries and the money and power they wield. As a parent, I felt it important my children knew their future was something worth fighting for. And that peaceful protest could be modelled with dignity and good humour. However, after several years I felt my efforts to create change only through this approach had been exhausted. I decided to switch tack, turning towards my colleagues in medicine.

It was heartening and motivating to discover an organisation of like-minded doctors. Doctors for the Environment Australia (DEA), a group of many hundreds of doctors and medical students, works to highlight the relationship between health and the natural environment. It's a diverse organisation, with members from all facets of the profession and a rich variety of backgrounds. Those from rural communities sit beside their urban colleagues. That doctors would see the interaction between nature and medicine is not a new idea, even though it wasn't on the curriculum during my time at university. The first physicians of the Western tradition had physic gardens where they cultivated medicines. And historically mental health and infectious disease hospitals were situated in the countryside for the fresh air and restorative benefits of nature. Still today, over half of all pharmaceuticals in use have come from the natural world. And it was doctors who highlighted the health dangers from environmental threats like exposure to coal, asbestos, industrial chemicals and nuclear weapons.

It is hardly surprising the medical profession is once again agitating for action on environmental dangers, climate change chief among them. The highly regarded medical journal, The Lancet, in their Commission on Climate Change in 2009 stated, "climate change is the biggest global health threat of the 21st century." What these experts were outlining was how the global environmental problem of climate change was a more significant risk to human health than infectious diseases, cancer, heart disease and the myriad of other illnesses and conditions preoccupying health systems throughout the world.

Our health depends upon us living in a stable climate because we have evolved within this planetary context. So, too, has the plant and animal life we rely upon.

The ecosystem services provided by nature are essential for life as we know it. Earth's vast and complex natural systems ensure we have clean air, plentiful fresh water and diverse land and sea ecologies which provide our food, medicines, and shelter. A warming shift in the planet's temperature has disrupted its equilibrium and the effects are devastating for all life. Climate change has increased the frequency and intensity of severe weather events like heatwaves, bushfires, droughts, floods, cyclones and storms. These catastrophes not only kill millions of people directly, they also cause secondary health harms by changing patterns of infectious diseases, contaminating air and water, reducing food sources and generating psychological distress. As well as these disasters, climate change has altered seasonal temperatures and rainfall patterns. In turn, flowering and fruiting times of plants have shifted, changing the behaviour of animals who rely on them for food. A warming Earth has also seen global loss of ice with shrinking polar ice caps and retreating glaciers. This is accompanied by sea level rise which threatens low-lying communities. In these many ways, global warming is a profound and urgent threat to the health of all people.

Alongside my medical practice, I worked for years with DEA to raise awareness of the dangers posed by climate change and coal pollution to the health of local and global communities. This involved collaborating with others to write submissions to government enquiries, articles for medical magazines and the mainstream press, meeting politicians and giving presentations to peers and the wider community. It was a marathon effort, and like an endurance race, it was exhausting. I started to feel burnt out, tired of trying to explain things to people they didn't want to hear. Of striving to get them to care about something vital and yet seemingly too complex and confronting for them to engage with.

During this period, I fell in love with the Tarkine/takayna rainforest in Tasmania. This incredible place is gradually being eroded by logging and mining projects. Ancient stands of myrtle beech and pristine rivers are decimated for minerals and timber with the encouragement of government. I travelled there twice, with two different environmental organisations, trying to raise awareness of its plight. My companions were other concerned citizens, everyday people from all walks of life. Together we made a short film, met with protestors living high in the canopy and shared our stories with the media and our networks. My middle son accompanied me on the first trip and we spent his thirteenth birthday deep within the cathedral-like forest. This experience was transformative, invigorating me to keep trying.

My focus shifted to biodiversity, the rich variety of life on Earth and how it forms the foundation for our wellbeing. The myriad ways wild places like forests, river systems and coral reefs provide, not only medicine and food, but also spaces for mental and physical rejuvenation. These beautiful environments are under enormous pressure from the destructive forces of people. The lens through which our society looks at a forest is clouded by a greed mindset. This sees timber and underground minerals, rather than ancient trees, pristine rivers and a complex interconnecting ecosystem containing millions of different species.

Nature itself, being all plants and animals held together in an intricate web of life, provides the basis of human health. Yet, I had come across few people in medicine who saw it this way. Even colleagues passionately working on environmental issues like climate change and pollution seemed to regard the loss of forests and other natural places as less urgent and somehow unrelated. Those talking about 'green' health care and 'green' hospitals tended to limit their thinking to energy, water, waste and transport. It can be hard to see much green in there at all. Despite scientific evidence for the healing benefits of contact with nature, suggestions to bring nature in, or encourage people to move outside, were often met by quizzical looks.

I was left pondering why my perspective was so different to others and how best to bridge this gap between nature and health in the medical setting. Could it be the negativity bias of our health system, where problems are sought to be fixed and patients are defined by their illness? Where the focus is on acute care rather than prevention. With surgery, drugs and intensive care funded instead of time, education and support. In our rush to fix people we had become blind to the importance of community and connection in healing and the wellspring of this offered by time outside, in nature.

I realised it was not so much that I was too connected to the beauty and diversity of the outside world, it was that our society had become almost completely removed from it. For most people, nature was simply beyond their physical and psychological sphere. There are many possible reasons for this. Those in urban areas with fewer parks and waterways have limited access to nearby nature. And people living with a disability may find it harder to get to such places. While demanding work and social pressures can make finding time to pause and notice nature a struggle. I also came to understand that the seed of nature connection was planted during my early years. Despite growing up in the suburbs, I had spent much of my childhood outdoors in bushland at the end of our street. In concert with my mother's love of birds and plants, the freedom to explore this place filled my life with nature.

As my first nature mentor, my mother had a powerful influence on my life, teaching me to notice and care for the living world, its birds, flowers and trees. I was taken outside from the earliest days of infancy when my pram would be placed in the garden, under a tree, so I could watch the leaves move in the wind. And a walk would see my pram filled with flowers. This fostered a love of gardening, bushwalking and camping and a feeling of wholeness when outside in nature and constraint when stuck inside. There is a deep love, an embeddedness and feeling of rich connection alongside a sense of stewardship and care. So, the drying of bushland near my home, and the panting of birds during a heatwave, evoke feelings of distress and a desire to help. My drive to fight for nature arose from this unbreakable bond, forged in childhood. I had a felt sense of the restorative value of time spent in nature. I wanted to see this reflected in the health care setting so others could experience its healing potential too.

Yet many questions remained. Primarily, knowing most people suffered from nature deprivation, what would be the best way to address the disconnection entrenched in society? Seeking answers, in 2010 I embarked upon further studies at the Centre for Sustainability Leadership. Here I joined with others to form the Kids In Nature Network (KINN), a cross-disciplinary collaboration to promote childhood outdoor play experiences. This matrix of nature-connectors has helped build a social movement to foster a love of nature through play. Through KINN, I have learnt how nature-time supports optimal child development, learning and health.

Since its formation, KINN has nourished connections and stimulated collaborations between large and small groups and provided a platform for sharing knowledge and inspiration. With the support of early childhood environmental educators at the Royal Botanic Gardens in Melbourne, the network's signature event, Nature Play Week, has become a staple in the calendar. First launched in 2014, the twelve days in April see nature play, in all its guises, celebrated. The event has spread globally and continues to thrive, with thousands of children benefiting from a social and cultural shift to bring them closer to nature.

As KINN has flourished, so too has our knowledge of the health benefits of time spent in nature. These positives are not restricted to children. Adults also enjoy significant improvements in their wellbeing by simply unplugging from their devices and getting outside. The exponential rise in research over the past decade has documented positive physiological effects and landscape-based health interventions are becoming widespread. Practises like shinrin-yoku (Japanese forest bathing) are spreading globally. And doctors are issuing nature prescriptions to address lifestyle-related health problems like high blood pressure, anxiety and depression. The gains are greatest with longer durations in lush natural areas but even the smallest nature doses are helpful. The key is slowing down and deliberately paying attention to the living world around us.

Even just looking out onto a natural view from your hospital bed speeds recovery. So we are now seeing innovations in healthcare design to bring nature in, with gardens, pot plants and aquariums. Programs like therapeutic horticulture, where people care for plants, are becoming a part of rehabilitation for those with severe injuries. This tending to living things helps patients feel a sense of agency rather than just being 'in care' themselves. For young people challenged by mental health and behavioural issues, novel approaches like Bush Adventure Therapy see them out in wild places developing healthy new ways to tackle difficulty. While nature-based counselling helps those with relationship problems and trauma.

Health programs may be based outside with a focus on environmental repair as well as improved wellbeing. Examples include restoration of degraded landscapes by small groups of people experiencing social isolation and mental illness. Facilitated by health professionals, these activities grow confidence and connection, not only between participants, but with the land itself. Approaches which combine these tandem benefits see human health within a broader context and seek to address immediate problems as well as those caused by ecological damage, like climate change. The many occupations in nature-based health care provision are the 'green jobs' of the future. Reimagining old-growth forests, beaches and other natural places as essential resources for our communities' health will see them valued and protected.

## What to expect from this book

*Nature, Our Medicine* is divided into two sections. In the first, the current state of life on Earth is explored, along with the trajectory humans and nature have taken to get where we are today. A brief scientific survey of the planet's water, soil and carbon cycles is also provided, along with how the web of plant and animal life interacts within this framework, which will support the following discussion of human health. Through this, you'll learn all the ways nature sustains us, from stabilising our climate to providing fresh air, clean water and healthy soils to grow our food. The intricate relationship between the inner-most workings of our body, our gut's microbiome, and the wider living world highlights our dependency on nature. I hope to teach you how to nurture this internal ecosystem.

Nature's other gifts include the many medicines we draw on in today's healthcare. There will be a focus on a few well-known agents and their surprising origins as well as promising new compounds. How protecting old-growth forests and their unique animals might hold the answer to contemporary health dilemmas like antibiotic resistance. The links between nature protection and future-proofing human wellbeing will become clear to you. Our beautiful planet also provides us with places of psychological and spiritual rejuvenation and of personal transformation. Naturally, this will be covered too.

Culture and philosophy influence our relationship with nature. I will cover concepts like Gaia, systems thinking, and some First Nations' perspectives. The First Australians have the longest continuous culture on Earth, surviving despite the ravages of colonisation. They have lived within the unique ecology of this continent for well over 60,000 years and have much to teach us about how our health sits within the wider frame of nature. Their wisdom is seeded throughout this book, alongside other First Nations' lessons.

The latter part of section one sees us turn towards the challenges for our planet and for people. How climate change and species extinction threaten human health and all life on Earth, is unpacked. This discussion will help you understand how environmental issues affect your health. Problems like pollution, pests and land clearing obviously damage nature but they ultimately hurt us too. Even infections like COVID-19 and HIV have arisen through the disruption of natural systems. We'll step through these issues in detail, covering the 'what' of our current predicament. Then we'll ponder the 'why' – the attitudes which have led to such widespread and sometimes callous destruction of nature. Contrasts between First Nations' philosophies of stewardship and care and the human-centric, extractive model of the Western capitalist system are contemplated.

At the end of section one, the state of today's relationship between people and planet will be clear. The diagnosis is not good. Natural systems are unravelling with climate chaos and ecological collapse destabilising the foundations of human wellbeing.

Part two focusses on health – the contemporary challenges we face and how reconnecting with nature provides a key part of the solution. Health problems fuelled by our indoor, sedentary lifestyle include obesity, diabetes, heart disease and depression. We are seeing these issues in younger and younger people along with behavioural struggles like poor sleep, attentional difficulties and anxiety. Despite great advances in our standards of living and life expectancy, many modern humans, in so-called 'developed' societies, are unhealthy and deeply unhappy. The environment we live in, often devoid of nature, is foreign to the world of our evolution. The COVID-19 pandemic highlighted the many vulnerabilities within our health systems and social structures and saw entire populations shut away. Many were cut off from friends and family and had no access to natural environments. The aftershocks of psychological distress are still with us and many will never be the same.

Fortunately, nature-based health interventions provide simple, inexpensive answers. Discover the benefits to be had outside for your physical and mental health and for children's learning and development. Learn how to incorporate a green hour into your day and how to write your own nature prescription. Discover the origins of shinrin-yoku. There is a whole world of health care out there, from surfing for autism through to Bush Adventure Therapy.

As nature can provide great relief for those suffering with grief and psychological anguish, I've devoted a whole chapter to this topic. Slowing down and mindfully connecting with nature to grow your green mind will help you weather life's inevitable storms. There is also a chapter focussing on children's need to grow up within the embrace of nature. Here you will learn about the joys of nature play and importance of greening our schools and suburbs. Every child has the right to time and space to play in nature. This provides the optimal environment for their growth and development, and for fostering their sense of wonder so essential for learning. Through wonder, children's curiosity and love of nature is born. This flourishes as they grow and kindles a sense of care for Earth. So the nature stewards of the future are nurtured.

We can work together to restore the ecology of our world and in doing so enhance our personal wellbeing and the health of humanity globally. But we must begin by acknowledging the harms done to date and the systems, attitudes and beliefs which have led us to this point. To start from a place of acceptance and understanding and then walk towards a new relationship with nature. No doubt this will take great courage and humility, particularly from those of us who have benefited from colonisation and environmental degradation.

Having a legacy of innovation, peace and stability, Aboriginal and Torres Strait Islander Peoples have an extraordinary relationship with Country. They understand how to live within the ecological parameters of this place we now call Australia and may guide us on how best to restore balance if we can respectfully listen and learn. I am profoundly grateful for the teachings I have received from First Nations people. These gifts have irrevocably shifted and enriched my world view. I share some of this learning in these pages hoping to move others towards a fuller and more reverential understanding of Aboriginal connection to Country.

I hope this book will provide the inspiration, motivation and tools to stimulate a reimagining of your relationship with the natural world. To bring nature into your heart and generate a meaningful change in the way you live. A shift towards a new way of being where you are healthier and happier and so is the astonishingly beautiful and fascinating world we share. A world where seals surf at sunset and our children's children can sit in the dunes to watch them.

# PART ONE

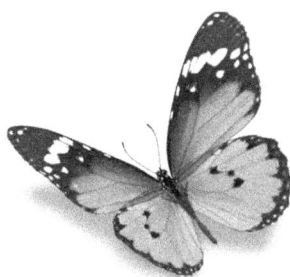

# The World

If nature is our medicine, then we should begin by exploring the natural world. Earth's biome—all the plants, animals and ecosystems we live within—is our life support system. Our evolution within nature's web has shaped our body's physiology, its intricate inner workings. From the microbes living in our gut to the essential minerals we obtain from the soil via plants, we rely on nature. Let's step back to view the entirety of Earth, the garden around us. Understanding this a little better will lay the foundation for appreciating how we care for ourselves by caring for nature.

This first section goes on to explore our relationship to Earth and where the trajectory of humans and nature has taken us. Some view our planet as a self-regulating organism, seeing connections and co-operation rather than competition. First Nations' knowledge systems incorporate the spiritual and challenge our notions of time, space and possession.

Where nature ends and begins, within and around us, influences our understanding of health. Nurturing our inner garden by attending to the way our food is produced supports wider biodiversity and personal wellbeing. Most of our medicines have come from nature. So ensuring ongoing rich biological diversity is essential for the discovery of future cures. Other gifts, bestowed on us by nature, are endless opportunities for learning, sparking creativity and transcendence.

# 1

# Earth's Biome

*"Biodiversity is the totality of all inherited variation in the life forms of Earth, of which we are one species. We study and save it to our great benefit. We ignore and degrade it to our great peril."*

~E. O. Wilson

Biodiversity, or biological diversity, is the scientific name given to the rich tapestry of life on Earth. Such a dry term to describe the beauty and wonder pulsing through our planet's reefs, forests, and rivers. Poetry or music seem a more appropriate, or intuitive, response and the natural world has undoubtably been the muse for much great art. Science is simply a tool with which we make sense of the life around us. It is through a scientific lens that this exploration of the natural world begins. Understanding biodiversity helps us appreciate how nature supports human health.

# THE GARDEN AROUND US

The variety of living things on our blue planet is extraordinary and almost incomprehensible. Despite some two million species currently identified, scientists predict between three and thirty million more remain unnamed. The overall figure could be higher still if some poorly known groups, like deep-sea creatures and micro-organisms, have more species than currently documented[1]. Even substances like soil, which seem ordinary at first glance, are in fact teeming with life. Just one teaspoon contains millions of different species, moving and interacting with one another, oblivious and yet connected to humankind.

Earth's biodiversity rests on a delicate balance, or homeostasis, having been maintained by key planetary systems for millennia. The global water, carbon and soil cycles circulate through all living things generating and sustaining biological variety and providing humanity's ecological 'life-support'. Our need for fresh water, clean air, and healthy soils in which to grow food is unequivocal. So, too, are the shelter, warmth and medicines provided by nature. Historically, doctors and scientists have studied plants and animals to develop cures for illness, while First Nations people have long recognised the healing role nature plays. The quintessential truth is that caring for and connecting to the natural world is necessary, not only for the continuation of life on the planet as we know it, but also for our individual wellbeing.

To understand the relationship between human health and nature, it's helpful to first investigate the planetary systems linking all plants and animals, both in the present moment and over evolutionary time. An exploration of water and how it moves around the planet, shape shifting through its gaseous and solid forms to transform and be transformed by all life is a good place to begin.

## *The story of water*

Earth is often described as the 'blue planet' because much of its surface is covered by oceans. This sets it apart from the other planets in our solar system which are mostly comprised of rocks and gas and thought to be devoid of life. Water is essential for all Earth's biodiversity. The abundance of fresh and saltwater ecosystems has allowed a rich variety of lifeforms to evolve. Water molecules cycle through liquid, solid and gaseous states and through plants and animals in a constant flow of movement and change. Clouds form when water droplets in the sky coalesce. They draw together, amassing within enlarging clouds until, through gravity's force, rain falls. Water hits the ground and is pulled down hill into gradually increasing flows – rivulets, creeks, and rivers. These run into one another, merging until they reach a large body of water such as a lake or wetland, or perhaps the sea. Some water seeps through the soil and that not taken up by plants or animals travels deep underground where it pools together to form large, ancient subterranean lakes, or aquifers. These may be located underneath very arid landscapes. For example, Australia's Great Artesian Basin, some 1.7 million square kilometres in area, contains water up to two million years old and is one of the largest underground freshwater bodies in the world. Standing on the dry earth in outback Queensland, you would never guess that deep beneath your feet is a vast, prehistoric pool.

Water from the surface of oceans, lakes and other large bodies evaporates into the atmosphere forming clouds, so the cycle continues. Plants play an integral part as they draw water up through their roots, trunks, and stems to their leaves. It is then released into the air via a process known as *transpiration*. In this way, forests generate clouds and ultimately make rain. The moisture in the atmosphere is pushed along by air currents, moving down wind of where it is produced. Scientists call this 'hydrologic space' and, while all plants produce water via transpiration, some ecosystems do it better than others. Forests and the vegetation in wetlands are the most effective and efficient, with crops and grasslands producing smaller amounts of moisture. Animals, including humans, have their own water cycle where they drink water, utilise it in various ways and then release it as waste. This effluent eventually runs into the broader water system. So all life is enfolded within the simultaneously intricate and vast phases of Earth's watery flow.

Given the fundamental need all plants and animals have for a reliable source of water, its availability affects the biodiversity of a given region. Interestingly, some areas with very low rainfall and nutritionally poor soils, like the south-western corner of Australia, have some of the most concentrated biodiversity anywhere on Earth. Also called the Kwongan, from a Noongar word for the sandplain, this area is about the size of England. Yet, while England has some 1,500 species of vascular plants (all plants except for mosses and ferns), the Kwongan has over 7,000. As this area evolved in relative isolation, with a stable climate, 80% of these plant species are regionally unique, or endemic. This contrasts with England where fewer than half the plant species are found nowhere else[2]. In the dry Kwongan landscape, plants have gradually adapted to arid conditions over millennia, adjusting their leaves, flowers, fruits and seeds in myriad and often spectacular ways. The slow evolution of their structure and behaviour enabled them to flourish until the changes triggered by colonisation in the early 19th century. This saw huge tracts cleared for agriculture, mining and forestry.

The gradual evolution into botanical richness seen historically in the Kwongan contrasts with rapid disruption of rainfall patterns occurring with climate change over recent decades. Without the long timeframes required for adaptation, plants and animals perish during prolonged droughts, and biodiversity is eroded. So, too, is human health as crops fail, riverine fisheries and water catchments collapse, and our collective psyche is traumatised through bearing witness to a languishing landscape. Human wellbeing relies on the ongoing stability of Earth's water system through its nurturing of biological diversity as much as its provision of our most precious elixir: water.

People have long interfered with natural water systems by draining wetlands and aquifers, damming rivers, and manipulating their flow. We have even learnt how to make fresh water by desalinating seawater, using large amounts of energy in the process. Yet our human efforts are paltry when compared to large forests, like the Amazon. This generates vast flows of water high up in the atmosphere, in hydrologic space. These rivers in the sky flow across continents and oceans. So, interference with a forest on one landmass may produce an effect in another, far distant place.

Scientists are still working to understand how water moves around the planet, whether through hydrologic space, across the land itself, or through ocean currents, glaciers, and polar ice caps. What is abundantly clear is that humanity is only just beginning to grasp the sensitivity of these planetary systems to change and the widespread consequences of our interference with them. Whether warming global temperature through altering atmospheric composition, or clear-felling huge tracts of rainforest, humankind is affecting the delicate balance of the water system. And risking our own survival in the process.

Like water, soil is fundamentally important for human health. We need it to grow our food, and it is from the earth we obtain essential micronutrients required for the intricate workings of our body. It also shifts through various phases and formations, from hard rocks and frozen tundra to the silty floor of a riverbed or fine dust lifted by the wind. This complex system, so full of life, remains poorly understood and threatened by humanity's actions to dismantle and displace it.

## The life-giving complexity and preciousness of soil

Soils are formed as rocks and plant and animal matter break down on their way to eventually form fossil fuels or rock layers in the planet's crust. Previously called dirt, the surface layer of Earth is now referred to as soil because it contains a rich array of life. Dirt is defined as displaced soil because it is no longer a complex, living ecosystem. For example, you might be digging into your garden's soil, alive with tiny plants and animals, but when you move inside and notice brown dust on your clothes and hands it is now simply dirt[3]. Soil contains living things much deeper than the top two metres or so where most plants are grown. Viruses, bacteria and fungi have been found at depths of over three kilometres; our planet has so much more life than we might at first think.

Soils are held in place by plants whose roots become fine and hair-like as they get smaller and smaller, impregnating the earth. Most gardeners will be familiar with this pattern and the extraordinary distance some roots travel from the largest, central taproot or the plant's stem. The interface between a root and the soil is as intricate and complex as between the air we inhale and the blood circulating through our lungs. Roots draw moisture and nutrients up out of the soil. Fungi and other small organisms assist in this process and also help plants communicate with one another through their roots. Various important nutrients are exchanged between the plant's roots within the soil. Some of these are taken into the body of plants and incorporated into their leaves, stems and flowers. This is how humans obtain essential micronutrients, like metals. For example, our red blood cells use iron to carry oxygen around the body, and zinc is used to produce new immune cells. We rely on the complex balance of life in soil to acquire these elements through the plants we eat.

Soil is important for the life it supports, the water it filters and holds, and the various gases it absorbs and emits. When land is cleared, the roots keeping the soil in place are removed. Soil becomes vulnerable to displacement by heavy rain or strong winds. In dust storms, large amounts of soil may be swept up into the atmosphere and deposited many thousands of kilometres away. Disruption of the stability of soil leads to erosion which can, in turn, lead to landslides and degradation of river systems. Soil loss is a major problem for many Australian farmers because, as the top layer of their pastures thins, underground water rises towards the surface.

Much of the soil in arid areas of Australia has relatively high levels of salt (primary salinity) which occurs because low rainfall stops the salt from being regularly flushed out, while high evaporation rates cause further concentration to occur. Almost thirty million hectares of this type of land is present in Australia, with naturally occurring salt marshes, salt lakes, flats and surrounding dry lands[4]. The plants growing in these areas have adapted to high salinity over thousands of years. These arid areas are richly biodiverse simply because the conditions are so challenging. Here, plants have developed deep root systems so as much water as possible can be taken up from the soil and they can survive despite little rainfall.

Land clearing for agriculture has seen these deep-rooted plants replaced by crops with their shallower growth pattern. Now, during times of high rainfall, water pours through the upper layer of earth to recharge the salty underground water table. This then rises to the surface dissolving still more salt from the soil and pushing it upwards. Ultimately, the land becomes super salty, resulting in secondary salinity. Crops are unable to be grown successfully in this degraded ground. If not addressed, the resulting lunar landscape is eventually abandoned. This problem has particularly affected south-western Australia's Kwongan area. Here, some farmers are responding by growing crops of native, salt tolerant plants to help pump the salty water out of the ground naturally[5]. Salt bush and pigface are a new type of crop for farmers and are in demand as restauranteurs discover Indigenous ingredients. It is hoped this regenerative type of agriculture will allow farmers to not only stay on their land and generate an income, but to also repair some of the damage destructive techniques of the past have caused.

It's a shame Australian farmers and policy makers hadn't paid attention to global history. The salinity crisis affecting Western Australia is following a similar pattern to that experienced in the United States in the Dust Bowl crisis of the 1930s. This ecological disaster was triggered by various government policies in the decades following the late 19th century decimation of native grasslands when large tracts of land were 'opened up' for agriculture. These immense areas had been used by First Nations people for millennia as a place where buffalo grazed and were hunted for food. As the buffalo were free to move over large areas, the soils were only lightly compacted, and the native grasses' deep roots stabilised the earth. Sadly, First Nations people were driven off their land and forced into reservations as their prime food source, buffalo, was hunted almost to extinction by the colonialists.

As the grasslands were cleared and crops grown, initially the nutrient-rich upper layer of soil resulted in good yields of corn and other crops. Strong prices for these grains from Europe during World War One stimulated further clearing and farming. However, as time went on the soils became depleted. Then, with a prolonged drought beginning in 1931, crops failed, and enormous dust storms resulted. These storms blew away the fields making thousands of kilometres of land uninhabitable. By 1934 an estimated 35 million acres of farmland had become useless for cultivation and another 125 million acres was losing its soil. The dust storms were devastating and became known as 'black blizzards'. Dust piled up throughout townships and caused serious respiratory health problems. It became impossible to live in these conditions and many people migrated out of the area. One major storm on 14th April 1935, a day known as Black Sunday, saw a wall of dust blowing from Oklahoma across the entire country. It is estimated some three million tons of topsoil blew off the Great Plains that day[6].

We now know the ancient grasslands cultivated by First Nations people would have stabilised the soil and maintained rainfall reducing the risk of drought. The murder and displacement of Native Americans, and the dismantling of their philosophy and systems of stewardship for the natural world, was catastrophic. It resulted in an environmental and humanitarian disaster.

Apart from filtering and storing water and nutrients, soils provide a repository of carbon and are an integral part of the global carbon cycle which stabilizes Earth's climate. A key element – carbon – moves between the atmosphere, land and water, and through all living things. An exhalation right now contains carbon that will move throughout the atmosphere and be used by plants and then animals, all over the planet. While the following inhalation may contain elements already breathed by dinosaurs, or our human ancestors. We have only ever had one atmosphere here on Earth. It may have changed in its composition, enabling the evolution of life, but it remains a fine, delicate layer of protection between us and deep space. The carbon cycle is crucial for the ongoing survival of all life on Earth. Its disruption through climate change, with ensuing human health impacts, is discussed in depth in chapter 5.

Just one handful of soil contains an abundance of life forms, from microscopic bacteria and fungi, invisible to the naked eye, through to wriggling worms and crawling insects. These provide food for one another, for the plants whose roots infiltrate the ground and the birds, reptiles and mammals who forage in the topsoil. The relationships between these different species of plants and animals are fragile and complex. An exploration of them is facilitated by looking to the field of ecology where biodiversity is investigated.

## *Understanding biodiversity – the web of life*

Each living thing interacts with and depends upon others, as well as its physical environment, within a network of relationships called an *ecosystem*. This describes an enormous variety of life. There are marine, freshwater, forest and woodland ecosystems; just about any natural environment imaginable can be understood as an ecosystem. These are then grouped together into much larger *biomes* depending on their geographic location. For example, an aquatic biome may contain ecosystems of coral reefs, seagrass meadows and kelp forests.

There is debate among scientists on how many biomes the planet is divided into and this may cause confusion. Some say there are just six biomes – forest, grassland, freshwater, marine, desert and tundra – while others suggest many more. Regardless, a biome is both general and global, and encompasses numerous smaller-scale ecosystems. For example, the tropical rainforest biome incorporates all that ecological community type across the planet from South Asia all the way through to South America. Within this biome, the rainforest of the Papua New Guinea highlands is a distinct ecosystem, in types of species, water flow and soil composition, from the Amazon Basin rainforests. The whole of Earth's ecosystem is called the *biosphere*[7].

Earth's biomes are interdependent, connected by vast planetary systems which maintain the stability that has enabled life to evolve. Some of these are the water cycle, as already discussed, the climate (or carbon) cycle, and land-based systems including those within which soil, plants and animals interact. The complex relationships between all these systems demonstrate the myriad ways our wellbeing rests on a natural world in balance. And how things which, at first glance, might seem unrelated are, in fact, deeply entwined.

Biodiversity is essential for strengthening ecosystems –the greater the variety of life they contain, the more resilient they are in the face of change. Biological diversity is measured from the tiniest microscopic level of genes through to species and then up to larger ecosystems. At each of these levels, variety, quantity, quality and distribution may be assessed. We can begin to understand how many life forms there are within each individual species, the number of different types of species, how robust they are and where they are located. Breaking it down in this way helps us to get our collective heads around the often-bewildering complexity of life on Earth.

Biological diversity is crucial for providing humankind with food and medicines. Having a larger number of species to choose from naturally increases the variety of possible compounds and nutrients available to us. Of course, there must be a reasonable quantity of each species and they need to be in the right planetary distribution to optimally support health. Having all the world's pollinators present, but only in one location, won't meet the needs of the plants that rely on them. Also, many ecosystem services are location specific, so human communities need to be nearby to benefit.

History provides many examples of periods where a limitation on the availability and variety of food sources has left people vulnerable to death via starvation. The potato famine in Ireland in the mid-1800s saw some one million people perish when the potato crop succumbed to a fungal infestation known as potato blight. Already suffering from malnutrition and poverty due to systemic oppression by British landlords, and reliant on this single vegetable for their sustenance, when several consecutive years of crops failed, a huge number of Irish people died[8]. Ultimately, keeping variety in any biodiversity component provides options for the future. Even if not all variants have an obvious role to play in the present.

Stepping in from looking at Earth's biomes to focus on one land mass, like Australia, highlights the role geographical isolation has played in the evolution of its distinctive soils, plants and animals. It also helps explain why land practises from other parts of the world, when applied crudely to an ancient and fragile landscape, have proved so destructive.

## Australia's unique biodiversity

Australia was once part of the super continent Gondwana, which connected it to Antarctica, South America and the islands of the Pacific and New Guinea. Over some 55 million years Australia separated from Antarctica as Gondwana broke up and the continental plate Australia sits on gradually drifted northwards to bump up against the Eurasian plate. Over the 65 million years in which Australia has been isolated from Antarctica there have been many changes in sea level. This created a shifting pattern of land bridges between Australia's coast and the islands of New Guinea and Indonesia, which sit on the same continental plate. Various plants and animals have moved over these land connections, dispersing and intermingling to create new species and ecosystems.

The extended timeframe of Australia's isolation has enabled regionally unique species to evolve. Those with the strongest and oldest links to Gondwana remain in moist coastal regions like the Wet Tropics rainforests of Queensland and temperate rainforests of Tasmania's takayna (Tarkine). Here, plants and animals are strikingly like those in other places with Gondwanan origins, like South America, Madagascar and New Zealand.

Following the break-up of Gondwana, Australia shifted northwards and began drying with fire becoming an important driver of the continent's biodiversity. Gradually, species who rely on fire for seed dispersal and germination evolved, including eucalypts and banksias. Over the tens of thousands of years in which Aboriginal and Torres Strait Islander people have looked after Australia, they have used fire to shape the landscape, working respectfully with this natural phenomenon to optimise conditions for the plants and animals they harvested. This landscape of fire and fire-stick farming is strikingly different to the environments of the northern hemisphere pre-18th century colonisation.

As a result of its gradual evolution in isolation, much of Australia's plant and animal life is endemic. This means it's found nowhere else on Earth. We are one of the seventeen megadiverse countries in the world which are home to 70% of Earth's species. Some 85% of our land-based mammals and over 90% of our reptiles, frogs and flowering plants are found only here. Australia has two of the world's biodiversity hotspots, areas where exceptional concentrations of endemic species are undergoing excessive loss of habitat. These are the south-west region of the continent, the Kwongan, and the forests of eastern Australia. We are in a unique position to gain from looking after our rich biodiversity and have much to love, celebrate and explore.

Among our natural wonders, within the forests of eastern Australia, we have the tallest flowering plant on Earth, the Mountain Ash. The tallest plant ever measured, the Ferguson tree, was 133 metres tall with its crown broken off. The crown's diameter was still one metre across, and it's thought that, had it still been intact when found, its height would have approached 152 metres. For some perspective, the tallest Egyptian pyramid is only 139 metres in height, and it took 100,000 slaves over 20 years to build. The Ferguson tree was found near Healesville in Victoria in 1872. As a measure of the myopic thinking at the time, it was logged for timber.

Living for 450 years, each Mountain Ash is a tower of life. An ecosystem in and of itself, supporting thousands of smaller creatures like insects, reptiles and mammals. Taking 140 years to form, large hollows develop in the most ancient trees in the forest. Many animals make these cavities home, including the dainty wollert (Leadbeater's possum). These petite marsupials live in communal family groups and nest in safety during the day. Venturing out at dusk, they scurry high into the canopy where they feed on insects and nectar. Only as large as a human hand span, this fairy-like possum was thought to be extinct until rediscovered in 1961. Although now the faunal emblem of Victoria it remains vulnerable due to ongoing habitat loss from logging and bushfires[9].

Alongside rich terrestrial biodiversity, Australia has unique marine ecosystems and is fringed by reefs. The iconic Great Barrier Reef, so large it can be seen from space, is renowned for its biological abundance and is the world's biggest coral reef ecosystem. It is home to thousands of species of shells, fish, corals, turtles, birds and large mammals like whales and dugong. Apart from coral reefs, the ecosystem contains over half of the planet's mangrove diversity, more than a thousand islands and thousands of kilometres of seagrass beds. While this enormous reef system is well known and much loved, Australia is also a global hotspot for seaweed biodiversity and has the world's highest level of seaweed endemism with most species found nowhere else on Earth[10].

Although plant-like, seaweeds are complex forms of algae. They anchor themselves to the ocean floor and grow upwards towards the sunlight, absorbing nutrients from the water in which they are immersed. Often arranged in large underwater colonies or forests, seaweeds form an important part of coastal ecosystems sheltering fish and other sea creatures. Seaweeds also stabilise and protect the shoreline from severe weather events and sequester carbon. Even when washed up on the beach, seaweed performs an important role as a source of food and shelter for many animals. Appreciating the role these organisms play in preserving the ecological integrity of a coastline recasts the site of seaweed piles along the beach as a marker of biological richness rather than an unsightly mess to be cleaned up.

From the enormity of the Great Barrier Reef and towering Mountain Ash forests, through to the minutiae of seaweed fronds, Australia's endemic ecosystems and species are essential for the healthy functioning of the planet. For, although they evolved in relative isolation, the large circulatory systems of the planet, the oceans and atmosphere, connect them to the rest of Earth. Mountain Ash and seaweed forests alike store carbon as part of the carbon cycle while simultaneously releasing oxygen into the atmosphere and oceans respectively. They are also linked through the water cycle as they discharge water vapour into hydrologic space contributing to cloud formation and rainfall. Consequently, they are as vulnerable to the disruption of these systems through climate change and pollution, as is all life. It is truly impossible to separate any living thing on Earth from all others. This applies to human beings as much as anything else.

## HOW NATURAL SYSTEMS SUPPORT HUMAN HEALTH

But how does this complex variety of life support human health? In simple terms, nature sustains our health in two key ways. First, through the huge planetary systems which provide 'ecosystem services' for us. These include creating and purifying the air we breathe and water we drink, stabilising our climate so we aren't exposed to weather extremes and nurturing the plants and animals we rely on for food. Second, specific plants and animals, by providing us with nutrition or medicines, help keep us well. These living things are found not only in the world around us, but deep within our own bodies, in the microbiome of our gut.

The Millennium Ecosystem Assessment (MA) provides a helpful framework to explore ecosystem services. Launched in 2005, the MA was developed over four years following a request from the United Nation's Secretary General and involved the work of thousands of social and natural scientists globally. As the Intergovernmental Panel on Climate Change (IPCC) seeks to provide a consensus scientific view on climate change, the MA aims to provide a shared statement on the condition of the world's ecosystems, the services they provide and the options to restore and regenerate them. The MA describes the following categories of ecosystem services: provisioning, regulating, supporting, and cultural.

The provisioning services are the essentials given to us by nature and include what we need for our food, water and shelter. From agriculture, fisheries, drinking water, fibre, timber and minerals come the building blocks for the communities we have built and in which we go about our daily life. Within each of these areas greater biodiversity provides strength and security. For example, highly diverse fisheries are more productive, yielding bigger catches and they have populations which are less vulnerable to disease.

Regulating services help maintain the larger systems mentioned above by air and water purification, waste management, crop pollination and climate stability and limiting the spread of diseases and pests. The old-growth Mountain Ash forests of Victoria provide a great example as they regulate the air and water flowing through and around them, the local weather and the stability of the soil. By drawing down carbon dioxide they are also part of the vast system which regulates the planet's climate. These forests have been found to store more carbon per hectare than any other forest studied in the world, including rainforests[11]. They hold an incredible 1,867 tonnes of carbon per hectare. So, they are involved in climate regulation both locally and globally.

Recent studies have shown that forests are important in producing rainfall for themselves, and for regions farther afield. The regulating role of forests through the water cycle is critical. Experts are calling for a paradigm shift in thinking about forests away from primarily their carbon storage capacity to emphasise their equally important role in the global water cycle. In his report for the United Nations in 2018, David Ellison, a researcher on forests and atmospheric moisture, states, "the (second) great challenge for the 21st century is to finally begin to understand and appreciate the broad range of forest-water interactions and their potential usefulness for human welfare."[12]

Vegetation within forests and woodlands helps buffer us from dust storms and landslides by keeping soils stable. Along the coast, mangroves and coral reef systems protect adjacent land from storms, tidal waves and associated erosion. Seagrass meadows, huge swathes of underwater grasslands, link the shoreline to deeper systems like reefs, and protect both people, reefs and fisheries from harmful bacteria. Studies have found seagrass beds halve the number of bacterial pathogens in the water so reduce disease levels of nearby corals[13]. These meadows, along with enormous kelp forests, not only provide shelter and nurseries for fish but also draw down carbon dioxide, contributing to Earth's climate stability.

The supporting ecosystem services act as enablers to all the other ecosystem assistances and include soil formation, seed and nutrient dispersal and cycling and plant photosynthesis. While the cultural services of ecosystems include the intangible, yet precious, sense of connection to place and spiritual fulfilment obtained only from nature. Mental health benefits gained by spending time in natural places fall under the banner of a cultural ecosystem service. These encompass lowering feelings of stress and sadness, improved sleep patterns and concentration and enhanced mood. The recreational, creative and educational opportunities afforded by nature also sit in this category.

Most ecosystems provide services to humans which bridge all these domains. For example, a wetland provides multiple services to us: purifying water, cooling nearby land, providing water and habitat for pollinators and food in the form of shellfish and fish as well as drawing down carbon dioxide and releasing oxygen. It is also a place to come and relax or play, and may have a cultural story for local people. Like most ecosystems, wetlands provide services both locally and globally as they connect through the atmosphere and waterways with the entire planet.

Everything on Earth is, in some way, linked to all else. The threads of connection are fragile and intricate, stretching like a web of life within which we humans are embedded. If we interfere with one strand of this web, all others are affected. Pulling on many threads at once risks a complete unravelling. We are as much a part of this web of life as any other species, nurturing various plants and animals and contributing to the water and other planetary cycles. Despite the intimacy and tenacity of our relationship with the rest of Earth's lifeforms, humanity seems to regard itself as somehow above the fray. The stories we tell reveal the lens through which we view nature. Our narratives have changed over time depending on various cultural forces. How we've come to see ourselves as so apart from the rest of Life is worth exploring. Let's turn towards this now.

## KEY POINTS

- *Biodiversity* (or biological diversity) describes the totality of all variation in Earth's life forms
- Each living thing interacts with and depends upon others, as well as its physical environment, within a network of relationships called an *ecosystem*
- A *biome* is a geographical grouping of ecosystems. Some scientists describe Earth as having just six biomes: forest, grassland, freshwater, marine, desert and tundra
- Biological diversity strengthens ecosystems making them more resilient
- Ecosystems are connected via large planetary systems like the water and carbon cycles
- Nature supports human health via *ecosystem services*
- *Ecosystem services* may be provisioning, regulating, supporting or cultural

# 2

# Our Relationship To Earth

*"Humankind has not woven the web of life.
We are but one thread within it. Whatever we
do to the web, we do to ourselves. All things
are bound together. All things connect."*

~Chief Seattle

Humankind has long grappled to understand its place within the broader network of life on Earth, using religion and other philosophical and cultural frameworks to seek clarity. Scientists have contributed to this process with Charles Darwin surely being the most famous to try to explain how the world's species evolved. His theory of natural selection was first published in the mid-1800s. It proposes individuals within a species with characteristics more suited to their environment are better able to compete for resources and produce young. Thereby the fittest survive and the weakest perish so that gradually, species change, evolving over time. More recently, other concepts have been put forward, with the Gaia Hypothesis being one of the most controversial.

## UNDERSTANDING GAIA

The Gaia Hypothesis was first proposed by chemist James Lovelock and microbiologist Lynn Margulis in the early-1970s as a scientific theory. Gaia was the goddess who personified Earth in Greek mythology, and the metaphor envisages Earth as a single, living organism. The scientists' idea, that Earth itself—its atmosphere, geology and organisms—was a self-regulating system, was radical at the time of its inception. They postulated that living organisms help regulate the planet's atmosphere, oceans and landforms to make it habitable and stable. While not accepted as true scientific theory by many academics, the Gaia Hypothesis has forced big-picture thinking across various scientific disciplines as we struggle to grasp the complexity of how life has evolved and how it continues to shift and change. Although a romantic notion, this metaphor is appealing because it focusses our awareness on the complexity and wholeness of life on Earth.

Controversially, Margulis believed evolution resulted from co-operation between species and ecosystems which ultimately achieved a state of balance for the whole planet. This was counter to Darwin's theory of competition. She said, "life did not take over the world by combat, but by networking."[14] Many in the scientific community are highly critical of the Gaia Hypothesis but loathe to dismiss it outright because Margulis has, quite famously, been right before. When Margulis proposed the inner working components of cells were originally living bacteria, she was derided. She reckoned these micro-organisms invaded cells and then evolved to perform functions for them in a symbiotic, or mutually beneficial, manner. We now know Margulis was correct. The mitochondria which generate the energy for all plant and animal cells were once separate organisms. The relationship between the mitochondria and the host cell is mutually beneficial because, in return for creating energy for the cell, the mitochondria receive protection within its walls. Symbiosis in cell evolution is now, quite rightly, regarded as one of science's greatest breakthroughs. Perhaps Margulis and Lovelock, and other Gaia proponents, are correct in regarding Earth as a self-regulating, complex system, much like the human body.

# HOW TREES COMMUNICATE

Margulis' cell symbiosis theory was paradigm shifting, jolting the scientific community's once steadfast thinking on cell structure. A similarly transformative discovery was that of the mycorrhizal networks through which trees in a forest share nutrients, water and carbon and communicate with one another for the wellbeing of the whole forest. Mycorrhizae are tiny, thread-like fungi which link with one another in a complex web around plant roots. In the 1990s, forestry Professor Suzanne Simard from British Colombia, along with other researchers, detected this 'wood wide web'. Simard also helped identify the 'mother', or hub tree, the largest tree in a forest. These huge and ancient trees have the most extensive mycorrhizal networks and use them to support young saplings, sending them beneficial nutrients and seeding fungi to help them thrive[15]. Like Margulis, Simard proposes the trees are working together for the benefit of the whole ecosystem they live within rather than ruthlessly competing against each other. This challenges the Darwinian idea of natural selection. As happened to Margulis, Simard's work is subject to criticism by the scientific establishment. Simard's research suggests a forest's motto may well be 'together we thrive', rather than 'survival of the fittest'.

In his book, *The Hidden Life of Trees*, forester and writer Peter Wohlleben lyrically describes the work of Simard and others to promote the understanding that trees communicate. Not only underground via mycorrhizal networks, but also through the air with scent signals like pheromone chemicals. An example of this occurs in the African acacia tree which emits ethylene gas when injured by grazing giraffes. Nearby trees sense this stress signal and respond by pushing tannins into their leaves. Poisonous in large quantities, the presence of tannins repels the giant animals and so protects the tree. Wohlleben summarizes, "it appears that nutrient exchange and helping neighbours in times of need is the rule, and this leads to the conclusion that forests are superorganisms with interconnections much like ant colonies."[16]

Extraordinarily, trees within a forest may be one enormous single organism rather than thousands of individuals. Perhaps the most famous example, Trembling Giant, resides in Utah, United States. Also called Pando, meaning 'I spread' in Latin, some 47,000 genetically identical trees grow in a vast grove of quaking aspens. Sharing a single root system and spreading over one hundred acres, Pando is awe inspiring[17]. First scientifically described by botanist Burton Barnes in the 1960s, Pando is thought to be one of Earth's oldest and most massive living organisms, perhaps 80,000 years old. Over centuries, as old parts of the giant plant die, new shoots emerge to continue its incredible legacy.

Even smaller plants, like Tasmania's King's Holly, may be ancient. With only one cluster remaining in the wild, this small shrub with a pretty red flower is thought to be over 43,000 years old[18]. Both Pando and King's Holly are precariously close to extinction due to pressures from humans. Their age highlights how stable Earth's environment has been for millennia and how quickly we have pushed it to the edge in a mere few thousand years. As the drivers of climate change and habitat destruction, modern colonising humans are truly the great disruptors, seeking to undo Gaia's work.

## THE TRICKERY OF PLANTS

The dance between species may be intricate, revealed only to those who have the curiosity required to spend hours in careful observation. One of Australia's most prolific and passionate naturalists was Victorian Edith Coleman. Even though she made one of botany's most extraordinary discoveries, Coleman's work only became more widely known through the writing of Danielle Clode in her book *The Wasp and the Orchid* in 2018[19]. Being a married woman in the first half of the 20th century, Coleman's career as a naturalist and scientist was delayed by the demands of raising children. So, it was not until mid-life that her discovery of pseudocopulation was presented to the scientific community. This occurred following years spent observing the behaviour of wasps and orchids in her garden and nearby bushland. Coleman noticed wasps entering certain orchids backwards and sought to explain this odd phenomenon by communicating with scientists and naturalists throughout Australia and the world. In the pre-internet era of the 1940s this meant trawling through scientific books and papers and corresponding via post, a process which took years.

Coleman had the additional difficulty of not being part of a scientific institution, like a university, and being a woman in a male-dominated field. She did, however, become a member of the Field Naturalists Club of Victoria, which enabled her to share her insights and keep abreast of the latest science. She was also a great scientific communicator, sharing her knowledge with the wider public through newspapers and magazines as well as the more traditional academic spheres. Apart from her work on orchids and wasps, Coleman studied spiders and echidnas. Despite the challenges she faced, Coleman was sure of herself and her place at the table, saying to The Age in 1950, "we nature lovers may open our windows on all aspects of nature even though we may sometimes abut on the preserves of the specialist".

What Coleman eventually found was that the orchids she was observing had evolved to look like a sexually-receptive female wasp so the male of the species would attempt to mate with it, a process called pseudocopulation. This was the backing in behaviour she had been witnessing. It was through this activity the male wasp pollinated the orchid. Pseudocopulation was an extraordinary discovery because it revealed how plants could entice an insect to pollinate it through sexual mimicry. Coleman was internationally applauded as her work explained a phenomenon that had puzzled scientists for decades, even Charles Darwin himself.

A little like Margulis and Simard, Coleman's thinking turned the scientific world on its head and shone a light on a new way of understanding relationships between tiny parts of the web of nature. Affiliations between organisms thought to be well known, between mitochondria and human cells, wasps and orchids and fungi and tree-roots were revealed to be different and perhaps symbiotic rather than competitive. As more is revealed about the complexity of life on Earth and the connections between biomes, ecosystems and species, the Gaia Hypothesis and other concepts of co-operation provide a stimulating framework for our understanding.

Knowing the ecosystem services provided by nature supports a richer conception of human health. Fields of study like One Health, ecohealth and planetary health see our wellbeing within this broader realm. These disciplines bring together the ecological sciences, veterinary and human health perspectives. It is only through cross-disciplinary thinking that we can repair the damage done to Earth by humankind over the past few thousand years. Defending the criticism her symbiotic cell hypothesis attracted, Lynne Margulis said her theory "crossed willy-nilly the boundaries that people had spent their lives building up. It [hit] some 30 subfields of biology, even geology"[20]. Today, more than ever, we need thinkers like Margulis. Those who are prepared to collaborate and work across disciplines and silos both within the scientific community and, more broadly, within civil society and between cultures.

## THINKING DIFFERENTLY

Perceiving Earth as one whole, living entity, as the Gaia Hypothesis does, enables comparisons to be drawn with the human body. This helps emphasise the interconnectedness of life on Earth, the sensitivity of the entire system to interference and the inevitable consequences of this for humankind, who are merely one part of the whole.

Just as our planet is comprised of multiple systems interacting with one another within the envelope of its atmosphere, our bodies hold a network of structures inside their skin.

It is helpful to utilise 'systems thinking', which describes linkages between interdependent and related parts of a larger entity, to investigate this metaphor further. And to stretch across scientific disciplines and into the realm of different ways of knowing.

Doctors understand the human body as a living organism containing multiple inner working components; a little like the ecosystems within the larger planetary systems of Earth as outlined earlier. We have a cardiovascular system, respiratory system, gastrointestinal system and so on. All of these have many parts and interact with one another and with the environment around us. For example, our heart and lungs—as key parts of our cardiovascular and respiratory systems—work together to move fresh oxygen around our body and to eliminate the carbon dioxide waste our cells generate.

Living systems are delicately balanced and rely on all their sub-parts working in concert. In turn, these components depend upon key inputs from their environment. Within the domain of the human body the role of iodine provides an apt example of how a system can collapse when a vital component is depleted. Iodine is a micronutrient found in soils and is used by the thyroid gland to make its hormone. Like all these compounds, thyroid hormone works throughout the entire body, so a deficiency affects many different parts. Initial symptoms seem benign and include weight gain, fatigue and a sensitivity to cold. However, if allowed to progress iodine deficiency may lead to heart failure, brain damage and, ultimately, death. It may seem surprising for a single micronutrient to be so essential. Yet it is, so delicately balanced is our physiology.

It is helpful to use this human body analogy when thinking about Earth's various living systems. We can think of forests as the lungs as they produce oxygen and draw down carbon dioxide, breathing for the planet. They can be underwater as kelp forests, or on land as temperate and tropical rainforests, woodlands or conifer forests. Mangroves, wetlands and seagrass meadows function as the planet's kidneys, cleaning water that runs off the land by removing pollutants. Nutrients and water move through the vast circulation systems of the planet in the flows and currents of the rivers, oceans and atmosphere. While plants, by using the sun's energy to transform carbon dioxide into their structure, provide food and fibre, and build soils. They are the reproductive system, creating new life in a constant process of generation.

As in the human body, if one of Earth's systems is damaged there are knock-on effects to others. This is clearly demonstrated by the ecological consequences of climate change occurring as the planet's atmosphere is polluted. Dramatic instances of ecosystem breakdown can also be seen in a more focal way. For example, if a river is contaminated, or its water flows significantly diminished, the rest of the system it is connected to will be harmed. The life along downstream riverbanks, the waterways the river runs into and ultimately, its delta and the ocean beyond. Just as the human body initially manages with iodine deficiency but ongoing depletion culminates in death, while at first the river may cope with reduced flows or pollution, eventually complete systemic collapse transpires.

## ANCIENT WISDOM

The philosophies of First Nations people encapsulate systems thinking and imbue it with spiritual and cultural meaning to guide behaviours that support future ecological richness. Authors Karl Erik-Sverny and Tex Sculthorpe, in their book *Treading Lightly*, explain how the complex belief systems of the Nhunggabarra people enabled their sustainable management of Country. The Nhunggabarra live in the north-western part of what's now called New South Wales in Australia. Tex Sculthorpe, an Elder, co-wrote his book with Karl Erik-Sverny to share the knowledge systems of his people more broadly. In the introduction, they explain how the book was birthed in 1999 when Erik-Sverny, a Finnish knowledge systems expert, asked Tex why his people didn't have a word for knowledge. Tex explained: "Our land is our knowledge, we walk on the knowledge, we dwell in the knowledge, we live in our thesaurus, we walk in our Bible every day of our lives. Everything is knowledge. We don't need a word for knowledge, I guess."[21]

Together they go on to outline, through the multi-layered meanings of ancient stories, how the Nhunggabarra had a knowledge-based society where value was placed on art, law, social welfare, spirituality, wellbeing and education, rather than physical possessions. They describe this society as being based on intangible values.

To help explain the recipe for ecological sustainability, Erik-Sverny and Sculthorpe describe how each Nhunggabarra person received an animal totem early in life. From a young age they were responsible for their totem and had to look after the habitat of all the plants the animal fed from. Great care was taken to ensure the longevity of species was ensured and so certain areas of country were off limits for hunting for periods of time. These First Australians had a carefully managed system of animal care and agriculture. Thought was given not only to the present but to future generations of people, plants and animals. This inherently sustainable model is seen in other First Nations communities and contrasts starkly with the legacy of colonisation seen globally as natural systems were disrupted. While First Nations' knowledge systems and philosophies regarded people as part of nature, European and British colonisers understood the world through a hierarchical structure where white men ruled from the top.

Many ecofeminists and philosophers describe the historical and ongoing abuse of the natural world as a manifestation of patriarchy and colonisation as righteous, white, 'man' dominates submissive, inferior, nature. Biologist and member of the Citizen Potawatomi Nation, Robin Wall Kimmerer investigates the differences in belief systems between her culture and the colonial/Western world view that predominates the United States today. She compares the stories of Creation held by the two cultures. In Christianity, the mother of man, Eve, is banished from the Garden of Eden for eating the forbidden apple and directed to control wild nature. The relationship between people and other living things is one of conflict and attempts at subjugation. Whereas in Potawatomi Nation culture, the Creator is Skywoman, who falls to earth and is saved by living creatures who then work with her to create all life on Earth. Here, women and all of nature are celebrated and collaborated with rather than punished, dominated and separated from the righteous man.

As Kimmerer writes: "On one side of the world were people whose relationship with the living world was shaped by Skywoman, who created a garden for the well-being of all. On the other side was another woman with a garden and a tree. But for tasting its fruit, she was banished from the garden and the gates clanged shut behind her. That mother of men was made to wander in the wilderness and earn her bread by the sweat of her brow, not by filling her mouth with the sweet juicy fruits that bend in the branches low. In order to eat, she was instructed to subdue the wilderness into which she was cast.

"Same species, same earth, different stories. Like Creation stories everywhere, cosmologies are a source of identity and orientation to the world. They tell us who we are. We are inevitably shaped by them no matter how distant they may be from our consciousness. One story leads to the generous embrace of the living world, the other to banishment. One woman is our ancestral gardener, a co-creator of the good green world that would be the home of her descendants. The other was an exile, just passing through an alien world on a rough road to her real home in heaven."[22]

The Christian view of nature flowed down through history from Europe and England and, by way of colonisation, to much of the rest of the world. In Europe, during the Age of Enlightenment in the 18th century, elements of nature were manipulated for the use and pleasure of the wealthy. Arising from the Renaissance movement centred around Italy, this intellectual and philosophical wave spread across the globe through the colonies. This had a profound influence on what was perceived as beautiful and of value within Western or 'civilised' societies.

We can see examples of this underlying philosophy today in the formal design of gardens from the Renaissance period where plants are grown into predetermined shapes or within rigid lines of garden beds. Standardised roses and rows of pleached, or espaliered trees interspersed by perfectly manicured lawns follow this pattern. There is no free-flowing messiness of wilderness, just order and symmetry. Gardens informed by this ideal can be found in places as diverse as regional Australia, Paris and Hong Kong. This aesthetic remains fashionable with many contemporary gardens having the same highly measured and controlled design. Plantings are restricted to only a few desirable species to be 'low maintenance', neat and tidy and to evoke this European archetype.

## THE INFLUENCE OF SCIENCE AND COLONISATION

The rise of scientific understanding also shifted how nature was valued and intersected with colonisation to effect most of the planet. In ancient Greece, where scientific thinking is thought to have originated, two famous scholars began a detailed study of the living world. Around 345BCE on the island of Lesbos, Aristotle and Theophrastus commenced their methodical Enquiries on nature. The former focusing on animals and the latter on plants. These two classical thinkers proceeded to share their knowledge through tutoring at early universities and writing detailed texts. Their work formed the foundation of the science of biology, the study of living organisms. Theophrastus' works, Enquiry into Plants and Causae Plantarum (Reasons of Vegetable Growth), explored plant classification, agricultural techniques and horticulture as well as ecology, or how plants interact with their surroundings. He was also interested in economic botany, the way in which plants could be taken from their natural surroundings and cultivated elsewhere for financial advantage[23].

Through the Middle Ages gardens were used for scientific learning and often attached to medical schools and universities where they were known as 'physic' gardens. When botany arose as a discipline in the 18th century's Enlightenment, it separated from the medical faculty of these institutions and directed its focus to understanding plant function and variety. Inspired by the classical texts of ancient Greece and with thousands of new plants discovered through colonisation, botanic gardens were established throughout Europe and England. The purpose of these places was ostensibly to expand the science of botany but an underlying economic imperative was strong, and many valuable plants were found as the 'new' world was conquered.

Botanic gardens were established along trading routes and in colonies to catalogue and study exotic plants to ascertain their scientific and agricultural value. Commercial crops like sugar, rubber, tea and coffee were uprooted from their rainforest habitat, analysed in botanic gardens, and subsequently established in plantations elsewhere. The rubber tree originally only grew in the rainforests of South America where Amazonian tribes had used its special sap for generations. In 1839 Charles Goodyear, an American inventor, realised the milky sap's potential for industrialisation. This information made Amazonian rubber highly sought after and expensive to import to Europe and England. In 1876 an English collector supported by the British government, Henry Wickham, smuggled thousands of seeds from tropical South America to Kew Botanic Garden in London. Although only a few survived, the botanists at Kew successfully germinated them, cultivating plants for dissemination according to directives given by the British government. These rubber plants were sent to the Botanic Gardens in Sri Lanka (then part of the British Empire and known as Ceylon).

Rubber eventually became a key crop for this small island country and large areas of native rainforest were cleared to make way for plantations. Other nearby countries also cleared rainforest to grow rubber. Today almost all rubber is produced in Asia, and huge areas of biodiverse forest have been transformed into rubber farms. The forces of colonisation, commodification and 'free trade' have seen many different species of plants uprooted and taken far from home to become a cash crop, or perhaps a noxious weed, in a foreign ecosystem.

In Australia, the legacy of colonisation is manifest in the major disruptions to natural ecosystems and the associated massacres and displacement of First Nations people. In his book, *The Bush*, writer Don Watson painstakingly explores the relationship between non-Indigenous Australians and their country. He describes the fear of the bush felt by the colonisers as they attempted to farm in an environment so very different to that left behind. Anxiety about the new land with its strange plants and animals and 'hostile natives', led to a reactionary attack where country was slashed, cleared and fenced off, and often outright slaughter ensued.

To impose order and control and to make it seem more like home, native plants and animals were shunned and those from England brought in. Very little effort was made to understand what was already here, and indigenous flora and fauna were quickly dismissed as strange, useless or dangerous. Watson describes "myriad accounts of European behaviour since settlement began, of serial psychopathy: of men and women hacking and gouging; hurling themselves at rival kingdoms, plant and animal alike; poisoning the ground; uprooting, planting, and uprooting again; crashing and roaring about, making fortunes and going broke, shooting anything that might move against them and never stopping to watch the clouds except to look for rain – in general obeying the demands of every neurosis peculiar to our species, and, for trying to survive their furious assault, declaring nature treacherous."[24]

This ecocidal behaviour has continued into the present with the killing of wildlife and the annihilation of entire ecosystems for mining, logging, agriculture and urbanisation. Although presented as 'development' essential to our economy, the destruction of nature is often thoughtless, violent and unnecessary. Perhaps this ecocidality is best epitomised by the detonation and ruin of an ancient sacred site in Juukan Gorge in north-western Australia by mining giant Rio Tinto in May 2020. In their rush to gouge iron ore out of the ground, the London-based company destroyed Deep Time rock shelters believed to be over 46,000 years old on the lands of the Puutu Kunti Kurrama people. This occurred with full knowledge of the cultural and archaeological significance of the site by both the company and relevant government bodies.

The contrast with First Nations' philosophies could not be starker. The natural world is revered and tended with kindness. In describing Yuin lore, writer Bruce Pascoe says: "Any Australian can climb Gulaga Mountain and visit the seven chapters of Yuin lore. Women can walk to the summit if they wish, but men can go no higher than the gallery of granite tors. It is on the walk through those tors that the gentleness of Aboriginal culture is most apparent. You enter by the forms of Nyaardi, the woman; you pass Tunku, the man, who is second, and then you pass the pregnant woman, and it is culturally appropriate to rub her swollen belly. The next chapter is the baby being carried on its mother's back. Look at that child's eyes and, if you are a parent, allow yourself to be engulfed by the memory of your own children's births. Where are the swords and war machines, where are the gilded halls of selfish men, where are the severed heads of people who disagreed with the king? On Gulaga Mountain you are invited to rub the belly of a pregnant woman."[25]

It may be difficult for descendants of colonisers to confront the legacy of this history, the ways the natural world and First Nations people have been harmed. However, facing this truth is necessary to fully comprehend the interdependence of all life on Earth. And how best to repair and regenerate our planet. Aboriginal musician Archie Roach succinctly captured the interconnectedness of people and nature and the place of humankind within the embrace of a living ecosystem in his memoir. He wrote, "In the bush, a thousand years ago, every sensation was part of a whole; part of an ecosystem. Every sound and smell was useful, part of a story of rising and falling, life and death. We blackfellas were part of that story, but just a part. A thousand years ago, everything was part of everything; everything was connected. You were in nature, and everything in nature was part of you."[26]

If we embrace this First Nations' perspective to see ourselves as a part of nature, then we will be mindful of how it is treated. For by looking after the natural world, we are caring for ourselves, our families and our communities, human and non-human. Conversely, actions which damage the ecosystems around us are, in fact, ultimately acts of self-harm. Archie Roach's insight that human beings are one part of a larger whole and that nature is within us as we are simultaneously inside nature itself captures a true appreciation of health and wellbeing.

Let's move on to unpack this further, seeing nature within ourselves.

## KEY POINTS

- ❤ The *Gaia Hypothesis* proposes that Earth is a self-regulating system
- ❤ Trees share nutrients, water and carbon via *mycorrhizae*
- ❤ *Mycorrhizae* are tiny, thread like fungi which link together around plant roots
- ❤ Trees communicate via these networks for the benefit of the whole forest
- ❤ 'Systems thinking' describes links between interdependent parts of a whole entity, like the human body or Earth
- ❤ First Nations philosophies encapsulate systems thinking and see people as part of nature, rather than separate from it
- ❤ Colonisation and science have disrupted Earth's biomes
- ❤ Regenerating our planet requires a shift in our thinking

# 3

# Human Health Within Earth's Biome

*"Look deep into nature and you will understand everything better."*

~Albert Einstein

Western science has only recently caught up with the idea that nature not only resides within us but also directs our body's functioning. The expansion of research into our gut's microbiome, our inner garden, has proved paradigm shifting. The interplay between this internal world and the workings of our body is intricate and complex. As with other ecosystems, the greater the diversity of our microbiome, the healthier it is and, consequently, so too are we—physically and emotionally. One story which encapsulates the sometimes-surprising role bacteria and other microscopic organisms play in our body's functioning is that of Helicobacter pylori. It also demonstrates how new information can completely shift scientific thinking and expose entirely different ways of understanding both the generation of illness, and the foundations of wellbeing.

# NATURE WITHIN US

Late last century, a controversy challenged the way stomach ulcer disease was understood. Australian scientists Barry Marshall and Robin Warren hypothesised a bacterium—Helicobacter pylori—as being the causative agent of ulcers rather than stress and cigarette smoking as was believed at the time. In this debate, there were essentially two opposing camps, the H. pylori 'believers' and the 'non-believers'. This second group was comprised of two often opposing specialties, surgeons and physicians. The surgeons had honed their skills in gastric surgery over many years and performed a variety of operations in which part, or all, of the stomach or small bowel was removed to stop the catastrophic haemorrhaging caused by untreated ulcers. And the gastroenterologists, physicians who diagnosed stomach inflammation and ulcers, treated patients with acid-lowering medication in the hope that surgery could be avoided. The idea a mere bacterium had the power to alter acid secretion such that ulceration and life-threatening bleeding resulted was widely derided by physicians and surgeons alike.

After years of being ridiculed by the medical fraternity, in the true spirit of science, Barry Marshall put his own health on the line and drank a liquid containing the bacteria. As he and Warren had predicted, the bacteria caused stomach inflammation, a precondition of ulceration. They were vindicated, and further research led to the development of simple breath tests for diagnosis of H. pylori infection and antibiotic regimens for its treatment. Ulcers seldom cause death now and in general practice we routinely test for, and treat, Helicobacter infection. Marshall and Warren's work not only helped prevent ulcer disease, it also almost eradicated stomach cancer in the Western world, a disease also caused by H. pylori. Rightly, in 2005 Marshall and Warren won a Nobel Prize for their work.

Today, we are experiencing a similar paradigm shift in understanding the role microbes play in the functioning of our body beyond the gut. We now know, even though they reside in our gastrointestinal tract, these microscopic communities affect our immune and nervous systems. Through their role moderating inflammation, it is likely they also affect our vascular system, and through this, our whole body. Rather than simply causing disease, these microscopic organisms are crucial for the body's healthy functioning and development. The burgeoning research into our flora challenges the idea that we are separate from nature and that the organisms living in and on us are mere hitchhikers. We have an inner microscopic ecosystem with all the diversity of a rainforest.

Humans have bacteria both on our skin and hair and deep inside us, in our whole gastrointestinal tract and in the vaginas of women. It is likely we have lived with these micro-organisms since the Palaeolithic age, evolving together in a bodily ecosystem. We have some one hundred trillion gut bacteria or gut microbiota of up to one thousand different species, and scientists are finding the more different species we have, the more biodiverse our gut flora is and the healthier we are[27]. These microbiotas interact through the surface of our gut with the millions of nerve cells located there. Some researchers describe this complex as our second brain, it's so important. We also have 60-70% of our immune cells located within our gut tissues. There is a complex interplay between our immune, gastrointestinal and nervous systems occurring in our gut and this affects the workings of the rest of the body.

Functions attributed to our microbiota include assisting food digestion, manufacturing vitamins K and B, helping nutrient absorption, regulating our immune system and fighting against pathogens. As the uterus is thought to be mostly sterile, we receive our gut microbiota from the first bacterial communities or 'seeding' bacteria we encounter in early life; from our mother and the environment we are born into. The diversity of our microbiota increases over the first year of life and stabilises around the age of three. In addition to bacteria, our microbiota includes viruses and other microscopic organisms. The variety of life inside us is as complex and varied as that of a tropical rainforest, and surely worth tending.

Our microbiota's composition is influenced by early life exposures, including how we were born, and first fed. Babies born vaginally receive their seeding bacteria from their mother's birth canal. The composition of the maternal gut and vaginal microbiomes reflect one another and seem to change over the course of pregnancy. As birth approaches, the vaginal microbiome becomes more populated with lactobacilli whose metabolic products, like hydrogen peroxide, are anti-infective. Some strains of this bacterium protect against infections like gonorrhoea and make the vagina more acidic, so reducing bacterial overgrowth. This is important, as vigorous bacterial growth could ascend to the uterus and infect the pregnancy.

Breastfed babies receive microbiota from their mother's nutrient-rich colostrum and then breast milk[28]. Colostrum is the first substance produced by a lactating breast and is like a living medicine for the newborn infant's gut. Our mother's diet, the level of cleanliness into which we are born, and antibiotic usage all influence the microbiota we are seeded with. Stable microbiotas are resilient to sudden environmental challenges; this stability is called compositional homeostasis, our steady state.

## OUR IMMUNE SYSTEM

This inner rainforest plays a crucial role in the development of our immune system, which controls the way our body fights disease and infection. If this complex malfunctions, various illnesses develop. These may be *autoimmune* where our immune system attacks other parts of the body, or *allergic*, where external substances provide the trigger. In multiple sclerosis, a well-known autoimmune disease, the nervous system is damaged and progressive loss of brain and nerve function may occur. If our gut contents are attacked, the bowel wall becomes swollen and painful causing inflammatory bowel conditions like Crohn's disease and ulcerative colitis.

In allergic disorders such as asthma, hay fever and eczema, harmless things are fought by our bodies, instead of tolerated. An allergen is any substance that elicits an allergic reaction and includes pollens, animal hair and some foods and chemicals. The cascade of immune and inflammatory reactions triggered by an allergen see various chemicals released as cells are activated in the airways or gut, or on our skin. This response varies in severity from mildly irritating to life-threatening.

The slippery linings of the gut, vagina and upper airways form the mucosal system, the key interface between the environment and our internal tissues and organs. The microbiotas in these places facilitate the interaction between our body and the substances we take in through our food and drink and the air we breathe. There is geographical variance in microbiota. Allergic sufferers in different countries differ in their microbiota composition, much like natural landscapes change from one place to another. This is reflective of dietary and environmental factors, which are location dependent. What is especially interesting is that in developing countries, where people have greater exposure to bacteria in the natural environment, there are lower rates of allergic disease. Could it be that in our zeal to prevent infectious diseases, we have inadvertently stripped away the microscopic building blocks that stabilise our immune system?

## OUR 'OLD FRIENDS' FROM NATURE

Since the 1950s the prevalence of immune diseases like asthma, multiple sclerosis and Crohn's disease, has increased in Western countries. This correlates with infectious diseases like typhoid becoming almost unheard of. The Hygiene Hypothesis was first proposed by Strachan in 1989 and poses the idea that overall microbial exposure is beneficial for our immune system and that the excessive reduction of bacteria in our environment may be harmful to health[29].

A variation on this theory, used to explain the rise in allergic and immune-mediated illnesses which has correlated with a change in the way we live, is the Old Friends Hypothesis[30]. The rationale for this thinking is that our collective move into an urbanised and sanitised environment has reduced our contact with the various organisms we have evolved with, our Old Friends from nature. These Friends include microbiota, infections acquired during birth and the environmental organisms from animals, mud and untreated water we were in daily contact with for millennia. Living near other people promotes microbiota variety and those with domestic pets have lower rates of allergic disorders, and richer microbiota in their household dust. Humans have lived with dogs as domestic companions for thousands of years. We have most likely co-evolved with our pet's Old Friends, perhaps even relying on them for the development of our immune system.

As modern humans have moved indoors, away from nature and our Old Friends, we have also adopted a lifestyle led increasingly apart from people and animals. Our houses have become larger and we have retreated to our rooms to spend time on devices in virtual worlds. The opportunities for interaction between the dynamic ecosystems of our bodies and the wider world have diminished. The consequences of this dramatic change, over a relatively short period of evolutionary time, are seen in the rise of non-communicable, autoimmune and chronic diseases.

It is thought our Old Friends, through their interaction with the immune and nervous complexes in the gut and other mucosal tissues, helped us develop *immunoregulation*. This describes how the immune system switches off and on in response to environmental threats. Well-functioning immunity rapidly swings into action when threatened by an infection or other insult, and then switches off as soon as the event is over. If our immune system is constantly on, our bodies enter a state of chronic inflammation. This can be exhausting and result in illness.

Medical microbiologist Professor Graham Rook uses the analogy of a computer with minimal data to describe our immune system at birth[31]. Through exposure to our Old Friends, data is incorporated into the body's memory cells so they can rapidly recognise harmful substances and respond appropriately. The process of exposure also establishes rules within the immune system. It learns not to attack itself, harmless molecules in the air or the contents of our gut. These Old Friends are working to build up the memory and capacity of our immune 'computer'. If the process goes awry, this malfunctions to attack itself causing various autoimmune diseases. If it attacks benign air molecules, hay fever and other allergic conditions occur or, if it attacks gut contents, inflammatory bowel diseases may arise. Much like when our electronic computer crashes, the consequences can be dire.

If a computer is constantly working when not needed, using up valuable processing capacity and data, it is more prone to break down. This is analogous to our bodies being in a state of constant background inflammation predisposing us to heart disease and other health problems. The sorts of conditions relating to this state of persistent, low-grade inflammation are those seen with increasing frequency in modern, urban communities and their healthcare settings.

Research in mice supports the Old Friends Hypothesis with studies showing animals bred in sterile conditions have abnormal immune tissue structure and increased susceptibility to allergies. These problems may be fixed by seeding the intestine with healthy strains of bacteria, but the timing is important with success occurring only if this is done in the first six weeks of life[32,33]. While these experiments were done in mice, scientists think similar changes may occur in humans. Also, other research has found children with eczema have different microbiota to those who don't and these differences seem to arise prior to the onset of allergic disease[34,35]. It may be the case that changes in microbiota predispose children to allergies. Other experiments have shown allergic risk can be transferred by putting disease-associated microbiota into healthy mice and conversely, that disease protection can be given by transferring healthy microbiota[36].

This work may mean infants at high risk of developing allergic diseases can be given microbiota as a preventative health strategy. It also suggests we should be encouraging vaginal birth where possible and supporting breastfeeding where able, to optimise healthy seeding of the infant microbiome, especially when there's a family history of allergy. Also, given antibiotic treatment of a pregnant woman can alter her vaginal and gut microbiomes, the use of these medications in pregnancy should be restricted to when absolutely necessary. Research is underway to find out whether probiotics taken during pregnancy will help support a healthy maternal microbiome, and if so, which ones. In situations where a vaginal birth is not possible, some doctors and scientists are recommending the newborn be wiped with a cloth carrying its mother's bacteria. While not yet a formal recommendation, this could become a simple and inexpensive way to reduce the risk of allergies for babies born surgically who are otherwise at higher risk of these conditions[28].

The new knowledge of vaginal and gut microbiomes is causing a shift in antenatal care to a more wholistic model with a greater emphasis on lifestyle and health education. This includes encouraging women, where they can, to adopt a diet rich in high fibre, nutrient dense, whole foods including fermented items rich in beneficial bacteria. Providing information about the value of breastfeeding (where possible) and vaginal birth (should they be able) for their baby's future wellbeing will help women make sound choices. In all these ways, the inner rainforest of a child's microbiome may be tended well before birth giving them the best start in life possible.

## INFLAMMATION AND ILLNESS

Just as we are grasping the significance of our Old Friends from nature for the development of a healthy microbiome and optimal immunoregulation, the role chronic bodily inflammation plays in the development of disease is becoming clearer. The major causes of ill health in the Western world seem to share inflammation as a causative factor. These include non-communicable, or lifestyle-related diseases, like stroke, heart disease and depression.

The amount of inflammation occurring in the body can be measured by checking the c-reactive protein (CRP) level in a blood test. An elevation of this biomarker may be due to infection, injury or other disease processes. The CRP will be very high if we are seriously ill. Low grade inflammation is indicated by a slightly raised CRP and it is this which is associated with lifestyle-related illness. To continue with Rook's computer analogy, chronically raised CRP equates to this device being constantly on, with capacity and energy draining from the system.

Research into the ways inflammation affects the body is ongoing, with some scientists arguing it may be a key factor in the development of heart disease, a major cause of death and illness in modern societies[37]. It seems that the drag on the body from long-term, low-level inflammation sets the scene for this serious illness. Interestingly, some studies have found infants exposed to higher levels of microbes in their environment have lower CRP levels, less inflammation and fewer associated diseases in adulthood[38]. So, once again, exposure to living things in early life appears to be protective for human health.

Cardiovascular disease is now understood to have an inflammatory basis – the lining of blood vessels become irritated, making them sticky. Plaques of cholesterol readily attach to this tackiness, resulting in narrowing of the vessel and a restriction of blood flow[39]. If the blood supply to our heart muscle is reduced, we may have a heart attack; if the flow is restricted to our brain, a stroke may result. These conditions are very common in Western societies and predisposing risk factors include high blood pressure and cholesterol levels, diabetes, a family history of heart disease and smoking. Perhaps, given the causal role of inflammation, and the importance of our Old Friends in nature for its regulation, we should add a lack of microbial diversity to that list.

Like heart disease, depression is a condition causing enormous suffering in Western societies, rapidly approaching heart disease as the world's biggest global health problem. Community health professionals see many patients struggling with this illness and the anguish that spills out to affect all facets of their life. As with cardiovascular disease, scientists have found inflammation plays a role in the development of depression with raised CRP levels implicated as a predictive factor[40,41]. The relationship between CRP elevation, inflammation and depression is complex and the focus of ongoing research but one thing is clear, illness should be understood within the context of an individual's life story, lifestyle and social and environmental setting. This includes the amount of contact they have with the plants and animals of the natural world.

## NATURE ALL AROUND US

How exposure to nature improves mental health will be explored in a later chapter but it is apparent from the evidence accumulated so far, that interactions between our Old Friends and our immune system are an important part of the picture. If we wish to support the inner rainforests of our microbiota, we need to ensure we are surrounded by other living systems rich in biodiversity. Just as a tropical forest will not remain vibrant if it is encircled by a sterile, concrete wasteland. This *immuno-microbiological* view of the health benefits of nature adds weight to the argument for more public green space in our cities. Particularly numerous, highly biodiverse places spread throughout the urban footprint. These types of parks and reserves support high microbial quality which would enrich the air of our cities with an array of airborne microbiota. For rather than simply being an inert mixture of gases, the air we breathe contains its own collection of microscopic life.

Humans are exposed to air-borne microbes through the simple act of breathing when they become trapped in our upper airways and inhaled or swallowed. As we get down onto our knees to pull weeds or plant seedlings, we are also tending our inner garden, facilitating the interplay between the life in and around us. Viewing this interaction through the immuno-microbiological lens we can surmise that spending time in nature-rich areas will help lower bodily inflammation and associated illness. Even away from soil and gardens, in seaside or marine environments, the air is alive with microbes. The instinct many of us have to take deep breaths of 'sea air' may be as good for us as it feels given the likelihood each breath contains some bacteria to fortify our microbiome.

The composition of microorganisms in air varies enormously between urban and rural places and is influenced by their natural diversity. The types of airborne bacteria include those found in soils, on plants and in water. There is movement and interaction between the soil's microscopic communities, the air above and the rainwater flowing through. The richer an area's biological life, with multiple plant and animal species in healthy numbers, the more biodiverse its atmosphere will be. So, air in the country is more alive than that in the city and varies according to the type of farming occurring. It's likely country areas with vast plantings of one type of crop, or monoculture, have diminished diversity of air-borne microbes. This is because monoculture utilises pesticides and herbicides, chemicals designed to kill unwanted plants or insects. As these biocidal agents are sprayed on crops, they enter the nearby soil, water and air. They can be carried over significant distances on dust particles effecting large areas of countryside, diminishing biodiversity both on land and in the atmosphere. Ultimately, our Old Friends in nature are affected and consequently so are we.

As touched on earlier, just as the air we breathe is complex and full of life, so too is the soil vastly richer and more intricate in its composition than mere dirt. Apart from the myriad of microorganisms present, insects and other creatures constantly reshape its matrix. Canadian scientist and environmentalist David Suzuki describes soil as "a living community of organisms. It is a world that we barely know. In a single teaspoon of soil, we may find hundreds of millions to 3 billion bacteria and a million fungi, like yeast and moulds. There is a veritable zoo of creatures in soil".

Given our food comes from the soil, it would serve us well to treat it respectfully so future generations can grow healthy food too. Whether eating plants grown directly in the earth, or meat from an animal grazing on them, we are reliant on it for our nutrition. Looking after soil requires a shift to farming practices that support its living community of organisms. To this end, we need to stop using agricultural chemicals which destroy soil microbes and ultimately diminish our microbiome. Positive actions to grow food in a regenerative system that supports biodiversity at both microscopic and landscape scales are enormously beneficial to human health.

People who reside in cities are inextricably linked to those in rural areas through food systems and the planetary soil, water and atmospheric cycles. Not to mention the billions of creatures, like insects and birds, who move through both places. Decisions made on the farm effect those in the city just as choices by urban dwellers impact agricultural workers. All have a role to play in correcting the balance so biodiversity is restored.

## KEY POINTS

- ❤ We have bacteria both on our skin and inside our body

- ❤ Our gut contains a *microbiome* – a complex garden of bacteria and other microscopic organisms

- ❤ Our gut microbiome interacts with our immune and nervous systems and is vitally important

- ❤ This microbiome is born when we are, as we receive its first seeds from our mother's birth canal and breast milk

- ❤ Our microbiome can be damaged by antibiotics and a poor diet and nurtured by a healthy, plant-rich diet

- ❤ Exposure to our Old Friends in nature helps support our microbiome and immune system and reduce inflammation in the body

- ❤ Inflammation underlies many health conditions including heart disease and depression

- ❤ Our Old Friends include environmental organisms in water and soil and on other animals

- ❤ We encounter our Old Friends through our food and water, the air we breathe and the animals, plants and soils we interact with daily

- ❤ Keeping pets, spending time in nature and with others supports our microbiome

Apart from nourishing our inner rainforest, nature has provided many medicines to help heal our bodies when they sicken. Although their origin is often forgotten, over half of all drugs used in modern Western healthcare have come from the natural world. Novel agents continue to be discovered as scientists explore the chemical makeup of plants and various animal secretions, including toxins. Human health also benefits as nature provides researchers, inventors and designers with inspiration for innovation. In all these ways, the living world is of enormous value to people. Here are just a few examples to support the call for protection and valuing of biodiversity from a more, human-focussed, or *anthropocentric*, perspective.

## MEDICINES FROM NATURE

From the common aspirin, initially derived from the bark of the willow tree, humans are constantly turning to natural substances to soothe our pain and heal our body. Newer agents include Botox, which originated from a toxin called 'botulinum' toxin (BTX). Produced by bacteria, when eaten in contaminated food or absorbed into the body via an infected wound, BTX can make us severely unwell, even fatally so. The toxin blocks the transmission of acetylcholine and so prevents nerves from working properly, leading to progressive paralysis. However, like many poisons, BTX can be used in surprising ways to enhance human health.

Botox is commonly associated with the cosmetic procedure-injections to the face in pursuit of a youthful complexion. However, due to its ability to cause focal muscle relaxation, it also has many therapeutic uses. These include treatment of chronic headache and migraine, disabling conditions for which many sufferers become reliant on painkillers like codeine. Most of these drugs have problems with dependency and perversely, they may also trigger further headaches. Neurologists now carefully inject the scalp of severe headache sufferers with BTX to reduce muscle tension, helping thousands break free from chronic pain.

BTX is also used to reduce muscle spasm for those living with cerebral palsy (CP), a condition where muscle contractures have led to deformity and reduced limb function. Regular BTX injection, massage and exercise can see those living with CP gain more movement from their previously stiff and often painful arms or legs. Bladder irritability, a cause of incontinence or urine leakage, may respond to BTX treatment regimens too. Administered in a procedure called a cystoscopy, where a tiny camera is introduced into the bladder via the urethra, BTX is injected into areas of tight, spasming muscle. Once again, via inducing muscle relaxation, the toxin eases symptoms.

Another toxin, this time from the venom of a type of cone shell, *conus magus*, is now in use as a pain-relieving medication. Cone shells are found in coral reef systems, like the Great Barrier Reef, and kill their prey by injecting them with a paralysing toxin before ingesting them. This beautiful shell's venom contains chemicals known as *conotoxins*, some of which have been found to relieve severe pain in humans. While there are some 75,000 different conotoxins with potential medicinal purposes, only one is already in use. Marketed as the drug Prialt, this agent is injected into the fluid around the spinal cord by an infusion pump to relieve pain not responsive to usual treatments. It is extremely potent, around one thousand times more powerful than morphine, and comes without the problem of dependency which could lead to addiction. Unfortunately, it is complex to administer, and clinicians find it difficult to get the dose exact because the toxic and therapeutic doses are extremely close.

Scientists are working on other drugs from conotoxins which can be taken by mouth and have a safer profile. There are thought to be 700 different species of cone shell, most yet to be formally described. Sadly, they are threatened by climate change as warmer, more acidic seas impair shell formation. Cone shells are also highly coveted by collectors for their gorgeous shells. Coming in a myriad of colours and patterns, cone shells' beauty poses a threat to their survival as they are removed from the ocean and added to private collections[42,43].

Not all new medicinal agents come from the poisonous part of nature's larder. Many derive from fruits and the life-giving milk of mammals. The rind of delicious tropical fruit mangosteen contains a compound useful for the treatment of schizophrenia[44]. Mangosteen is native to the tropical forests of Malaysia and other South-East Asian countries where it is a staple food source for orangutans. Long recognised by Indigenous Peoples as having medicinal properties, its rind has been used in traditional medicines to treat abdominal pain, diarrhoea, cholera, wound infection and ulcers. Scientists have found it to have various pharmacological actions, being anti-inflammatory, antibacterial, anti-malarial and anti-oxidating. It can also modulate immune function and lower blood pressure. Some of mangosteen's key active ingredients are called *xanthones*, the most promising being alpha-mangostin. This compound has been used for the treatment of diabetes, high blood lipids and cardiovascular protection[45]. Sadly, like the orangutan, the mangosteen's native habitat is threatened by destruction as lowland forests are cleared for palm oil plantations.

Research in Australia has found the milk of Tasmanian Devils to contain compounds which may help combat antibiotic resistance. The Tasmanian Devil is a small marsupial with black fur and a strange gambolling gait. Increasingly known by one of its Aboriginal names, Purinina, it's the largest carnivorous marsupial in the world and is currently listed as endangered. Marsupials are mammals who suckle their young in pouches and are found predominantly in Australia. The Purinina is threatened by a cancer called facial tumour disease, as well as by human activity. Juveniles are suckled in their mother's pouch after being born at only twenty-one days of pregnancy. Being tiny with an immature immune system, they are extremely vulnerable to infection from bacteria in the pouch. They receive protection from small, potent antibacterial proteins, or peptides, in their mother's milk. These peptides are called *cathelicidins* and, while humans have only one type, Purininas have six. Two of the Purinina's cathelicidins are capable of killing bacteria which may be life threatening to humans, including Staph. aureus or 'golden staph'[46]. Other marsupials have high numbers of cathelicidins too, so research is ongoing into the properties of other Australian marsupial's milk, including koalas and wallabies.

The Purinina is a scavenger, so is attracted to carcasses of roadkill along rural highways. The facial tumour disease spreads when Purininas fight each other for food, often in the dangerous roadside environment. The last wild population of these animals is the Tarkine/takayna region of north-western Tasmania. This area is currently being destroyed by logging and mining. The loss of habitat from these industries, coupled with increased road traffic through its forest home, may see this wild Purinina population decimated.

The plights of the cone shell, mangosteen and Purinina demonstrate how destructive human activity risks extinguishing new, potentially lifesaving, medical discoveries. Action to look after these plants and animals, and their habitat, is therefore profoundly beneficial for our wellbeing. In this way, environmental protection and regeneration are preventative health actions. We save forests and other biodiverse ecosystems to save ourselves, as much as other living things.

# BUSH MEDICINE

Apart from appreciating how the natural world helps us from a Western medical and scientific perspective, it is also time to take a new and respectful look at Aboriginal Australia's knowledge of bush medicine. After all, these First Nations people have been skilfully practising their craft for millennia and had ample time to see first-hand the benefits and side effects of various treatments. Modern medical science seeks treatments which have been tested by a randomised, double-blind, placebo-controlled trial. This gold standard experiment involves two similar groups of people being randomly assigned to receive either a placebo or a test agent. Study participants are unaware (blind) as to which group they have been placed in, as are the researchers. Scientists can therefore measure the test medicine's effectiveness against the placebo. If found to be more beneficial, it is said to be therapeutic. Placebo on its own is thought to have around a 30% therapeutic effect. The randomised study is a very methodical and specific process. The strongest evidence is provided when results are replicated by other gold standard studies undertaken by different groups of researchers. The more people enrolled as participants, the better to detect rare side effects.

In contrast to this way of testing, First Nations Australians have, over at least 60,000 years, used trial and error to ascertain therapeutic benefit. If a bush medicine was found to help headache, for example, its use would spread, and its applications refined over many generations. There would be no point continuing with an ineffective treatment because it wouldn't support optimal health and longevity. While different to Western scientific methods, it is no less valid and may well be more useful because of the extraordinarily long duration over which a treatment can be monitored. This may be tens of thousands of years and multiple generations.

Many modern drugs may only have been trialled for five years before being released onto the market. This means adverse effects which take time to evolve are not discovered before thousands of people are affected. One famous example is diethylstilboestrol (DES), a synthetic form of oestrogen used to prevent miscarriage in pregnant women between the 1940s and 1970s. Tens of thousands of women were prescribed DES before its causative role in hormone-dependent cancers became apparent. This affected not only those taking the drug, but also their daughters, who had been exposed in-utero. While the mothers had an elevated risk of acquiring breast cancer, their daughters received this increased risk as well as a 1/1000 chance of developing a rare vaginal and cervical cancer called clear cell adenocarcinoma.

Many Australian indigenous plants are both a food source and a medicine. The ground cover commonly called 'pigface' has a delicious, edible fruit and its inner leaf exudes a jelly-like liquid which helps relieve sunburn and other skin conditions. It's a food and medicine in one[47]. This plant is found over large areas of southern Australia, so has several Aboriginal names. Known as Katwort by the Gunaikurnai people of the area now called Gippsland, swathes of the countryside become covered in its hot pink blooms when it's in flower. Apart from soothing skin inflammation, the leaf juice can relieve stomach upset and throat infections. There are estimated to be some seven thousand bush foods in Australia and it's likely many also have medicinal properties.

The usefulness of plants for First Nations people extends far beyond food and medicine to include building materials and clothing. Seaweeds especially have multiple applications and been used over millennia for nutrition, clothing, shelter and cultural and fishing purposes. From seaweed, ropes, fishing nets, water containers, cloaks, and even shoes, were made[48]. Scientists are just beginning to understand the complexity of these plant-like algae and are looking to Aboriginal knowledge systems to better learn how they might be used in today's modern society.

Historically, First Nations knowledge has been dismissed by Western scientists as primitive and simple, but in their illuminating paper on seaweeds, Ruth Thurstan and others took a new, more respectful approach. They reviewed historical records to unearth valuable insights into the multitude of uses First Nations people have for seaweeds. These learnings were not possible with the myopic lens used by earlier scholars. Thurstan's group found the strong, leathery, bull kelp from southern Australia's coastal waters can be used for "roofing material for shelters, footwear, moulding of cups and water-carriers, and a 'highly nutritious' food that was suitable for preservation and transport."[48]

Aboriginal and Torres Strait Islander culture is living, not simply historical, and is ever evolving and innovating. A great opportunity exists for non-Indigenous people to learn from First Peoples' deep and continuing knowledge of the natural environment. The scope for unearthing 'new' treatments and technologies is astonishing, if we listen carefully to the custodians who hold this wisdom. Given First Nations people have an oral culture, where knowledge is passed down verbally through stories and songs, listening respectfully to Elders is the most effective way to receive these insights. This means learning is best done on Country rather than in a lecture theatre or laboratory. Non-Indigenous people can seek out Elders and other knowledge holders through First Nations organisations across Australia and the Torres Strait.

One such organisation is Living Culture, located on the traditional lands of the Boon Wurrung/Bunurong people of the Kulin Nation, an area now called the Mornington Peninsula, in Victoria. Its founder and well-known teacher is Lionel Lauch, a Gunditjmara Kirrae Wurrung-Bundjalung man with an encyclopaedic knowledge of local plants and animals. Lionel has the blessing of the local Boon Wurrung and Bunurong community to share traditional knowledge and stories on Country[49]. Keen to impart his wisdom to those willing to join him out in the forest or along the rugged coastline, Lionel has a gift for teaching. Walking with him through bushland as he explains the many medicinal uses of various plants is a revelation. Sap from the 'grass tree', known as Baggup in Woi Wurrung, can be heated and used as a glue to repair wounds. Like the Histoacryl glue currently used in medical clinics and emergency departments, but without the bright blue dye and plastic packaging.

Lionel challenges popular beliefs about the common bracken fern. Its toughness and pervasiveness as an understorey plant see it frequently regarded as weed-like and not to be nurtured. However, for Aboriginal people, this woodland fern, Muulaa (Djab wurrung), is a true super plant, both in its enormity and utility[50]. Muulaa is, like the King's Holly, all one plant, connected beneath the surface of the forest through its rhizome root system. It is also likely to be ancient. Muulaa's rhizomes were once a staple food for the Boon Wurrung and Bunurong people. A rich source of starch, they can be baked into cakes or roasted. On his walks through the forest Lionel demonstrates how Muulaa's young fronds can be squashed into a paste to alleviate the sting and irritation of insect bites. When the season is right, he also points out delicious native raspberries rambling through the understory[50]. These fruits look much like their European cousins albeit slightly smaller with a softer flavour.

Walking with Lionel facilitates a richer understanding of the forest's bounty. Bushland previously loved for its beauty and peacefulness transforms into a pharmacy and supermarket once you know where and when to look. Opportunities for this kind of experiential learning abound and are an essential part of developing a richer connection to Australia's natural and cultural heritage. They may also provide inspiration for the development of new treatments in collaboration with First Nations people.

Apart from providing us with medicines and sustaining us physically, nature stimulates our learning. It also provides for our spiritual enrichment. Let's look towards these intangible gifts of nature next.

# KEY POINTS

- More than half of medicines in use today were derived from nature
- New agents are being discovered from plants and animals all the time
- Future cures are at risk from the destruction of nature
- Protecting habitats like reefs and forests safeguards these potential medicines
- First Nations people have a deep understanding of natural medicines
- First Australians describe many plants as being both food and medicine
- The best place to learn about Bush Medicine is on Country

# 4

# Nature's Gifts

*"The great book, always open
and which we should make an
effort to read, is that of Nature."*

~Antonio Gaudi

Human beings have a unique capacity for learning and our first and best schoolroom is the natural world. This is where our curiosity is piqued, our sense of wonder stoked. We watch and notice the lifeforms around us. How they are formed, how they function and how they interact with their environment. Vast landscapes provide us with a sense of perspective, of our place within the wider web of life. They evoke feelings of awe and the contemplation of connection to a force larger than ourselves. Together, awe and wonder are perhaps nature's greatest intangible gifts. Let's see how the natural world helps us learn, create, and contemplate. From the pragmatic workings of body systems and medical devices through to places of worship and enlightenment.

## LEARNING DESIGN FROM NATURE

Most of us have sat for a while and wondered about the behaviour of animals, whether it's our pet dog, or the ants marching across the ground outside. Nature, in all its forms, stimulates our curiosity and prods us to think what, how and why? Over hundreds of years scientists and doctors have learnt from studying, not only the chemistry of plants and animals, but also their behaviour and structural design. One example of the complexity of nature is the now extinct gastric brooding frog. Once found in southern Queensland, this frog had evolved an extraordinary capacity to temporarily convert its upper stomach into a uterus. This transformation only occurred in the female and involved the acid-secreting mechanism being switched off for the gestational period. The mother frog would swallow up to twenty fertilized eggs and keep them in her stomach until they were ready to be regurgitated as young froglets.

When this species was first studied in the late 1970s, it fascinated scientists. Investigation of the frog's stomach and its contents found an acid-secreting inhibitor called prostaglandin E2 produced by the larvae of the developing froglets[51]. In switching off the acid production in their mother's stomach, the baby frogs altered their environment so they could survive and grow. Once they were expelled from the stomach, the prostaglandin E2 was no longer present, so the organ recommenced secreting acid for food digestion. This discovery helped researchers working on treatments for stomach ulcer in humans, where an excess of acid burns through the stomach's lining potentially causing catastrophic bleeding. They realized prostaglandin E2 had the effect of inhibiting acid secretion in the stomach and so had potential as an ulcer-healing agent. As has often been the case, scientists in the field of biology, and other related sciences where nature is explored, discovered something that could help relieve human suffering. This was well before H. pylori's role in the generation of stomach ulcers was realised. So, the use of prostaglandin E2 analogues provided interim relief until the true causative agent was known. The gastric brooding frog demonstrates the capacity within nature for transient structural and functional change to occur to facilitate reproduction of species in a most remarkable way.

People have used nature as a source of inspiration for solving complex problems for millennia. *Biomimicry* is the imitation of the designs, systems and elements of nature. It covers historical examples, like studying birds to develop human flight in aeroplanes, through to modern buildings which have copied design elements from termite mounds to optimise temperature regulation. We see this in healthcare with researchers finding inspiration from the way a mosquito painlessly sucks blood to develop new needles which hurt less.

A mosquito uses several techniques to extract blood without us noticing. First, it secretes a numbing substance onto the skin. It then pierces the surface with a vibrating proboscis which is serrated along its shaft and flexible at the tip. The design features of vibration, serration and flexibility mean less than one third of the force required by an artificial needle is needed to pierce the skin. So, it's less deformed as the proboscis passes through[52]. This makes a mosquito bite almost painless. It's our body's immune response to mosquito saliva that renders the puncture site annoyingly itchy. Hopefully researchers will acquire the funding needed to bring this innovation to market, especially for young children with illnesses such as diabetes, where multiple injections are required. Beyond healthcare, designers look to optimize human interaction with nature because, as well as being aesthetically pleasing, it evokes positive feelings.

Many urban dwellers, whether at work or home, feel more relaxed and comfortable when they can see outside. Even catching a glimpse of the sky or a distant treetop is restorative. Similarly, being in a room with natural light, fresh air from an open window, indoor plants and/or a water feature, feels good and enables better focus and friendlier interactions with others. Architects, interior designers, and town planners who are switched on to our inherent need for this contact with nature use *biophilic* design principles when creating places for us to live and work.

Biophilic design is underpinned by the principle of *biophilia*. The Biophilia Hypothesis describes an inherent love of nature baked into us as we evolved in sync with the natural world. It will be explored in detail later when we investigate how contact with nature supports mental health. Biophilic design itself is not a new idea, rather our language for it is new. As the great Spanish architect Antonio Gaudi said, "anything created by human beings is already in the great book of nature". Gaudi noticed that in nature there were no straight lines, or sharp corners, so his buildings had soft, organic shapes everywhere. Doors, windows and furniture were all curved and naturally sculpted.

Stepping into the Sagrada Familia, Gaudi's famous cathedral, is an awe-inspiring experience. Compared to other churches which are often dark and cold, the Sagrada is flooded with rainbows of light through tall, multi-coloured windows. The walls are curved and gigantic 'trunks' of stone form a forest to support the canopy-like ceiling. The inspiration of nature is almost tangible in this place despite it being constructed from stone, glass and concrete.

While we can't all travel to Barcelona to marvel at Gaudi's genius, we can be inspired, as he was, by nature and look to it for ideas, comfort and peace. For many, immersive experiences in nature can be both healing and transformative, affecting the body, mind and heart.

## NATURE – A PLACE FOR TRANSCENDENT EXPERIENCES

Nature can provide a place of deep connection to the earth and offer transcendent experiences, like those attained with meditation or prayer where one feels connected to something greater than oneself. Well known Australian environmentalist Bob Brown was arrested and imprisoned in 1983 during the campaign to save the Franklin River wilderness area in Tasmania. In a letter from his prison cell he wrote, "for several years I have returned to it (the south-west) to watch the interplay of forests, rivers and sky by day and to listen to the animals stir at night when the stars are ablaze, and the scintillating blue specks of glow-worms pierce the forest floors of blackness. I am not a conventionally religious man, but in the wilderness, I have come closest to finding myself and knowing the universe and accepting God-by which I mean accepting all that I don't know. The wilderness is my best place on Earth. It is at least as important to me as a place of refreshment, inspiration, and fulfilment as is the house of worship to many other Australians. Now I have been made a trespasser in the cathedral of my choice."[53]

It is clear from Brown's writing that when in the south-west wilderness he feels a connection to something greater than himself. Within this place of trees and rivers, he has a spiritual home, akin to a place of worship.

Brown's reflections mirror my own as I too, feel an inner peace, a sense of being truly at home when in wild places especially when surrounded by ancient trees as in the Tarkine/takayna rainforest. Looking at my diary from a visit there in 2012, I am reminded of the transcendent feeling of immersion within the larger living world. I wrote: "Time stands still here, there's a sense of peace and tranquillity and it feels like I'm connecting to an ancient way of knowing. All is green, everywhere I look. Moss and lichen on logs and rocks, a myriad of verdant shades with different textures, from gossamer-like hanging threads and luxurious velvet mosses on logs, to rings of flat lime lichen on rocks. Patterns upon patterns of living things. Metallic jewel beetles, more precious than any mined substance, are tucked within moss cushions, and enormous fallen trees have a metropolis of spider webs in their undersides. I am bathing in green, restored and healed- 'forest bathing'". Reading this now I realise that I was using the term forest bathing well before I had learnt of the Japanese practice, shinrin-yoku. I recall feeling as if I had been truly immersed in nature and, akin to a baptism, transformed by it.

Psychologist Abraham Maslow used the term *peak experience* to describe 'non-striving, non-self-centred, purposeless, self-validating, end-experiences and states of perfection and of goal attainment.'[54] Famous for his 'hierarchy of needs' first introduced in the 1940s, Maslow was interested in understanding what made people happy and fulfilled. Depicted as a pyramid, the hierarchy held basic physiological necessities at the bottom. These were followed by needs for safety, love and belonging, self-esteem and then, at the apex, self-actualisation. According to his theory, without meeting the basic requirements, higher needs of personal growth could not be reached.

Self-actualisation is the culmination of complete personal development where an individual's full potential has been reached and is considered quite rare. Maslow thought peak experiences played an important role in self-actualisation but could be experienced by anyone, even those yet to reach their full personal growth. I consider my experience in the Tarkine/takayna rainforest to be a peak experience, a time of pure joy and elation, a turning point. Subsequent psychologists have identified peak experiences as holding the characteristics of personal significance, fulfillment and a sense of being at one with the world[55]. They might include falling in love, gaining a key insight or a feeling of deep contentment. Peak experiences often occur in nature and nourish us when we return to our regular lives. By recalling the sights and sounds of our special place, sensory memories evoke positive emotions. We are soothed and calmed by these transcendent experiences long after we have left their source.

Prolonged time spent in nature, away from the stresses and routines of regular life, has been a part of humankind's story for millennia. From monks and ascetics retreating to mountain caves, to pilgrims journeying to sacred places, people everywhere have sought the peace and space of the natural world to grapple with existential questions. Many of these encounters would be described as peak experiences using today's academic language. Weeks spent living simply, walking from place to place, either alone or with others, allow gentle rhythms to develop. This is the path of the pilgrim and offers insights into our common humanity.

## NATURE – A PLACE FOR PILGRIMAGE AND RECKONING

There is a long history within many cultures of pilgrimages for spiritual enlightenment and these usually occur through a grand natural landscape. Today, there is a resurgence of people seeking these types of experiences to reconnect with themselves and reflect on life's meaning and purpose. Many Christians, as well as the nonreligious, choose to take the Camino de Santiago, a long walk over some four to six weeks in northern Spain. While journeys to Mecca, the River Ganges and other religious sites continue to be an aspiration for the devout. For First Nations people, spirituality is embedded within nature itself.

First Australians have wound spiritual meaning into their knowledge of the landscape through their Songlines. These are pathways which have been journeyed for many thousands of years for cultural and survival purposes. Clans have walked through the landscape, the timing of their journey dictated by the seasonality of plants and animals. Many roads we now drive along are the modern manifestation of colonisation of these sacred paths. First Nations Australians taught white arrivals the best ways to move through their country, often threading beside and between fresh water sources. This knowledge was exploited as the newcomers took over, progressively widening and shaping the way, until we now have eight-lane freeways running beside major waterways.

This has occurred along the Yarra River in Melbourne. Called Birrarung in Woiwurrung and Boonwurrung languages, the river is a Songline leading from the mountains to the sea. It now has a major freeway running alongside its lower section, a large tunnel burrowing underneath and bridges of concrete straddling it. Cars crawl alongside, underneath and over this ancient river.

In her book *The Comfort of Water*, Maya Ward recounts the extraordinary journey she took along Birrarung from the sea to its source high in the mountains, walking the Songline. This was her way of more deeply understanding the country she lived in and her place within it. She writes "these two different traditions; religions originating overseas, and local, ancient practices – neither tradition was mine. But for me to go on a pilgrimage in Australia, with all of this history in mind, felt like bringing them into some sort of conversation. I was interested in what, if I listened carefully, I might overhear."[56]

Before setting out on her journey, Maya sought the permission of Aboriginal Elders and learnt the story of Barak, the Ngurrung-gaeta of the Wurundjeri, a man of power and influence within his community at the time of early colonisation. Barak fought hard for the rights of his people, walking from the mountains along the Songline to the developing city of Melbourne, many times. He had seen his country despoiled, his people's communities scattered and fractured. Maya felt that walking along this ancient Songline as a pilgrimage was a way to pay tribute to his memory. She was walking a path trodden for thousands of years and throughout her journey she met Barak's descendants as well as those who now live alongside the river.

Maya lyrically describes her quest, and it is clear how moving this journey was for her. She was not only seeing the river landscape slowly, in close up, but was also using the time to journey inward and make sense of her place. As she set out, she wrote: "A Songline is a path of the Dreaming, a narrative of the ancestors, which mapped the land in song. I imagined how stories would be alive in places all along the way, days and days of walking and chanting, walking and chanting, woven together into neural pathways, the brain grooved to the shape of the land. Paths of mind, heart and country, traversed over a lifetime. Stories passed down the generations, regenerated each time the song was sung. The ancestors, the people, the land, becoming one thing, enchanted through chant, grown together through song, and each singing made them anew. The singing of hills (now flattened), bends (straightened), billabongs (drained). To imagine such a web of meaning once alive in this place, to have read of its dismemberment and its forgetting, yet to be stepping out on a fine morning with the wind and the words of kind people, was to be emptied and filled, blown clear through, free and indebted and with the chance to be true. May I breathe through my feet, lay my skin open, and be there to meet it all. All that is left, and all that is new."[56]

Having travelled for weeks, Maya and her companions were dismayed to discover the upper catchment was out of bounds to the public. This was because it was ostensibly being protected by the state water authority. Resourcefully, her group found a way to walk to the very edge of the restricted area and were shocked by coming face to face with a recently logged section of forest. The ground was still smouldering from the burning done after an area is denuded, or clear felled. The harsh reality of what our society has done, and continues to do, to the sacred Songline of Birrarung was there for her to witness. She writes "the journey had been a path of healing, of living in beauty, an enchantment that could make me strong enough to bear this. That path was the means of bringing me there, on the twenty-first day of our pilgrimage, to the 21st century where I live. The journey was saying what needed to be said over and over again."[56] Her companion described it as being their moment of reconciliation, of facing the truth of what colonisation has done and continues to do to this ancient land. It was a profound realisation of this truth.

As happened with Maya and her companions, time spent in the bush may evoke conflicting emotions for non-Aboriginal Australians. While being in nature often provides experiences of wonder and rejuvenation, there may also be a sense of discomfort as the legacy of colonisation is confronted. In national parks on the urban fringe, the presence of landscape degradation, weeds and feral animals are a pervasive visual reminder of the lack of care for nature held by our society. There may be poignancy and sorrow as we reflect on what would have been. How this place was before its original inhabitants were murdered or displaced. Apart from the abundance of plants and animals, the chatter, laughter and music of language as the people of the land went about their life, singing up Country, would have rung out across the continent and nearby islands. The erosion of First Peoples' language and culture, forms another layer of loss sitting with the vanishing of ecological richness.

Of course, this phenomenon is not confined to Australia, it is global. The attrition of First Nations people's knowledge and stewardship for the natural world and the attempted eradication of their culture has far-reaching consequences for us all. The history and the future of all humankind are inextricably linked, wherever we live on Earth. And we are tied together within the pulsing of all life, whether we agree with the concept of Gaia or not.

## KEY POINTS

- Humans are inspired by the designs and structures they see in nature
- *Biomimicry* describes how this inspiration flows into human creativity
- *Biophilic design* is inspired by nature and creates places we feel safe and comfortable in
- Nature provides places for *peak experiences*
- *Peak experiences* are a joyful state of non-striving and goal attainment
- Prolonged time deeply immersed in nature allows for self-growth and spiritual fulfilment

# The Challenge

The first section of this book has explored the natural world from the minutiae of our inner rainforest, our microbiota, to the vast biomes which make up planet Earth. The relationships between living things, be they airborne, aquatic, or earth-bound, have been investigated and their significance for human health contemplated. We have seen how global water and soil cycles intersect with one another and all life on Earth. And we have considered the myriad ways in which nature supports our wellbeing, providing us with food, medicine, shelter and, most fundamentally, air and water. The intangible gifts we receive from nature include moments of transcendence and insight and enduring, profound, spiritual meaning. The wisdom of First Nations people has been respectfully acknowledged and the legacy of colonisation touched on.

While the impact of humankind on planetary ecosystems has been mentioned, the looming, catastrophic, twin sequelae of climate change and mass extinction has yet to be deeply interrogated. How these global threats have evolved will be covered next, beginning with an overview of the basic science of the carbon cycle to foreground an exploration of climate change. Given the foundations of human wellbeing rely upon nature's ecosystem services, their disruption poses a dire risk to humanity. Discussion of the health impacts accompanying Earth's evolving climate chaos and diminishing biological diversity will naturally follow, bringing us to the present.

# 5

# Nature and Health Today

*"They keep saying that climate change is an
existential threat and the most important issue
of all. And yet they just carry on like before.
If the emissions have to stop, then we must stop
the emissions. To me that is black or white.
There are no grey areas when it comes to survival.
Either we go on as a civilization or we don't...
You would think every one of our leaders and
the media would be talking about nothing else,
but no one ever mentions it... Nor does hardly
anyone ever mention that we are in the midst of
the sixth mass extinction, with about two hundred
species going extinct every single day...
We already have all the facts and solutions.
All we have to do is to wake up and change."* [57)

~Swedish teenage climate activist, Greta Thunberg, addressing
'The Declaration of Rebellion' rally in London on 31 October, 2018.

Planetary systems, like those regulating Earth's climate, water and soil cycles, are undergoing a dramatic shift due to humanity's actions. Since the Industrial Revolution's 'dig it up or chop it down' mindset was unleashed there has been a wave of devastation breaking all over the world. That we are amid the sixth mass extinction event is widely accepted by scientists. So, too, is the knowledge that global warming's effects are being felt everywhere. The future in the Anthropocene epoch we find ourselves in is uncertain and, quite frankly, frightening. In this section, the various threats to nature are explored, as well as the inevitable consequence for human health. Following this, some of the factors contributing to people's collective apathy for remedying the situation will be teased apart – the 'why' to pair with the 'what', if you like.

I felt conflicted about including a detailed description on threats to nature, wanting the thrust of this book to be a positive celebration of how the natural world supports human flourishing but daily reminders of the strain people are placing on Earth compelled me to include these details on climate change and other harms to biodiversity. We need to act urgently to repair the damage, and this requires massive shifts in how we live. Without understanding why such big disruptions are needed it's difficult to compel people to change their way of life.

As Greta Thunberg says, we must all begin to talk about what's happening. It needs to become a key focus of our attention, defining the prism through which we make all our decisions. Everything really is black and white. Either our choices help Earth's biosphere or they do not. As these words are being written, Europe is suffering through a heatwave with temperatures never seen before, the polar ice is melting at an unprecedented rate and record temperatures have been found to be the cause of a dramatic decline in mammals in Queensland's Wet Tropics World Heritage area. Not including the topics of climate change and the sixth global mass extinction event would be complicit with the denial much of humanity is currently caught in. As Einstein said, "the world will not be destroyed by those who do evil, but by those who watch them without doing anything." Let's not simply stand by, let's stand together and step up to the challenge. Let's be Gaia's gardeners, not her gold-diggers.

# THE CARBON CYCLE
# AND CLIMATE CHANGE

To begin, the carbon, or climate, cycle requires exploration. The impacts of climate change are felt globally and profoundly affect biodiversity and human health. The rapidly escalating climate crisis is due to humankind's interference in the climate cycle. Establishing a foundational understanding of this area of science provides important perspective.

When thinking about the carbon cycle it is helpful to start with forests which, as with the water cycle, are key. Millions of years ago, vast forests of primitive plants, alive with strange insects and rich in carbon, covered the earth. After they died, they were gradually crushed under rock and soil to form underground reserves of fossil, or very old, fuels such as oil, coal and gas. It is paradigm shifting to truly appreciate that fossil fuels, like the petrol in our cars, took millions of years to form. When considered within the context of the relatively short human life span, fossil fuels are non-renewable, or finite. Once consumed, their stocks cannot be replenished.

When we mine and burn fossil fuels to run our homes, planes and cars, the stored carbon is released as the gas carbon dioxide ($CO_2$). This mixes into the air around us becoming part of Earth's atmosphere. Much of the carbon dioxide in the atmosphere is taken in by plants—above and underwater—in places like forests, wetlands, grasslands, seagrass meadows and kelp forests. Tiny plant-like life forms in the oceans called phytoplankton absorb $CO_2$ and are taken in by fish larvae and other minute creatures. As they break down and fall to the sea floor, tonnes of carbon are pulled into the depths. This process is called *drawing down* and takes $CO_2$ out of the atmosphere.

The places where carbon dioxide is drawn down are called *carbon sinks*. All living things containing carbon are sinks, as well as oceans and soils. Plants, through the process of photosynthesis, use the sun's energy and water, to turn the carbon in $CO_2$ into the building blocks of their structure. At a molecular level, these blocks are called carbohydrate. To the bare eye, they are the leaves, stems, roots, fruit and nuts of plants.

Oxygen is released in this process, which is neat for us because we need oxygen to breathe and function. Of course, we also like to eat plants, or the animals who eat plants, so our wellbeing is absolutely dependent on the ongoing, healthy functioning of the carbon cycle.

During respiration, we exhale carbon dioxide as one of our waste products. There is a beautiful symbiosis between us and plants as what we exhale, they absorb and what they release, we inhale. We breathe together. As scientist and writer Tim Flannery explains, "carbon is everywhere on the surface of planet Earth. It is constantly shifting in and out of our bodies as well as from rocks to sea or soils, and from there to the atmosphere and back again."[58]

Animals are an integral part of the carbon cycle. The planet's largest mammals, whales, function as carbon sinks. Their embodied carbon drops to the bottom of the ocean when they die. In a process known as a *whalefall*, tonnes of carbon are taken out of wider global circulation and out of the atmosphere. One whale has been estimated as equivalent to over a thousand trees in terms of carbon sequestration. An unrealised consequence of centuries of whaling is the diminishment of this aquatic carbon sink.

### The basics of the carbon cycle

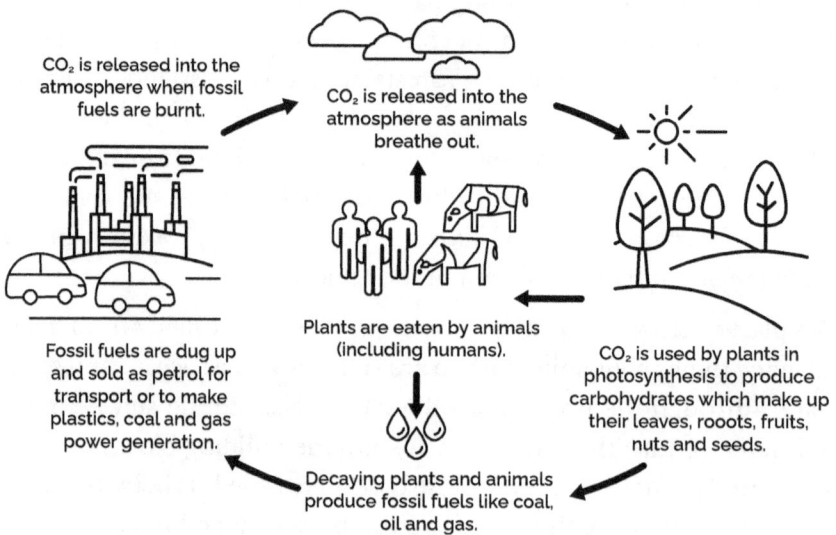

$CO_2$ is released into the atmosphere when fossil fuels are burnt.

$CO_2$ is released into the atmosphere as animals breathe out.

Fossil fuels are dug up and sold as petrol for transport or to make plastics, coal and gas power generation.

Plants are eaten by animals (including humans).

$CO_2$ is used by plants in photosynthesis to produce carbohydrates which make up their leaves, rooots, fruits, nuts and seeds.

Decaying plants and animals produce fossil fuels like coal, oil and gas.

Most of the heat hitting Earth's surface from the sun is reflected out into space. However, carbon dioxide, together with other greenhouse gases, works to form a kind of heat blanket around the planet. As it retains some of the sun's warmth, this action is called the *greenhouse effect*. A greenhouse is a small glass shed people living in cold climates use to grow plants. In the greenhouse, plants are sheltered from cold air and winds and yet the sun's light can still reach them, so they flourish. The glass acts to keep the heat inside just as greenhouse gases keep our planet warm.

### The Greenhouse Effect

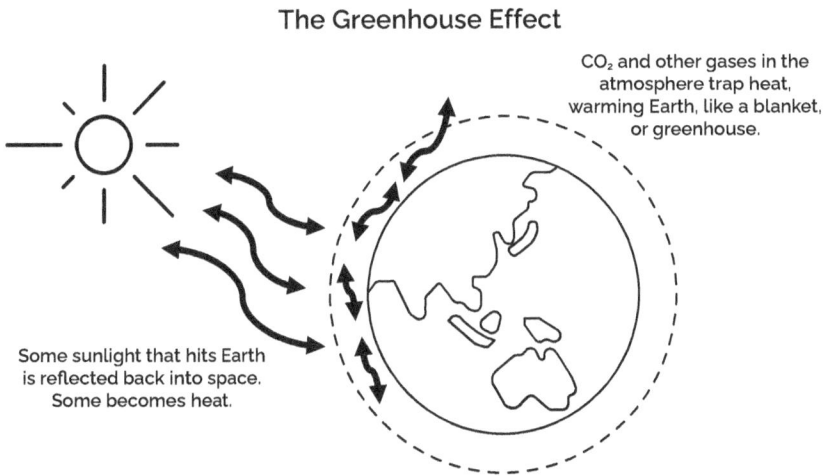

CO₂ and other gases in the atmosphere trap heat, warming Earth, like a blanket, or greenhouse.

Some sunlight that hits Earth is reflected back into space. Some becomes heat.

The current problem we are facing with global warming is the dramatic increase in the atmosphere's carbon dioxide, the most abundant greenhouse gas after water vapour. The mining and combustion of fossil fuels since the industrial revolution, in concert with the destruction of Earth's carbon sinks, particularly its forests, is responsible for this rise. Carbon dioxide takes between twenty and two hundred years to be cycled out of the atmosphere. The heat-holding capacity of Earth's greenhouse has been accelerating as new $CO_2$ is added faster than older gas can be removed by natural processes. We humans are fortifying the greenhouse.

Our species, Homo sapiens, largely evolved over the past 150,000 years, within the latter part of the Pleistocene epoch of geological time.

During this period, atmospheric $CO_2$ levels stabilised between 160 and 280 parts per million (ppm). Even Homo erectus, our primitive human forebears who evolved over some 2 million years, experienced $CO_2$ levels averaging below 300 ppm. So, most life as we know it, and certainly humankind, has only ever experienced Earth with relatively low $CO_2$ levels in its atmosphere.

With the onset of the industrial revolution in the late-1700s, and its upsurge in the mid-1950s, the concentration of $CO_2$ has risen dramatically. The industrial revolution saw a societal transformation which began in London and spread through Europe to the Americas and Asia. The key invention was the steam engine, which burnt coal to boil water and generate steam. This pressurised vapour was manipulated to move turbines and power large machinery. In factories this coal-fired energy was used to manufacture goods, while the technology was adapted for transportation in steam trains and boats. Demand for this new energy source saw tonnes of coal mined and combusted. The processes' gaseous $CO_2$ waste product silently mixed into Earth's atmosphere.

Initial increases in $CO_2$ were relatively slow as the level climbed to 315ppm in 1959. But over the past 60 years the upsurge has been exponential. Atmospheric $CO_2$ levels have increased almost 50% since the first coal-powered steam engines sprang to life in Britain. At the time of writing, in 2022, the level is 420 ppm. Global temperatures follow the same curve as $CO_2$. From a pre-industrial baseline of zero around 1850-1900, the Earth is currently sitting at +1.2 degree Celsius. Somewhat confusingly, there isn't always clear consensus amongst climate scientists and policy makers about this baseline. For simplicity's sake the level referred to here is that referenced by the Intergovernmental Panel on Climate Change (IPCC)[59].

A level of +1.2 degrees Celsius might sound insignificant but, as in the human body, small shifts in temperature profoundly affect the living system. We have a stable body temperature of 37 degrees Celsius and are said to have a fever if it moves over 37.8 degrees C. Levels above 40 degrees C., are potentially life threatening.

Current estimates see average global temperatures reaching +1.5 degrees

Celsius in the 2030s. This measure is Earth's average, which means some regions will have much greater temperature changes with unprecedented extremes. Without urgent action to reduce atmospheric $CO_2$ levels, planetary average temperature rise is expected to be +3 degrees Celsius by the end of this century. Most climate scientists agree that global warming over this upper level would be catastrophic for all life on Earth and possibly not compatible with humankind's survival. There is an urgent need to not only cut $CO_2$ emissions to zero, but to move beyond this and draw excess carbon down from the atmosphere. To plummet $CO_2$ levels from over 400ppm back towards 280ppm as soon as possible.

## *The other greenhouse gases*

It's helpful to know a little about the other naturally occurring greenhouse gases because humankind's manipulation of them imperils Earth further. These include water vapour, methane and nitrous oxide. Sometimes known as laughing gas, nitrous oxide ($N_2O$) is the gas that helps women cope with the pains of labour. It is often used as an anaesthetic agent and is piped into many hospital wards and operating theatres. Once in the atmosphere, $N_2O$ persists for around one hundred and fourteen years. Just one hour of using $N_2O$ as an anaesthetic gas in surgery is equivalent to driving a fuel guzzling Hummer (16 litres petrol/100km) for one hundred kilometres. There are alternative agents which are just as effective for patient care but not nearly as damaging to the atmosphere.

Alarmingly, over the past forty years global nitrous oxide emissions rose 30%. The major source of this gas is synthetic nitrogen fertiliser use in agriculture. While fertilisers have increased crop yields, the large-scale farming process in which they are generally used sees excessive nitrous oxide released. Techniques to carefully titrate fertiliser use, minimise soil tillage and improve soil microbe communities are being found to help. These approaches not only reduce $N_2O$ release from farms but improve biodiversity and air and water quality.

Methane is a very potent greenhouse gas with high heat-holding ability. Although about sixty times more powerful than $CO_2$, methane doesn't last as long in the atmosphere, usually around twelve years. It is produced by microbes who live in oxygen-starved environments like swamps and animals' guts. Methane is released from animals when they discharge wind, usually through belching. Cows and other ruminants like sheep and goats, do this frequently. So, copious amounts of methane are produced by animal farming. This is partly how reducing dietary intake of meat and dairy products addresses global warming. Most natural gas is methane. A fossil fuel sucked from deep underground and used in our homes for heating and cooking. Methane is also the fugitive gas which leaks out around coal seam gas wells, escaping directly into the atmosphere and rendering gas as carbon intensive as coal.

There are also some man-made greenhouse gases, namely the hydrofluorocarbons (HFC) and chlorofluorocarbons (CFC). The latter were once used in refrigeration and aerosols and are ten thousand times more potent as a greenhouse gas than $CO_2$, lasting for centuries in the atmosphere. This high potency means only small amounts of these gases in the atmosphere can cause far reaching impacts. In the 1970s scientists realised these man-made gases were damaging the ozone layer, a thin slice of the atmosphere which protects Earth from the sun's ultraviolet (UV) radiation. CFC's chlorine molecule is highly damaging to the ozone. One atom can destroy 100,000 ozone molecules. It works best at very cold temperatures, so damage to the ozone layer was greatest over the south pole. As the CFCs wore a hole in the southern ozone layer, people living in lower latitudes like Australia, New Zealand and South America became concerned about possible health risks. This region has about 15% higher levels of UV radiation than northern parts of the globe due to lower air pollution levels and Earth's trajectory around the sun. Concern that the depleted ozone layer would further increase UV levels and associated skin cancers fuelled the call for these chemicals to be banned.

Eventually, despite push back from the makers of CFCs, namely industrial giant DuPont, global recognition of the risks to human health saw the Montreal Protocol signed in 1987. This agreement by developed nations to phase out the use of CFC gases was successful and now we have seen a shrinking of the ozone hole. This is a good news story demonstrating how, when people get together to take environmental issues seriously, we can make positive changes to reverse damage we humans have inadvertently caused. It is currently estimated the ozone hole is at its lowest level since 1988 but ongoing vigilance is required as some countries continue to produce problematic chemicals. A global investigation found factories in ten Chinese provinces were illegally using CFC-11 as a blowing agent for making foams to insulate buildings and appliances[60].

## The role of forests, oceans and polar ice

There are a several other factors to consider when thinking about global warming. First, along with the burning of fossil fuels following the industrial revolution, the destruction of forests and other large areas of vegetation has diminished the carbon sinks within the system. Much of Europe and the Americas were covered with forests. It is estimated over two thirds of central and northern Europe was forested. This was reduced to approximately one third over thousands of years as land was cleared for farming. In America the process was much faster, as clearing the land to 'civilise' was a colonial imperative. Prior to the arrival of colonisers, some one billion acres of the United States was covered in forests, this was reduced by 286 million acres, or just over one quarter, over the next few hundred years[61]. In Australia, land clearing for agriculture and logging was also rapid with over 44% of forests and woodland having been cleared since colonisation began. It is an ongoing activity and a major contributor to our carbon footprint. On a planetary level, tropical rainforests such as the Amazon, have been important carbon sinks. Scientists have found these areas are now reaching their sink saturation, meaning they are unlikely to be able to draw down as much $CO_2$ in the future.

Second, the oceans also act as carbon sinks because they take in carbon dioxide as it dissolves into the water. This phenomenon has occurred for millennia but because the Earth is now rapidly warming, this ability to absorb $CO_2$ is reaching its limit. Just as a soft drink loses its bubbles of carbonation when it warms and goes flat, warming sea water can't hold as much carbon dioxide. The oceans have absorbed over 90% of the increased energy in the climate system due to $CO_2$ emissions as heat, with the seas gradually warming. This capacity, too, is reaching its ceiling. Once passed, there will be a net transfer of heat from the ocean into the atmosphere, further warming the planet.

Third, the loss of ice from the polar ice caps at the north and south poles is fuelling further climate change. Being white, polar ice reflects warm light from the sun back out into space. This is called the *albedo effect*[a]. Around one third of the sun's energy reaching Earth is reflected by the planet's white surfaces. As Earth has warmed, these ice caps have been melting, their whiteness transforming into the sea's deep blue. As dark-coloured objects take up heat, these frozen areas of the planet, once pale and reflective, are darkening as they thaw. This process further warms the oceans.

Through all these means, the planet, or globe, is becoming hotter. Hence the term *global warming*, which is often used interchangeably with climate change. There is a call among some scientists and environmental advocates for these terms to be replaced with *climate chaos* or *climate emergency* because this more accurately describes the planetary consequences of climate disruption. As with other complex, living systems, the interconnectedness of life on Earth means sequelae from climate destabilisation are unpredictable, extensive and often catastrophic. Chaos seems more apt a descriptor than the moderate, measured language preferred by scientists, policy makers and international negotiators to date. As we move on to explore how natural systems are being unravelled, it will become clear how prescient a shift to this more emotive language is.

---

a    From Latin, where 'albedo' means 'whiteness'.

# KEY POINTS

- Carbon dioxide ($CO_2$) is the second most abundant greenhouse gas after water vapour
- Humans have evolved with an atmospheric $CO_2$ level of around 280ppm
- Atmospheric $CO_2$ level was approximately 420ppm in early 2022
- Earth's temperature rises as $CO_2$ levels rise
- Global temperature is currently +1.2 degrees Celsius above pre-industrial levels (2022)
- Burning fossil fuels releases $CO_2$
- Destroying plants (in the oceans and on land) reduces Earth's ability to take $CO_2$ out of the atmosphere
- The ocean's ability to absorb $CO_2$ is reaching capacity due to warming
- Polar ice is melting so the cooling poles are shrinking, accelerating global warming
- Methane is a potent greenhouse gas produced by mining and by farming cows and sheep
- Methane ('natural gas') is 60 times more powerful than $CO_2$
- Without urgent action Earth's temperature will reach +3 degrees Celsius by 2100
- +3 degrees Celsius is probably not compatible with humankind's survival

# HOW CLIMATE CHAOS DISRUPTS NATURAL SYSTEMS

It is important to take some time here to examine the profound effect climate change is having on human health. As more energy enters the atmosphere and Earth warms, the global systems upon which our wellbeing depends are being irrevocably altered. Major shifts in the water, soil, carbon and other natural cycles risk overstepping the planet's ecological boundaries. It may be impossible for balance to be restored.

## *The warming ocean*

Changes in the water cycle have seen precipitation such as rainfall and snowfall become unpredictable, with deluges causing floods. While increasingly powerful storms, cyclones and hurricanes are occurring globally with greater intensity. The ocean is warming, and worldwide currents are changing their course. This effects rainfall patterns and the distribution of plants and animals in the seas. As the water warms, it expands, so sea levels rise making some countries uninhabitable. Global sea levels have risen by over 20cm since 1880, and this rate is accelerating. People living in Pacific Island nations like Tuvalu and Kiribati are suffering the dual challenge of diminishing fresh water supply from less rainfall, as they simultaneously lose their land due to the encroaching ocean. They are also facing more intense storms and cyclones. Island leaders are in the awful position of looking to other countries to assist with relocation of their communities. Despite these Pacific Islanders not being responsible for the increased fossil fuel emissions which cause global warming, they are profoundly affected by the consequences. In losing their homelands and becoming climate refugees, they suffer greatly.

Oceans around Australia have warmed by around 1 degree Celsius since 1910 contributing to more frequent marine heatwaves and rising sea levels causing coastal inundation. Given major population centres like Melbourne, Brisbane and Sydney are located where major rivers flow into the sea, many Australians are likely to be affected by sea level rise. Although they will not need to move to other countries as some Pacific

Islanders have, potentially millions of Australians face the loss of their homes and subsequent displacement.

Warming of the planet's oceans is variable and unpredictable. A United Nations report on climate change and fisheries released in 2018 found that Australia's tropical oceans are warming nearly twice as fast as the global average, and three to four times the global average off the south-west and south-east of the continent[62]. Consequently, the distributions of over 100 Australian marine species have started to shift south towards cooler waters. This impacts fish stocks and related fishing industries and communities.

Shellfish, like oysters and crayfish, are especially vulnerable to climate change because the oceans, in absorbing large amounts of carbon dioxide, have become more acidic. It is estimated that seawater has become 30% more acidic in the last two hundred years. The calcium carbonate shells are made of is dissolving, making these sea creatures sick as their protection is weakened. This has affected their size and ability to reproduce[63]. There has been a dramatic reduction in the number of these sea animals, with the knock-on effect of reducing the food supply to communities where they are a staple food source.

## *Coral reefs are in peril*

Large reef systems like the Great Barrier Reef have a coral skeleton composed of the same calcium carbonate. This makes their structural integrity vulnerable to ocean acidification. Also, the coral animals living in this skeleton are expelled by the reef when it's under stress from ocean heatwaves or cyclones. These coral animals, or microscopic algae (zooxanthellae), have a symbiotic relationship with the coral, providing it with food in return for shelter. If they leave the coral, its major food source is removed. It turns very pale and is more vulnerable to disease. It is these zooxanthellae which give the reef it's wonderful colours. When an ocean heatwave causes a widespread expulsion of zooxanthellae, the result is a mass bleaching event. Diversity of the colours and forms that make the Great Barrier Reef famous, are lost. It becomes a dull, white structure with few fish. The effect of sequential bleaching events is devastating. This occurred when one third of the reef was bleached by a marine heatwave in 2015 and a further fifth damaged in another event the following year. As the exposed skeleton is eventually covered by algae, the reef transforms from a colourful, complex wonderland to a monotonous, rocky structure.

Usually, after a mass expulsion episode, most of the remaining adult coral animals spawn trillions of larvae annually to repopulate and replenish the reef. Unfortunately, this restoration is not occurring as effectively as it previously did. There is less and less time between bleaching events for new corals to grow. Over the past few decades, climate change has caused an increase in the frequency and severity of bleaching. The two consecutive events in 2015 and 2016 were the first time sequential bleaching had occurred. Prior to the 1980s, bleaching occurred, on average, every 27 years. After the 1980s, the rate increased to every six years. The frequency is now accelerating at an astronomical rate. New corals need at least ten years to recover – time they no longer have. This reduction in recovery capacity is confirmed by the finding that the amount of baby corals born on the reef dropped by 89% in 2018. Scientists think this was due to a depletion of adult populations from the preceding bleaching events[64]. Given the increase in frequency, it's unlikely the Great Barrier Reef will ever return to its former glory, if it survives at all.

The higher, more delicate table and fan-like corals are more vulnerable to bleaching than flatter corals, so the diversity of coral species is diminishing, and the reef is becoming lower. Rather like chopping down the canopy in a rainforest and leaving the understory exposed. This, in turn, alters the habitat for fish and other sea creatures, so the reef's overall biodiversity is dwindling. Climate scientists expect the world's coral reefs will be unable to survive more than 2 degrees Celsius of global warming given the major impacts we are seeing at just over 1 degree Celsius.

Global warming is affecting the reproduction of some marine animals in surprising ways. The northern Great Barrier Reef's Green Sea Turtles are born mostly female, with a ratio of female to male 116:1. If the sand in which they incubate is over 29 degrees Celsius they remain female, whereas cooler sand causes them to become male. With continued warming and only female turtles hatching, the species will become extinct. A unique collaboration between researchers, World Wide Fund for Nature, and the Queensland Government is exploring ways to cool turtle nesting areas in an attempt to address this threat[65].

## Mangroves and kelp forests are perishing

Along the shorelines, huge mangrove ecosystems have perished in marine heatwaves as very warm seas cook the root systems of mangrove plants. A marine heatwave occurs when seawater temperatures exceed the usual regional temperature's upper threshold for at least five consecutive days. These events coincide with reef bleaching. In 2016, along a 1000-kilometre stretch of the northern shoreline of Australia in the Gulf of Carpentaria, a mass death of mangrove forests occurred. The huge band of mangroves usually form a continuous canopy of rich green foliage that provides the interface between tropical seawaters and the serpentine river systems of the north. The heatwave transformed them into a pale, grey gash of skeletal forms along the water's edge. Images of the dead forests are shocking. Yet it was local tour operators, alarmed by the unprecedented event, who alerted authorities. There has been a failure of governments to monitor and protect these vulnerable, ecologically important areas during times of extreme marine weather events. This is despite their importance to local communities and industries like tourism and fishing[66].

Mangrove ecosystems provide a nursery for fish and other aquatic animals and a physical buffer from storms. They also form an important carbon sink. Their loss impacts both the variety and number of marine species and makes coastal areas more vulnerable to erosion and sea level rise. A recent research paper found 45% of Australia's coastline has already been affected by extreme weather events due to climate change. This includes the bleaching of coral reefs and loss of mangroves in tropical waters and the death of kelp forests and seagrass meadows in temperate, southern waters. The scientists studied extreme climate events (ECEs) between 2011 and 2017. These included marine heatwaves, droughts and flooding from tropical storms. They concluded, "these events are changing ecosystems in profound ways that in some cases are unlikely to be reversible. ECE impacts also suggest that while climate change may be viewed as gradual, in many cases it manifests through a series of often extreme and abrupt changes. ...ECEs will have significant consequences not only for coastal marine ecosystems but also for the human economic, social, and political systems that depend on them."[67]

In southern seas, the warming ocean has caused a significant change in kelp forests. With their giant leaves some 20 metres long, kelp provide diverse habitat for an enormous array of plants and animals and support fisheries and other coastal industries. The monetary value of kelp forests to Australia has been estimated at over $10 billion annually. Kelp forests have been affected by both the gradual warming of the ocean and by marine heatwaves. They also face pressures from overfishing and marine pests. During the 2011 marine heatwave off the coast of Western Australia ocean temperatures were over 3 degrees Celsius warmer than average for 60 consecutive days. Consequences of this extreme event include the extinction of some species of kelp over a 100-kilometre area of coast.[67] Seaweeds, fish and sharks were also affected, as their habitat shifted southwards.

## Strife at the poles

As the globe has warmed, the polar ice caps have shrunk and their melting has fed sea level rise. So far, there has been a dramatic reduction in the size of the north pole. In summer the sea there is now navigable by ship. Some countries are recklessly planning on using this opportunity to plunder the depths in a search for oil despite it being a major fossil fuel. It is estimated the sea-ice extent in the Arctic Ocean has decreased 4% per decade since satellite records began in 1979[68]. As mentioned earlier, the loss of white polar ice reduces the albedo affect where the sun's warmth is reflected into space. This results in the dark blue of the northern ocean absorbing more heat and accelerating warming further. So, the poles are warming faster than the rest of the planet. The image of a polar bear stranded on a melting iceberg has become symbolic of climate change because of the significance of the loss of this northern ice. Simultaneous loss of ice in the southern, Antarctic region with major ice sheets calving ice bergs into the sea during the warmer months is also worrying.

## Changes on land

Climate change impacts seen on land include increases in severe weather events like heatwaves, bushfires, droughts, floods and high intensity storms and cyclones. In Australia, alongside these catastrophes we are experiencing more gradual shifts in climate. Occurring progressively over decades, scientists have observed a change to fewer very cold days, a large increase in extremely hot days and a general rise in temperature throughout the year. Heatwaves here are becoming hotter, longer, and more frequent due to climate change. Overall, Australia's climate has warmed just over 1 degree C since 1910[68]. The changes in rainfall have varied across the continent with rainfall increased in the north and reduced in the south. Associated changes in streamflow see less water running in southern rivers and more in northern waterways.

In south-western Australia there has been an overall longstanding drop in May to July rainfall of around one fifth since 1970. While in south-eastern Australia the drop has been around 11% between April and October since the late 1990s and snowfall over the alps has diminished and is no longer reliable. Rivers in the south are reducing their flow and, in some instances, drying up altogether[68]. These changes have pushed some animal species to the brink of extinction while others have shifted their habitat to cooler places. It is not always possible for animals to move where they need to due to the fragmentation of habitat by roads and other human developments. Their ability to adapt to climate change is impaired by us.

The ongoing drying of already fragile landscapes has seen progressive erosion and salinity increase in large areas of south-western and central Australia. This has reduced the productivity of farmland. Less reliable water supply and excessively warm temperatures have placed pressure on pollinators, like bees and other insects. This has further compounded difficulties for cropping farmers and is a global problem. In Puerto Rico, there was a 2 degree Celsius increase in the temperature of the Luquillo rainforest between 1976 and 2012. This has resulted in a 10 to 60 times drop in the number of insects with an associated reduction in the birds, lizards and frogs who were dependent on them for food.

The scientists who researched this data were shocked to discover 98% of ground insects and 80% of canopy insects had gone[69]. Biologist Brad Lister, who has been studying the forest for decades, said, "We knew that something was amiss in the first couple days. We were driving into the forest and at the same time both Andrew and I said: 'Where are all the birds?' There was nothing... It was a true collapse of the insect populations in that rainforest. We began to realise this is terrible – a very, very disturbing result."[70] Given this particular forest has long been protected, factors like insecticides and habitat destruction are not responsible for the decline. Instead, it is the elevation of temperatures to levels well over those the forest is adapted to, which is to blame. And ultimately, climate change is responsible for this.

Certain bioregions of Earth are more vulnerable to global warming, often because their plant and animal species are adapted to very specific climatic conditions. Tropical rainforests are located either side of the Equator and are notable for their high rainfall. Many receive over 2,000mm of rain annually. These forests have evolved within very narrow temperature ranges and are especially sensitive to shifts in climate. In far north Queensland, the Wet Tropics World Heritage area has been experiencing extremely warm periods, and this is affecting species like the lemuroid ringtail possum. These marsupials are adapted to temperatures of less than 29 degrees Celsius, but the 2019 summer saw an unprecedented 39 degree Celsius temperature reached on six occasions at Mt Bartle Frere. The highest mountain in the wet tropics, this peak is home to the largest population of lemuroid ringtail possums. Much of the wildlife in this tropical area is found nowhere else on Earth. It is thought that if warming continues at the current pace, over half of the rainforest's endemic animals will be extinct within decades[71].

With this in mind, the International Union of the Conservation of Nature has ranked the Wet Tropics as the second most irreplaceable World Heritage Area on Earth. Stretching from Townsville to Cape York along the mountainous spine fringing the edge of the continent, this is the oldest living rainforest on Earth and covers almost 9000 square kilometres. A recent report by the Wet Tropics Authority cited concerns about the lemuroid ringtail possum saying, "if the trends continue, populations at sites that previously had the highest density of lemuroid ringtail possums in the region could become locally extinct as early as 2022. This species is not currently even classified as endangered."[72]

## Precious pollinators: insects, birds and bats

Prolonged severe heatwaves in Australia have seen thousands of pollinating animals such as flying foxes and birds, succumb to heat exhaustion and, literally, fall from the sky. Consequently, populations of vulnerable species have shrunk. These animals are important for the healthy functioning of many ecosystems and perform valuable work for farmers, including crop pollination and pest removal. In November 2018, a heatwave saw the unprecedented mass death of spectacled flying foxes as 23,000 animals perished. Colloquially known as fruit bats, these animals are an important part of the food web as they fly huge distances to pollinate plants, which supports genetic diversity. Official counts, revealed in Queensland open data, found 1.4 million flying foxes of all species reported in the first quarter of 2016, but only 243,000 two years later. Perversely, rather urgently addressing climate change as the driver of extreme weather events, the Federal Government upgraded the status of the spectacled flying fox to endangered while simultaneously approving the controversial Adani coal mine[73]. This will be the largest coal mine in Australia and sure to exacerbate climate change.

The ability of many bird and bat species to reproduce is harmed by progressive warming and associated changes in rainfall. This is partly due to a shift in the flowering and fruiting patterns of the plants that form the basis of their diet. If a species' main food source starts flowering earlier in the season, or in a different location, it may not be able to reach it in time, or in adequate numbers, to meet a suitable mate. This changing plant behaviour compounds other challenges faced by pollinating animals like habitat destruction, predation by feral pests and insect decline due to biocidal chemicals.

## Alarming changes in fire behaviour

The Australian landscape was managed with fire for millennia by First Nations people. With colonisation, their sophisticated method of firestick farming was widely disrupted. So now, fuelled by the drier, hotter climate, we see major, very hot, catastrophic bushfires burning out of control and in areas they couldn't previously reach. In 2019, 190,000 hectares, or 3% of Tasmania, was burnt[74]. Hundreds of blazes, lit by dry lightning, coalesced into a huge firestorm. This unprecedented occurrence saw large areas of ancient Gondwanan rainforest burnt. Having evolved in the absence of fire, this habitat is unlikely to regenerate, so will be lost forever. These lightning firestorms are fuelled by low weather systems which are now occurring farther south than before. They are also more powerful and damaging than climate scientists had formerly predicted.

Severe weather events, progressive shifts in climate, ocean warming, and sea level rise are some of the mechanisms through which climate change is impacting Earth's biomes. Most worrying of all is the acceleration in the rate of change and the compounding effect of multiple systems being disrupted together. Climate scientists have been sounding the alarm about the urgency and complexity of global warming for decades. They are especially concerned with the unpredictability of climate destabilisation and the implications for all life on Earth. One key focus of their attention are the rapid changes occurring in the North Pole's tundra biome.

## Earth's tipping points

The frozen ground, or permafrost, of the Arctic region's tundra contains gigantic amounts of stored methane. As mentioned earlier, methane is an extremely potent greenhouse gas. When permafrost thaws, methane is discharged, fuelling climate change. This methane release is one of the tipping points climate scientists worry will trigger an unstoppable chain of events leading to a level of climate change unsuitable for life as we know it. The other tipping points are complete melting of polar ice caps, major shifts in global ocean currents and monsoonal systems, and loss of large forests like the Amazon. Sometimes referred to as 'known unknowns' by scientists, tipping points are unpredictable and have not been a significant focus in the latest report by the Intergovernmental Panel on Climate Change (IPCC), much to the concern of climatologists[75]. If these points are passed and runaway climate change triggered, Earth will almost certainly become uninhabitable for people.

## KEY POINTS

- Climate change is affecting the natural systems which underpin human health
- Warming oceans result in sea level rise and changes in global currents
- Polar oceans are warming fastest
- Ocean heatwaves cause coral bleaching and mangrove death
- Oceans are becoming more acidic, dissolving shellfish and corals
- Rainfall patterns have become unreliable causing droughts and floods
- Storms are more frequent and intense
- Fire behaviour is changing with firestorms and frequent, widespread bushfires
- Changes in weather alter flowering and fruiting of plants
- Food and water sources are no longer reliable for pollinators: insects, birds and bats
- Pollinator populations are collapsing
- Severe heatwaves kill animals who cannot escape the heat
- The Arctic's permafrost is thawing, releasing methane
- Tipping points are unpredictable, irreversible triggers within Earth's climate system
- Tipping points include permafrost thawing and complete melting of the poles

# CLIMATE CHANGE: A HEALTH EMERGENCY

As climate change disrupts these immense natural systems, all life on Earth suffers, including humankind. Just as other animals need reliable sources of food and water, and a habitat free from fire and flood, so do we. Despite what many in government wish to believe, the health effects of climate change are felt a long way from the power station where fossil fuels like coal, oil and gas are combusted. These health impacts are many and varied and affect all of us in some way or another, no matter where we live or how wealthy we are. They are categorized as being either *direct*, or *indirect*. In 2009, *The Lancet*, a world-renowned medical journal, described climate change as 'the biggest public health threat of the 21st century'. Yet it is often only spoken about in terms of its influence on the environment by decision makers[76].

## *The horror of bushfires*

The most obvious health problems due to climate chaos are the direct impacts caused by severe weather events. For example, bushfires are now more frequent, widespread and intense in Australia, parts of Europe and the Americas. These result in death and injury due to burns, smoke inhalation, heat stress and trauma from falling objects. The smoke from bushfires contains many different chemical pollutants which impair air quality and cause sickness many hundreds of kilometres away from the fire front. During the dreadful Black Summer of bushfires in southern Australia in late-2019 and early-2020 the major cities of Melbourne, Canberra and Sydney were shrouded in smoke for days. In a dystopian scenario, millions of people confined themselves indoors to avoid the toxic smoke and donned respiratory masks when venturing outside. Even thousands of kilometres from the flames the threat from the bushfires was palpable.

Once inhaled, microscopic, soot-like particles in bushfire smoke can penetrate deep into the body. Circulating from the lungs to the heart via the bloodstream they may cause fatal heart attacks and worsen respiratory disease. In Melbourne and Sydney, rates of heart attack, death from heart disease and admission to hospital with illness due to cardiovascular problems are elevated on high bushfire-smoke days. People with pre-existing health conditions, children, pregnant women and the elderly are more vulnerable. Over this same Black Summer, it is estimated that 445 people died from exposure to smoke, and over 3,000 were admitted to hospital with lung problems[77]. An extraordinary 80% of the Australian population were adversely affected by smoke.

Even after the fire has been extinguished there are potential health problems as the ash and debris often contain dangerous materials like asbestos and heavy metals. This might occur in previously built-up areas, or in water catchments and natural places where the soil or waterway has been contaminated by flying ash. Those workers involved in the clean-up and people and animals returning to burnt areas may be exposed to these toxins. Health effects from asbestos exposure can manifest many years later in the form of mesothelioma, an incurable lung cancer.

Other severe weather events like high-intensity storms, cyclones and floods are changing in their strength and frequency due to increased energy in the climate system from global warming. These disasters cause death and injury directly from drowning, or from the impact of rapidly moving objects in flood waters and landslides. Displaced wild animals, including snakes and spiders, may also cause harm, possibly fatally. In Queensland, a major flooding event in 2011 killed thirty-five people directly and adversely affected 2.5 million others. Enormous damage and disruption to health infrastructure ensued with 1,400 elective surgeries being cancelled and millions of dollars needed to repair damage[78].

More recently, sequential major flooding around the regional New South Wales town of Lismore has proved so catastrophic the entire town of 43,000 people may need to be rebuilt elsewhere. Long-time residents of Lismore are facing the dreadful choice of rebuilding or moving away from friends and family. Many homes were uninsured because of the flooding risk, meaning financial destitution and homelessness threaten many.

## Heatwaves, the silent killer

Sometimes the way natural disasters affect human health are less obvious. For example, heatwaves have caused more deaths and illness than any other natural disaster over the past century. Most people are unaware of the health problem posed by heatwaves, so they are often described as a silent killer. A heatwave occurs when there are three or more consecutive days of higher than usual temperatures, including persistent overnight heat. Without the respite of night-time coolness, the body is unable to recover from the day's heat. Heatwaves are often fatal because prolonged, elevated body temperature places a strain on the heart and brain. Also, the excessive loss of water through sweating leads to dehydration. People may then succumb to a heart attack, or organ failure. 'Climate change' or 'heat wave', although the underlying cause of death, won't be written on a death certificate as these factors cause death by exacerbating other problems and placing pressure on certain body systems. In this way, climate change as manifested through a heatwave, is causing 'indirect' health outcomes which culminate in illness and death. Climate change has led to heatwaves in unexpected places, and the number of people dying in this way globally is often surprising. For example, while we might expect heatwaves in Australia, the 2003 European event had a death toll of over 70,000 people. A staggering figure on a much cooler continent[79].

Heat related illnesses like dehydration, heat stress and heat stroke can occur in anyone exposed to very hot weather. Heat stroke is a medical emergency that occurs when the temperature-regulating function of the body derails and without prompt treatment death can ensue. People with pre-existing medical conditions, the elderly and those experiencing homelessness are at higher risk from these heat events because their bodies are already stressed and they are less able to adapt. Children and pregnant women are vulnerable because their immune, heart and breathing systems are more fragile, and cannot tolerate temperature extremes as well as others. Unsurprisingly, those living in remote communities and outdoor workers are also at increased risk. It is also noteworthy that city dwellers are vulnerable during a heatwave because of the *urban heat island effect*.

In a large city, structures like roads and buildings trap and maintain heat. When there are few areas of cooling green space, the overall effect is an island of heat within a comparatively cooler surrounding area. In Melbourne, this heat island effect adds some four degrees to the temperature experienced during a heatwave. As man-made materials retain heat absorbed during the day and slowly release it overnight, nocturnal temperatures can be especially elevated[80].

During heatwaves there may be associated infrastructure breakdown and, as was seen in Melbourne in 2009, it can be quite dramatic. Images of railway tracks buckling in the sun with ensuing transport chaos provide a stark reminder of the extreme heat the city endured. Power blackouts occur frequently during heatwaves and may leave entire suburbs without cooling, light or refrigeration for hours and sometimes days. All these factors combine to prolong vulnerable people's exposure to high temperatures. Their risk of succumbing to heat exhaustion, dehydration and organ failure rises correspondingly.

## Health systems strained by climate events

Climate change-induced severe weather events profoundly impact the provision of health care. Services may be overwhelmed as people call on ambulances and present to emergency departments and medical clinics seeking help. In the same heatwave in Melbourne, a 25% increase in emergency cases was noted by Ambulance Victoria. Power outages erode health service provision as clinics without back-up generators lose air cooling and refrigeration. This can interrupt the supply chain for vaccines and medications that need to be kept at specific temperatures to maintain efficacy. Also, health care workers may be unable to safely travel to work or may be rendered incapacitated when personally affected by the disaster.

The Black Saturday bushfires in 2009 are painfully etched in the memory of most Victorians. Images come to mind of flames racing across grasslands, towering infernos of fire and smoke and reports of embers flying kilometres ahead of the fire-front to bombard cowering communities. As we sat glued to the radio, television or our social media feed, stories flooded in. Some 173 people tragically lost their lives on that day and yet, far more died from the preceding heatwave. The morgue was already full of heat-related deaths by the time the first reports of the fires aired on the Saturday. Over southeast Australia, the 2009 heatwave resulted in almost 500 excess deaths[81]. As is often the case with the increasing frequency and severity of climate-related disasters, they often occur together, compounding the devastation. Both direct and indirect health effects occur and interact with one another. On this occasion prolonged drought, a heatwave and then bushfires occurred in rapid succession with catastrophic consequences.

## *Psychological and social harms from climate events*

There are many other indirect health consequences from climate change. These include psychological and social problems resulting from witnessing and experiencing severe weather events. The list of these is long and includes Post Traumatic Stress Disorder (PTSD), depression, anxiety, survivor guilt, grief and the associated fracturing of communities and families due to loss of homes, schools and jobs. Certainly, the trauma may be long lasting and intergenerational. In one study, children were surveyed six months after the 2003 bushfires in Canberra. Rates of behavioural and emotional problems were elevated and almost half had symptoms of PTSD[82]. As affected individuals go on to have their own families, behaviours and attitudes shaped by the traumatic event may affect future generations. The scars on the psyche of millions of Australians after the 2019/2020 Black Summer bushfires will undoubtedly be profound. So many people watched their precious forests and coastal bushlands decimated by bushfires, anxiously waited as loved ones were evacuated from danger areas and felt bereft as the death toll of wildlife crept into the billions.

Prolonged droughts and other extreme weather events can lead to rolling crop failures, year after year. This has far-reaching effects on rural communities, leading to mental health issues, family and community breakdown and, possibly, armed conflict. Displacement due to natural disasters may lead to fighting as people who normally would not live near one another are forced into close proximity. This was seen in 2011 after flooding resulted in the Warmun community of north-eastern Australia being relocated to Kunununurra where they had to live in compounds away from their Country. This displacement meant many Gija people were exposed to alcohol for the first time. Along with homesickness, some experienced conflict and associated mental and physical trauma. Overseas, the war in Syria has been widely attributed to prolonged drought in the region leading to displacement of large numbers of people and subsequent fighting. The physical and psychological trauma wrought by conflict due to displacement and dispossession from climate-induced natural disasters are all indirect health effects. The number of affected people is likely to be many millions.

## Changes in infectious diseases

The disruption of rainfall and temperature patterns from global warming affects the life cycle of insects and microbes, which in turn changes infectious disease sequelae for humans. By shifting the habitat zones for insects like mosquitos, climate change is altering subspecies distribution. So, diseases spread through this vector are changing. The most common mosquito-borne illness in Australia, Ross River Fever, has previously been generally limited to the tropics of northern Queensland. Now more cases are being reported farther south. The mosquitos that spread the virus live and breed optimally at 26 degrees Celsius. With climate change causing a rise in temperatures throughout Australia, the mosquito's original habitat may become too hot. While the more populous, southern regions are already proving favourable. As the climate warms and periods of heavy rain intensify, plentiful freshwater pools provide reservoirs for mosquito breeding. Rurally these may be in wetlands and waterways, while within built-up areas, puddles, bird baths and pot plants provide breeding sites[83]. A reduction in the number of frogs, birds and other animals due to loss of habitat means there are fewer predators to counter this increase in mosquito numbers.

Alongside the climactic and habitat changes which support the proliferation of mosquitos, shifts in human behaviour see people become more vulnerable to insect bites. With warmer weather, they are more likely to be outside, dressed in clothing where their skin is exposed for longer periods of time. Ross River Fever, while not life-threatening like malaria, causes significant disability with fever, headaches and joint pains that may be prolonged and severe. Some 2,000 to 9,000 Australians suffer with this illness annually and treatment is based on symptom relief only. Even those living in cooler, southern Australia have been advised to take measures to avoid mosquito bites. Over the summer of 2018 the government issued health directives because Ross River Virus had been detected in mosquitos in Victoria's Gippsland Lakes for the first time[84]. So, climate change, in making southern Australia's habitat more suitable for mosquitoes, has led to the once tropical disease of Ross River Fever becoming a health threat for southern populations.

Global warming is implicated in the genesis of other infectious diseases including those spread through contaminated food and water. Damage to infrastructure from severe weather events may result in inadequately stored or spoiled foodstuffs causing gastrointestinal sickness. Other illnesses, like hepatitis A and E, leptospirosis and parasitic and skin infections may occur in the aftermath of a major flood or cyclone.

Like the changing pattern of infectious diseases, illness due to the incidental ingestion of poisons may be a silent sequela of climate chaos and its floods and storms. Toxins like pesticides and heavy metals may be displaced by deluges and enter water used for drinking, washing and food production. While airborne asbestos fibres and moulds, released during the climate-induced natural disaster, may be inhaled and can cause illness and death many years later.

### Changes in allergies and asthma

Often the health impacts of climate change are unexpected and only noticeable to public health experts after years of observation and study. The warmer temperatures and higher levels of $CO_2$ in the atmosphere from global warming, increase the potency, production and release of allergens like pollens and spores[85]. These aggravate allergic diseases, including asthma, a common problem in Australia. Some 10% of Australians suffer from asthma and 20% have an allergic disease. Rates of these conditions have been rising globally, as Earth has warmed. These conditions majorly impair quality of life and may be fatal, or cause significant disability by interfering with a person's ability to participate fully at school, work or in their social lives.

The dramatic *thunderstorm asthma* event which hit Melbourne in November 2016 took healthcare workers by surprise. The spring thunderstorm weather triggered the shattering of billions of ryegrass pollen grains which were propelled through the air by gusty winds. Thousands of people, many of whom had only ever had very mild asthma or hay fever, presented to emergency departments and called ambulances for help. Sadly, ten people died. It is expected these types of events will become more frequent with further climate change, as we are already seeing the hay fever season lengthen. There are more days of high pollen load, and the frequency and severity of storms is rising.

All severe weather events may disrupt infrastructure inhibiting access to medical care and making food, water and power provision difficult. This, in turn, can lead to malnutrition, food insecurity and a breakdown in the routine provision of health care like childhood immunisations and pregnancy checks. Illnesses and deaths resulting from these climate-induced disruptions to medical attention are amongst the many human costs not currently accounted for when world leaders discuss climate change.

The social determinants of health include underlying economic and social conditions like education, employment, housing, transportation and access to nutritious food and clean water. These are all underpinned by ecological systems which are vulnerable to disruption from climate change. One example, touched on earlier, is the way oceanic warming is seriously damaging aquatic ecosystems like kelp forests and reefs. As the fisheries dependent on these underwater nurseries are eroded, communities who rely on the fishing industry are affected. The social disruption from changes in natural fisheries and their dependent industries like fishing, boating and tourism can result in psychological health problems as affected people lose their income, occupation, and sense of purpose. Similar patterns of social erosion are seen in outback rural communities following prolonged droughts, the severity of which is amplified by climate change.

# SOLASTALGIA

Some indirect health effects from global warming may be difficult to measure scientifically, being of a spiritual, or deeply emotional nature. They are also hard to describe, requiring new words to capture the hurt. The term *solastalgia* was first used by Australian environmental philosopher Glenn Albrecht in 2003 to describe a mixture of sadness and nostalgia for a place that's meaningful to us, our home, as we experience its demise. Put simply, it is "the homesickness you have when you are still at home".[86] This profound sense of loss for the natural world, as it once was, resonates deeply for many of us trying to prevent further destruction of nature.

Although originally solastalgia was said to affect those living in or nearby their beloved home, surely a form of it may affect those farther away too. Memories of a personally meaningful place, and the knowledge it remains there for future solace can steady us in the tumult of life's many stresses. Consequently, knowing these places of comfort are being harmed is deeply upsetting. Perhaps the concept of solastalgia can help non-Indigenous Australians understand the distress First Nations people feel when their Country is suffering, whether or not they are physically there to witness it.

Solastalgia may lead to pervasive low mood, and even depression in people who care deeply about the natural world. And it is likely to be a key factor in the burnout felt by environmental advocates and activists. Whether acting on climate change, biodiversity loss or plastic pollution in the oceans, a sense of feeling overwhelmed by the massive scale of the ecological catastrophes we are facing globally can simply become too much to bear. This problem (and its siblings, climate anxiety and climate grief) seem worse each year and could certainly be dryly described as indirect health impacts of climate change. As Glenn Albrecht wrote in 2012, "Regional solastalgia is produced under the impact of gas fracking, mining, and agribusiness, as they bring unwelcome damage and pollution on a huge scale to ecocultural and bioregional landscapes. However, as bad as local and regional negative transformation is, it is the big picture, the Whole Earth, which is now a home under assault. A feeling of global dread asserts itself as the planet heats and our climate gets more hostile and unpredictable."[86]

Even those rejecting the scientific assertion that climate change is anthropogenic, or man-made, may be experiencing solastalgia as the natural places around them suffer. It was Albrecht's time in the Upper Hunter region of New South Wales that stimulated his thinking on how best to describe the deep unease and chronic stress people around him were feeling. This region, once rich farmland, has been irrevocably transformed by massive open-cut coal mines and prolonged drought. He says, "I realised that there was no concept in the English language that adequately described the distressed state of the Upper Hunter residents. The melancholia of nostalgia (nostos: to return home) was close but had the obvious disadvantage that these people were still living in the place they called home, so were not 'homesick' in the traditional nostalgic sense......I defined 'solastalgia' as an emplaced or existential melancholia experienced with the negative transformation (desolation) of a loved home environment."[86]

We see solastalgia manifested in the high rates of mental health issues and suicide in rural communities as they experience the consequences of climate change firsthand. Severe weather events like prolonged drought, bushfires, floods, and cyclones may come year after year in a relentless pattern. Despite many farmers denying these changes are due to climate change, they are vulnerable to psychological stress as they experience waterways drying up, stock dying from starvation and repeated crop failures. Having to shoot your herd because you can no longer provide enough food and water for them is confronting and there may be guilt and shame at this failure. Given many farmers are socially isolated and live with a stigma that sees mental illness as weakness, they are often reluctant to seek help. Suicide can seem like their only option.

There is no doubt climate change forms yet another layer of loss and trauma for First Nations people everywhere, especially in Australia. Along with the dispossession and displacement from Country experienced through colonisation, the climactic shifts and associated extreme weather events are degrading sacred places and harming animal totems. The impact of severe bushfires and other disasters is evocatively captured by Aboriginal artist, Clinton Naina in his work *Stolen Climate*. In an interview for the Big Weather Exhibition's launch in March 2021, he succinctly stated, "Stolen climate is just another part of colonisation, imperialism, capitalism."[87] Conciliation between First Nations people and other Australians cannot occur without the regeneration of natural ecosystems and action to address global warming.

Through its disruption of humankind's ecological life support systems, climate change is profoundly harming health. This may be in direct and shocking ways through cataclysmic severe weather events and their associated injury and loss of life, or more gradually via the erosion of psychological stability and spiritual connection to place. Either way, Earth's climactic destabilisation affects us all in some way. Global warming also jeopardises the planet's biodiversity as it unravels natural systems, untangling the complex web of relationships between species. This, too, has repercussions for our wellbeing.

# KEY POINTS

- Climate change harms human health both directly and indirectly
- Direct effects include severe weather events: bushfires, floods and storms
- Indirect harms are physical, psychological and social
- Altered weather patterns are shifting infectious disease distribution
- Climate change alters pollen release increasing asthma and allergies
- Droughts, storms and pollinator decline threaten agriculture and food supply
- Severe events disrupt routine and emergency health care
- Vulnerable populations suffer most – those living in poverty or homelessness
- Heatwaves are the most severe, silent climate killer
- The elderly, children, pregnant women and those with chronic diseases are especially at risk
- Severe weather events cause prolonged psychological suffering
- Emotional distress may manifest as PTSD, depression or in suicide
- *Solastalgia* is deep sadness and nostalgia for your place/land/Country as it was before
- Witnessing the suffering of the natural world from climate change is a cause of solastalgia

# CLIMATE CHANGE ERODES BIODIVERSITY, HURTING HUMANITY

The damage to global biodiversity from climate change is far reaching and interacts with the other threats to living systems posed by people. These include habitat destruction, the introduction of pests and pollution. A loss of worldwide biological diversity profoundly harms human health because it undermines our foundational needs – clean air and water, stable, healthy soils and the myriad of foods and medicines we rely on.

At the current level of global warming, we can hardly keep up with impacts on biodiversity. It can be difficult, perhaps impossible, to attribute species loss to one factor alone given the interconnecting issues of habitat loss, chemical and other pollution, and pests, as well as climate change. But in some instances, climatic shifts are clearly fundamental. One Australian example which encapsulates the devastating decline in an extraordinary species through the stacking on of environmental insults, loaded by climate change, is the decline of the Bogong moth.

## *The story of the Bogong moth*

Like the Monarch butterflies of North America, the Bogong moth is an iconic species renowned for its exceptional ability to navigate huge distances as part of its life cycle.

The Bogong moth migrates from lowland areas of southern Australia up into the caves and rocky crevices of the alps to *aestivate* (hibernate or rest) over winter before returning to breeding grounds in autumn. Historically, billions of moths have made this journey annually and scientists have documented the density of insects in the alpine caves at an incredible 17,000 moths per square metre. Unlike its American cousin, the Bogong moth travels at night and relies on various sensory stimuli as well as being the only insect to use the Earth's magnetic field to navigate from breeding grounds to places of hibernation.

Covering distances of up to 1000 kilometres, the moths' journey may last weeks and includes multiple stops along the way for daytime rests and feeding. As they fly at night, they are highly sensitive to the light pollution radiated by urban development. Migrating Bogong moths have been known to congregate in highly illuminated spaces and have famously descended on night-time sporting events, including the 2009 Australian Open tennis tournament in Melbourne and the Sydney Olympics. In the latter event, a swarm of millions of moths, attracted to the giant stadium lights, was originally thought by weather forecasters to be a raincloud until an insect landed on the famous soprano performing the Olympic hymn. Fortunately, most moths continued to their destination.

This remarkable insect was once a prized food for First Nations people from the alpine and surrounding regions of south-eastern Australia. Various clans annually harvested Bogong moths in the warmer months. Much more than the simple extraction of a food source, huge harvesting festivals brought people together for inter-tribal gatherings. As this nutritious insect was prepared and shared, important ceremonial and social interactions took place. In her book, *The Moth Hunters*, archaeologist Josephine Flood collates records from early scientists and historians to build a picture of these activities. Numerous accounts describe the moths being roasted to eat whole, or ground into cakes, and as having a delicious, nutty flavour. One source quoted by Flood is the anthropologist, Richard Helms who was guided up Mt Bogong, along with colonial traveller George Bennett, by several Aboriginal men in 1832. Helms and Bennett reported the Bogong feasting took place over a period of some three months and that the moth cakes were sometimes smoked and cured for later consumption[88].

Another early record, recounted by journalist John Gale in his 1927 book on the history of the Australian Capital Territory, is that of an early pastoralist, Mrs John Mc Donald. Her family took up a landholding on the Murrumbidgee River in the 1830s. In conversation with Gale, Mc Donald described many "blacks and gins" and their "piccaninnies" gathering to feast on the "boogong moths" [sic] that "swarmed" the mountains nearby. She also recounted how a large flat rock on the property was heated to cook the moths and that the feasting, centred around the rock, would last many weeks. According to Mc Donald, this stone was called "urayarra" by local Kamberri (Ngambri) people and meant 'running to the feast'. She described the nutritious benefits of the moths thus, "the ebon skins of the eaters literally shone, and their bodies showed a plumpness quite in contrast with the leanness of normal times."[89]

These accounts were supported by the 2019 discovery of an ancient grindstone encrusted with Bogong moth residues in a cave in the southern foothills of the alps. On the land of the Krauatngalung clan of the GunaiKurnai people, this ground-breaking discovery highlighted the importance of insect foods for First Nations people in Australia. In the spirit of true collaboration, scientists and Traditional Owners worked together, marrying ancient knowledge with modern science. As the researchers said, "the results of our study indicate that Aboriginal peoples of south-eastern Australia were harvesting, preparing and cooking Bogong moths for food 1600-2000 years ago, allowing for the scheduling of the associated summer feasts going back at least 65 generations."[90] In a press release at the time of the discovery GunaiKurnai Elder Russsell Mullett said, "historical records are witness to our people going to the mountains for the Bogong moths but this project tells us that it also happened in the deeper past. Because our people no longer travel to the mountains for Bogong moth festivals, the oral histories aren't shared anymore, it's a lost tradition."[91]

The oral history accounts from First Nations people align with colonial archives and modern scientific discoveries in describing the presence of many millions of Bogong moths for millennia. So it is deeply concerning that a dramatic decline in numbers of moths is now being observed. In 2019, at one cave near Canberra where moth numbers were previously recorded in the millions, only three individuals were found. Ecologist Dr Ken Green, who has been monitoring the moths for some forty years, said, "They haven't just declined. They've gone. We have done mountains from down to the Victorian border all the way to Canberra. We have checked every cave we know."[92] He hypothesises the devastation as being due to prolonged droughts, evinced by climate change, in the moth's breeding areas throughout south-eastern Australia.

A knock-on effect of the precipitous drop in moth numbers is the starvation of the endangered mountain pygmy possum. This marsupial relies on the protein and fat-rich Bogong moths to feed its young when it emerges from hibernation. The mountain pygmy possum is Australia's only hibernating marsupial and spends between five and seven months dormant, under snow. When it emerges from hibernation it is very thin, so it relies on a predictable food source to regain a healthy weight in time for breeding and before the following winter. Researcher Dean Heinz describes finding dead litters of baby possums in the pouches of females in twelve different locations in Victoria. He says, "it's a widespread event. The concern is that over time, if this happens more frequently, we will see declines in the adult population as well."[92] A recent interview with reproductive biologist from Zoos Victoria, Dr Marissa Parrott, reported the spring of 2018 found 95% of surveyed female possums had lost their young, reducing the population to two thousand. What is being described here, in the understated and circumspect way typical of scientists, is the collapse of an ecosystem.

By causing prolonged drought in the Bogong moth's breeding grounds, climate change has been a key cause of its decline. No doubt the use of fertilizers and pesticides, poisonous to the moth, were key contributing factors. While fragmentation of habitat and light pollution along its migratory path, consequences of human 'development', further undermine its resilience to climate change. As the Bogong moth and the plants and animals it supports have perished, people's health has inevitably suffered. This is especially true for those who have strong nutritional, spiritual and cultural ties to the moth – the First Nations communities.

As the Bogong moth was so plentiful over many thousands of years, a great number of plant and animal species have evolved in concert with it and are therefore dependent upon it. Whether serving as a pollinator, or food source, this insect is central to the healthy functioning of multiple ecosystems. This makes it a *keystone species*.

## Keystone species

Ecologists often use the word *keystone* to describe a species which is central to the survival of many others. Classical examples are apex predators, like the wolf or coyote. These apex predators sit at the top of the food chain and hold the ecosystem in balance. They do this by maintaining correct numbers and distribution of other animals. A famous case is that of the north American wolf which was eradicated from Yellowstone National Park in America in the 1930s. The result was an explosion in the numbers of elk who damaged waterways and decimated certain plant species, especially willows that grew along the water's edge. Erosion of riverbanks led to contaminated water sources and a loss of plant variety and ground cover with diminished ecological richness of the entire landscape. The beaver, which used willows to make its home along the riverbank, was rarely seen. A concerted effort to reintroduce the wolf into the park has resulted in a rebalancing of the ecosystem as the elk move away from the water's edge into thicker forest for protection. This has enabled willows and other riparian plants to flourish and the beavers' numbers to rebound. The dams and ponds of their colonies are now seen along waterways throughout Yellowstone.

We have seen a similar situation here in Australia with farmers shooting dingoes. As an apex predator, the dingo was not only keeping numbers of grass eating animals under control but also moderating numbers of introduced pests such as foxes and feral cats. The loss of dingoes and subsequent upsurge in numbers of feral cats has contributed further to the loss of iconic species like the Bilby. A feral cat kills up to thirty animals per day and there are approximately four million feral cats in Australia. Just doing the maths is upsetting[93]. Given it is not always possible to tell which is the keystone species in an ecosystem, all need to be valued. This is especially important with the increasingly unpredictable climate to which plants and animals are having to adapt.

Climate change drives biodiversity loss directly, and amplifies other factors. We are already seeing the effect on biodiversity with changes in animal migration, habitats and reproduction rates, and widespread coral bleaching. The global extinction rate due to climate change is expected to increase from the current level of 2.8% to 5.2% with a 2-degree Celsius rise in global temperature or, with a worst-case scenario of a 4.3-degree rise, to 16.8%. As global temperature increases, it is expected that extinction rates will not only increase, they will accelerate[94]. Given current policy settings globally, we are on track for the direst of these predictions. This loss of biodiversity through climatic destabilisation is having a profound effect on the very things that sustain us:- our food, our medicines, and our communities. Inevitably, our health is harmed.

Globally, many leaders and organisations are calling for biodiversity to be addressed with equal importance to climate change given the intricate connections between the two issues. This is translating to calls for clear biodiversity targets for Earth to sit alongside climate targets. President Biden's pledge for 30% of the planet to be protected by 2030 is one such goal and is energising the environmental movement. For this to be achieved, not only is urgent action on climate change required, but other environmental challenges need solutions too. These include various forms of pollution, land clearing and introduced pest species. Alongside eroding Earth's biodiversity, each of these factors impinge upon human health. So, let's gather ourselves for an exploration of the dark side of mankind's industrial expansion and quest for comfort and riches.

## OTHER THREATS TO BIODIVERSITY

Apart from climate change impacts, Western cultures today are driving loss of biodiversity through our carelessness and greed to make more money and consume ever more 'stuff'. Our tendency to use poisonous chemicals, chop down trees and throw out, or let go, things we no longer want, has irrevocably changed the natural world. These behaviours manifest in various forms of pollution, the destruction of habitat and the introduction of pests. Within a given ecosystem these problems diminish the variety of plants and animals and disturb the natural balance.

The widespread use of man-made chemicals poison soil and water, killing insects and those species who depend on them for food, like birds, reptiles, and small mammals. Solid pollution mainly includes plastics. Ubiquitous in our throwaway society and often casually discarded, this rubbish ultimately ends up contaminating waterways, oceans, and landscapes. Widespread habitat destruction involves land clearing for extractive industries like logging and mining, and large-scale agriculture. While the urban sprawl of new suburbs, built in ever-expanding rings around super cities, sees progressive loss of natural areas.

In the oceans, fishing has become industrial as mega-trawlers scrape the sea floor and use enormous nets to take huge quantities of life from the seas. Intensive aquaculture sees pens of fish, like Atlantic salmon, constructed in once pristine environments. Fed antibiotics and colourants along with animal meal, these farmed fish have been described as 'battery hens of the sea' by environmental and animal welfare advocates. The seabed underneath their cylindrical aquatic feedlots is choked with fish excrement and other waste.

Introduced pests are an immense problem as they invade habitats and kill native animals. They do this by eating them directly, competing with them for food, or interfering with breeding cycles. In Australia, these pests range from small creatures like cane toads, feral cats, and rabbits, through to huge animals such as like camels. Cumulatively, their effect on biodiversity is shocking. Pest species include plants too. These unwelcome environmental weeds encroach upon indigenous plants' natural territory, competing for water and the pollinating attention of insects and birds.

While it is clear from this summary how damaging humankind's actions are to nature, the links to our own self-harm may be trickier to envisage. An examination of synthetic chemicals will help illuminate how blinkered we've been to the widespread harm we've inflicted on ourselves, one another, and future generations.

## Drenching the world in chemicals

With the widespread use of chemicals in industrial scale agriculture, we are making ourselves sick by spoiling food sources and medicines as we kill or injure plants and animals. We are also poisoning ourselves more directly by contaminating the water we drink and air we breathe. The insecticides we liberally spray over crops to kill insect 'pests' become part of our food supply, then part of us. The endocrine-disruptor chemicals present in these commonly used agricultural agents have the potential to accumulate in the fatty tissues of our body. There, they may upset our hormones and contribute to conditions as diverse as infertility, cancer, and diabetes.

Sometimes we release poisons inadvertently. The coal we mine and combust to generate electricity releases mercury and other toxins into the air. Mercury falls back to earth in rain, dissolving into the oceans. It eventually enters our food sources through the fish we consume. Small fish are eaten by larger fish, so mercury accumulates up the food chain. When we eat large predatory fish like shark or swordfish, we are getting some mercury along with the healthy protein and oils fish contain. This is such a problem that pregnant women need to limit their intake of large fish to reduce the risk of mercury damaging their developing baby's brain[95].

Where mercury pollution is a side-effect of coal power, the use of agricultural chemicals intentionally kills insects and has far-reaching consequences for all of nature. American scientist, Rachel Carson, alerted the world to the damaging effects of man-made chemicals with her ground-breaking book, *Silent Spring*. This was published in 1962 after Carson noticed the lack of birdsong in her rural home following the use of DDT by nearby farmers. An insecticide developed as a weapon of war, DDT (dichloro-diphenyl-trichloroethane) was used globally in cropping from the 1940s. Carson described the situation, "over increasingly large areas of the United States, spring now comes unheralded by the return of the birds, and the early mornings are strangely silent where once they were filled with the beauty of bird song."[96] Rachel Carson was pilloried during her lifetime and died of breast cancer soon after *Silent Spring* was published. She was fifty-six.

As a woman daring to question the testosterone-driven gallop of post-war industrialisation, Carson was heavily criticised by chemical companies, politicians and some scientists. However, she had the support of many life scientists—biologists like herself—who were aware of the interconnectedness of nature. She also had the backing of the public who were noticing the effects of chemicals on the animals around them too. By waking the world up to the influence of chemicals on nature, Carson had a profound effect on many people. David Attenborough, the famous British naturalist, has described *Silent Spring* as the most important book since Darwin's *Origin of Species*.

In *Silent Spring* Carson warned, "it is our alarming misfortune that so primitive a science has armed itself with the most modern and terrible weapons, and that, in turning them against insects it has also turned them against the earth."[96] In defiance of her words, chemicals like DDT continue to be used throughout food systems and in many everyday products like cosmetics, cleaning agents, dyes, and plastics[97]. Concurrently, we are witnessing a global collapse of insect, reptile, and bird species.

Many of the chemicals Carson was concerned about can be grouped together as *persistent organic pollutants (POPs)*. They are characterised by their toxicity to human and non-human life forms, their ability to remain in the environment for an extended period and to pass from one species to another via the food chain. Carried by wind and water, they affect regions great distances from where they are used. POPs have been found in what are often thought of as pristine natural environments, like the Arctic. Here, monitoring has found chemical residues in soil, air, water, plants and wildlife. Their use is truly a global problem. The most dangerous POPs are referred to as the 'dirty dozen' by the United States Environmental Protection Agency. The most well known in this list are DDT, dieldrin and dioxins. Most Western countries have banned or severely limited the use of these agents. But chemical companies continue to manufacture them in jurisdictions with less oversight and to push for novel products to be endorsed.

Industry giants defend the use of their products, describing newer agents as safer, despite a lack of independent studies to support their claims. Much like the corporate powers who continue to fight tobacco control, these businesses influence governments, so curtailment of chemical use is slow and clumsy. In Australia, the regulatory framework for assessing chemicals and their risk to human health provides little oversight and the very real risk of increased public health problems.

Over 99% of new chemicals are not assessed for threats to human or environmental health with the government relying on overseas data or industry itself. With over 10,000 new chemicals introduced in the year prior to 2017 alone, the chemical onslaught is impossible to keep up with. This is especially true if a government views the precautionary principle as 'red tape' to be gotten rid of[98].

## Flavouring ourselves with chemicals

As chemicals accumulate within our bodies over years, they may affect the hormonal systems that regulate growth, reproduction and development. They also upset the immune system's ability to respond to infection or inflammation. Some agents, like organophosphates and the newer *neonic* pesticides, are thought to damage brain development and are implicated in childhood neurological problems including autism spectrum disorder and memory difficulties. Measuring these effects can be challenging, and research is ongoing.

There is a strong scientific case that long term environmental exposures to synthetic chemicals are contributing to rising infertility and increases in certain hormone-dependent cancers like breast and testicular cancer, as well as diabetes. Various scientific studies have found sperm counts have approximately halved over the forty years between 1973 and 2011 in many Western countries[99]. Reproductive epidemiologist Shanna Swan explored this topic in great detail in her recent book *Countdown*[100]. Swan predicts human beings ultimately being unable to reproduce naturally if current trends in diminishing fertility continue. This is because the effects of endocrine-disruptor chemicals (EDCs) on fertility take decades to manifest. The chemicals' actions on a boy's developing testes begin in utero and continue throughout childhood, yet low sperm counts are only realised once adulthood is reached. There is an inbuilt lag in the system, a little like the delayed effect of carbon dioxide's impact on global warming. Alongside waning sperm counts, other abnormalities of the male reproductive system likely to be due to EDCs are being documented. These include deformities in penis structure, testicular development, onset of puberty and testicular cancer.

Harmful effects of EDCs have also been described in the female reproductive tract. While research in this area is complex and ongoing, it seems the timing of chemical exposure is a key determinant of outcome. Whether it occurs in utero, childhood, puberty, or later in life, manifestations of toxicity vary. Research suggests modern common gynaecological conditions like uterine fibroids, endometriosis and Polycystic Ovarian Syndrome (PCOS) may all have EDCs involved in their genesis [101,102,103].

Many EDCs double as carcinogens – chemicals known to cause cancer. As the American Endocrine Society says, 'we know how some EDCs harm us, but it's estimated that more than 1,000 of the over 85,000 man-made chemicals may be EDCs based on how they interact with our endocrine system. However, most of those 85,000 man-made chemicals have never been fully tested for safety, so the problem may be even more far-reaching than current research shows.'[104] EDCs and other synthetic chemicals may accumulate within our bodies, particularly in tissues high in fat, like the breast. Many also cross the placenta into the developing foetus, or to the infant via breastmilk. People living in modern societies are virtually flavouring themselves with these types of compounds. Although present in just tiny amounts, they are very potent and so have biological effects. Much like a few flakes of chilli can turn a bland dish spicy. In one study of a reference population in the United States, over 95% of participants had the EDC Bisphenol A (BPA) in their urine[105].

Synthetic chemicals may enter the body via the food chain, through inhalation, or skin absorption. These compounds are ubiquitous in modern society, being present in plastics, fuels, and the various products we use for cleaning, grooming, and cooking. Alongside the array of chemicals we use for these activities, in our zeal to banish unwelcome animals from our lives, we release still more into the environment directly via insecticides and pesticides. Despite the known risks to all life, DDT remains in use. Those countries where malaria is a major cause of illness are sanctioned by the international agreement overseeing DDT's use globally as a pesticide. The Stockholm Convention on Persistent Organic Pollutants accepts DDT being used for this indication in many places, including various African countries, India, and North Korea. While these nations have decided the risk of chemical exposure is a tolerable cost of malaria prevention, the implications of their decision are far reaching. DDT spreads effectively throughout the atmosphere, so it is likely harming wildlife and human health well beyond a given country's borders. Despite Rachel Carson's warning over half a century ago, humanity's recklessness with chemicals continues, albeit in new ways. And all life on Earth is affected.

## *Thinking about insects*

That we are amid the sixth mass extinction event in Earth's history is widely accepted by scientists. While it's been easier to see this in large animals, the global decline in insect species is of grave concern because they provide the foundation of the food chain. Scientists have recently completed the world's first global scientific review of all studies looking at insect numbers and the results are sobering. They found over 40% of insect species are declining and their extinction rate is eight times faster than other animals such as birds, mammals, and reptiles. The current rate of total mass of insect decline is 2.5% annually. So, they could conceivably vanish altogether within a century[106]. You don't need to be a scientist to understand that if insects vanish, so too do humans. This global analysis backs up other alarming studies, like the Puerto Rican project discussed earlier which revealed a 98% reduction in ground insects over 35 years[107]. Concurrent studies of insect numbers in Germany's protected nature reserves found a 75% drop over a 27-year period[108]. What's especially concerning about this latter analysis is that it measured insect numbers in conservation areas where habitat is preserved. If insect numbers are dire in these places, surely their plight is critical elsewhere.

The authors of the global analysis asserted the major cause of insect decimation to be intensive agriculture. This type of farming sees vast fields of crops exclude trees and other plants which would otherwise support biodiversity. Industrial scale plantings of one type of plant (monocultures) are drenched in synthetic fertilisers and pesticides. Such compounds sterilize the soil and leach into waterways contaminating life elsewhere. Other factors include light pollution from human developments, like roads and buildings, whose bright lights attract insects, pulling them off course. The insects then fail to reach their natural destination, ultimately dying before pollinating or mating, as would previously have occurred. As with the Bogong moth, climate change is a major influence, altering the habitat of insects and interfering with their reproduction. Changes in weather patterns make water sources and the flowering of plants unreliable, threatening the survival of insects which rely on them.

The plight of Earth's insects adjusts the lens through which everyday activities are viewed. It no longer seems reasonable to spray poisons around the home or onto one's skin to prevent insect bites. It is safer and kinder to cover up with light clothing. And solastalgia arises when embarking on nocturnal road trips as the loss of insect life proves unsettling. In decades past such activity required the judicious use of detergent in the windscreen wash water to see safely such was the abundance of insects accumulating on the glass. The profusion of these creatures was at once incidental and mildly bothersome. Today, because there are so few insects, this is seldom necessary. While the decline in insect numbers may pass unnoticed by many, especially those without memories of prior abundance, the implications for human health are profound. By pollinating our crops and sustaining other life forms, insects are essential for our wellbeing. We ignore their demise at our peril.

Just as the widespread use of chemicals has underpinned the collapse of insect populations globally, humankind's tendency to produce and discard plastics is choking the seas. The concept of single-use products, touted to make life simpler, easier, and cleaner, is seductive to modern society. The myth which underlies plastic use is that these items can be thrown 'away' after just one use. There is no such place on Earth. As we will see from an exploration of the world's oceans, solid pollution in the form of plastics, is irrevocably changing the nature of the aquatic environment.

## The problem with plastic

Perhaps the most graphic example of humanity's obscene polluting abilities is the way we treat our oceans. Images of the Great Pacific Garbage Patch (GPGP) are shocking and powerfully encapsulate the problem with single use plastics. Situated midway between Hawaii and California in the once pristine Pacific Ocean, this swirling mass of man-made refuse slowly and inexorably expands. Water currents and prevailing winds have led to the GPGP's formation which was first noted in the 1970s. As we carelessly discard what we no longer want, the GPGP continues to grow like an oceanic cancer. The GPGP covers a surface area of 1.6 million square kilometres and it's estimated the 1.8 trillion pieces of plastic in the patch weigh approximately 80,000 tonnes[109]. Some 80% of rubbish in the GPGP is washed out to sea from North America and Asia. It takes six years for debris from North America to reach the patch, while garbage from Asia needs only a year. The remaining 20% of rubbish comes from offshore oil rigs and ships, and is mostly fishing nets[110]. These are a big problem, trapping seals, turtles and large marine mammals who drown when unable to break free.

There are four other offshore plastic accumulation zones in the world's oceans. No country or corporation will take responsibility for them. While these patches of garbage are clearly visible, most plastic in the oceans is less obvious. Microplastics, fragments less than five millimetres long, are found throughout the world, even in the remote Antarctic. Most rubbish in the sea comes from land after it's washed into waterways and storm water drains. Sometimes the route is more direct, with ships simply dumping their rubbish overboard. Studies have estimated between 1.15 and 2.41 million tonnes of plastic enters the ocean each year from rivers. Approximately a quarter floats and the tougher plastics travel great distances to accumulate in the huge garbage patches. On its journey, the plastic fragments into mostly small pieces, readily ingestible by birds and sea creatures. Eventually, the garbage patch becomes a massive column of plastic fragments, much like a toxic, peppery soup.

Sea birds suffer from plastics in various ways. They may become entangled and drown or suffocate. Or they may eat the fragments, mistaking them for food. This is problematic in several ways. First, the birds feel satiated and so fail to meet their nutritional requirements; eventually starving to death with a belly full of plastic. Second, sharp pieces may perforate their internal organs causing fatal bleeding. Finally, smaller fragments may accumulate in the bird's gut and other tissues. Over time the plastic's chemical toxins affect bodily functioning. Just as in humans, endocrine-disruptor chemicals and persistent organic pollutants can affect the bird's reproduction, growth and survival. It is especially worrying when adult birds inadvertently feed their chicks plastic. Juveniles are even less able to deal with these man-made substances, having a smaller gut and more sensitive physiology.

Below the surface, other animals struggle to cope with the legacy of our profligate lifestyle. Almost all marine life is affected in similar ways to seabirds. Large mammals, like whales and dolphins, as well as turtles and all fish are vulnerable to entanglement or poisoning by man-made plastics. Apart from the cruel and unethical suffering we inflict on these creatures, given the reliance we have on sea life to meet our nutritional needs, we harm it at our personal cost.

Just like the atmosphere where we pump waste without a second thought, our beautiful seas suffer for our collective selfishness. In the 1970s it was socially acceptable in Australia to throw rubbish out the window when driving through the countryside. This action now seems unthinkable. But we seem to be stuck still mindlessly discarding our waste into the air or sea, wilfully blind to the consequences. Polluting the natural environment, whether it's the water we drink, the air we breathe, or the oceans our seafoods live in, ultimately harms our health. Inhaling or ingesting toxins from decomposing plastics and chemicals can have far reaching and long-lasting health impacts. The legacy of this cumulative poisoning of Earth is reflected in many modern diseases yet is rarely acknowledged as a causative factor.

Humans are not only generating plastic and chemical pollution, we are also steadily denuding the landscape. Today, the human population has reached an historical high. There has been an accompanying surge in the number of middle-class consumers whose appetite is voracious. Never has so much been taken from the natural world. As our cities, mines and farms expand to produce food and commodities, richly biodiverse natural places are destroyed. While some animals can move to other habitats, most cannot, so humanity's expansion comes at an enormous cost to other species. Many people would expect high rates of deforestation in the so called 'third world', or 'developing' countries. However, it is right here, in Australia, where land clearing and deforestation are racing ahead, stripping away our unique biodiversity. Continuing our exploration of the dark side of 'progress' let's move on to survey how the land is being forever changed.

## The devastation wrought by land clearing

In Australia we are seeing an explosion in land clearing with the eastern part of the country considered a global deforestation hotspot. The only one in the developed world, according to the World Wildlife Fund (WWF). At our current rate of land clearing, Australia sits alongside New Guinea, Indonesia, Congo, and Brazil in the top ten of WWF's global deforestation hotspot list. WWF estimates Australia will lose between three and six million hectares of trees by 2030, an area at least half the size of Tasmania[111]. It can be difficult to grasp the enormity of what's happening, so journalists often use analogies to get the message across. When it comes to land clearing, we are using huge chains strung between enormous bulldozers to knock down every living thing at a rate of 1,500 football fields per day. And that's just the estimate for Queensland in one year, 2015.

Apart from the plants destroyed in this process, the suffering caused to native animals is mind boggling. It is calculated some fifty million mammals, birds and reptiles are killed annually because of land clearing in Queensland and New South Wales alone[112]. The distress animals experience may be prolonged as they try to survive in the newly denuded environment, or nearby habitat, before they die. Presently, decisions to allow land clearing don't consider harm done to animals despite this being an embedded promise of such plans. Perhaps lawmakers should insist those wanting to clear native vegetation first estimate the numbers of animals to be killed by their actions. That way we, as a community, can more fully understand the costs of land clearing. Not just in simple financial terms, but in terms of loss of life, of suffering. This may help shift perceptions about whether so much land needs to be cleared for agriculture. As the author of a study estimating animal distress from land clearing in Australia says, "while it's unlikely that someone who wants to clear land actually wants native animals to suffer, suffering will nevertheless be an inevitable consequence. The relevant question is not *whether* animals will be killed and harmed when land is cleared, but *how much* of that harm will occur, how severe it will be, and whether it ought to be avoided".[113] If we care about animals and donate to charities protecting the habitat of orangutans in Malaysia, or elephants in Africa, then we would be right to be deeply distressed about what is happening right here in Australia.

Similarly, if we care about culture, we should be worried about the damage to Aboriginal and Torres Strais Islander sacred sites wrought by this rampant land clearing. Much of it is occurring on crown land, or pastoral properties, where there is very little oversight. A recent report from north-western Australia cites claims by Nyikina Mangala Traditional Owner, Wayne Bergmann, that an area ten square kilometres was cleared without native title approval. The Chinese super-company Shanghai CRED forged ahead with clearing and, according to Mr Bergmann, "they've knocked over important trees and places where our people historically have been buried. There's been no heritage survey or clearance or approval by Traditional Owners".[114] Shanghai CRED owns some 80,000 square kilometres of cattle stations across three Australian states and the Northern Territory so, if this same reckless land clearing is occurring in all their land holdings, the scale of cultural and environmental damage is likely to be enormous. The image of a battling farming family struggling on the land is often what's presented as the public face of farming but huge, multinational conglomerates rule. They seem to have no connection to the land and no sense of stewardship, just a focus on profit at all costs.

The knock-on effects of land clearing include the pollution of rivers and oceans as soil sediment enters waterways. In turn, this harms habitat for species within fresh and saltwater systems. Run-off from land clearing in Queensland enters coastal waters, smothering corals and clouding the water. This reduces the amount of light reaching the plants and animals that make up the Great Barrier Reef. It is estimated that of the 700,000 hectares of forest and bushland that were destroyed in Queensland between 2016 and 2018, almost half were in catchments of the Great Barrier Reef[115]. An accompanying increase in nutrients entering the water stimulates algal growth on the reef, causing coral disease and stimulating outbreaks of invasive pests, like the crown-of-thorns starfish.

In freshwater systems, high nutrient loads from land clearing can lead to algal blooms. This is especially the case in warm weather, and so is occurring more frequently with climate change-induced heatwaves. The algae produce toxins harmful to humans if ingested directly, or through eating contaminated fish. In the past decade, summertime algal blooms in the Victorian lakes system have episodically turned the water a sickly pea-soup colour. Apart from giving the lakes a ghoulish appearance, the presence of algae made the water off limits for popular activities, like swimming and fishing.

The consequences of land clearing extend far beyond ground and water systems. Air quality is affected when displaced soil enters the atmosphere. As described earlier, this can have far reaching effects on human health. Just like the great dust storms of 1930s America, nearby communities suffer physically and psychologically when the land is shrouded. Dust entering the airways may trigger asthma and other lung problems, while vision is impaired as eyes are irritated. Dust storms can also spread harmful organisms. One recent example is the 2018 listeria outbreak. This occurred in the aftermath of storms in the Riverina region of New South Wales where crops of rockmelons were contaminated by bacteria-impregnated dust. This resulted in deaths and miscarriages in people who ate contaminated melons many thousands of kilometres from the farm.

Forests and woodlands form an important part of the water cycle as they release vapour into the atmosphere, generating clouds and stimulating rainfall. So, land clearing is linked to an increase in duration and intensity of droughts. As discussed earlier, these severe weather events effect human health in many ways. Clearing also causes changes in the water table, with the rise in soil salinity making huge areas unsuitable for ongoing farming or habitation. This jeopardises long term food production and threatens the viability of many agricultural communities.

## COVID-19 – A consequence of nature's collapse

A frightening outcome of habitat destruction and the subsequent erosion of natural buffers between people and animals is the emergence of new infectious diseases. Scientists call infections which jump from an animal species to humans, *zoonoses*. As we destroy habitat, animals are forced into proximity with species with whom they would naturally never interact, including people. The wet markets of Asia, where exotic species from vulnerable ecosystems are traded, slaughtered, and eaten, are a petri dish for new infections. So too, are the encroachment of human developments into richly biodiverse places like rainforests. Diseases such as COVID-19, AIDS, Lyme disease, and those caused by Hendra and Ebola viruses, are well known zoonoses. Images of thousands of people sick and dying are evoked when we hear these names, and such illnesses seem infrequent and exotic. However, new infectious diseases are arising in humans at the astounding rate of one every four months and not all of these will reach the headlines or cause such widespread suffering[116].

Some people would rather destroy the species involved in the generation of novel zoonoses than address contributing human behaviours. This attitude is ill-informed and overly simplistic when we understand that some three-quarters of all emerging infectious diseases are spread by non-humans[117]. Where would the killing stop and what would be the result of such losses? Surely a far better approach is to restore damaged habitats, address climate change and quash the hunting and trading of rare species.

Land clearing seems such a benign term for the myriad of insults it encapsulates. The brutal and extensive destruction of flora and fauna, the shredding of Earth's soil matrix, and its displacement via air and water. Not to forget the downstream effects whereby waterways are choked and poisoned and the sea's coral gardens smothered. In this multiplicity of ways, humankind shatters natural systems to facilitate their expansion. Ultimately, this armamentarium of harmful behaviours serves to inflict a variety of illnesses on people everywhere. While they may seem unrelated, conditions as disparate as AIDS, listeriosis and dust-related lung disease share a common link – they all ultimately stem from humanity's unrelenting quest to dominate the landscape.

## The problem with pests

Sitting alongside this tendency to conquer and pillage is our unsettling propensity to discard what we no longer need. While the abandoned item is often inanimate 'rubbish', as outlined above, sometimes it is other living things. Animals and plants people have finished using are often carelessly released into the wider natural world. We collectively turn our backs on these lifeforms then label them 'pests' when their increased numbers interfere with the healthy balance of ecosystems, or with our agricultural and farming endeavours. The disruption caused to the complex and delicate relationships between species by a single pest may be profound. And while there are many examples currently playing out across the globe, let's begin with an Australian case: the feral camel.

The vast desert region near Australia's iconic Uluru has suffered significant biodiversity losses due to the explosion in the feral camel population. It is estimated one million of these huge animals roam the centre's rangelands. One of the camel's favourite foods is desert quandong, or wild peach, known to the local Anangu people as mangata. Once one of their staple foods, at the time of writing, there is only one known mangata plant left in the entire Uluru National Park.

The delicious, bright-red mangata are eaten straight off the tree by the Anangu. The fruit's oily kernels condition and strengthen human hair, which the Anangu use to weave belts[118]. Mangata are like the Australian version of the acai and goji berries and have been an invaluable food and medicine for the Anangu for generations. Various species of quandong are found across Australia and are culturally and nutritionally important for First Nations people, yet some species, like the mangata, are vulnerable to being lost in the wild.

Some 20,000 camels were imported from India between 1840 and 1907, and used by early explorers to traverse the desert. Camels forage over seventy kilometres per day and live in groups of around fifty animals, with herds of up to one thousand being reported. As a five-hundred-kilogram animal with a huge appetite for plants, camels have dramatically altered the ecosystems of a vast area of central Australia. Apart from decimating various plant species, camels foul water holes, damage cultural sites and potentially carry disease. Envisioning hundreds of these beasts descending on a waterhole, with their voracious appetites for food and water, hard hoofed feet and copious excrement, it's not difficult to imagine the damage they have wrought. Particularly upsetting is comprehending how grossly they have defiled many sacred sites, which are often near water sources. Traditionally, Aboriginal children were born near water, so these sites are often especially sacred to women.

Given the areas impacted are immense and remote, out of sight and mind for most Australians, efforts to remove feral camels have been piecemeal and inadequate. A Federal Government project to reduce camel numbers which involved culling animals across both pastoral and Aboriginal lands ran for four years and was wound up in 2013. Concerns regarding transparency of the process were raised as the agency tasked with culling camels was also responsible for monitoring numbers. The fox in charge of the hen house maybe? Unsurprisingly, they recorded a dramatic decline and concluded their own great success. Others were not so impressed, with one Senator describing the drop in numbers as 'miraculous'![119]. Since that time, with no ongoing, co-ordinated management plan or monitoring of camel numbers, the population has rebounded with consequent large-scale landscape degradation. Without a transparent monitoring of the camel population, it's impossible to say what current numbers are but central Australian pastoralists are describing a huge increase[120].

The feral camel problem is a legacy of colonisation and its associated displacement of Aboriginal people and their land care practices. The damage wrought by pest species extends well beyond camels to include foxes, cats and rabbits. All these creatures have been intentionally introduced into the Australian landscape. Rehabilitation of the central

Australian rangelands by addressing the feral animal problem is a clear responsibility of government and part of the conciliation process. By ridding the region of feral animals and restoring the land, staple foods like the mangata can return and be a key part of closing the gap in improving Aboriginal health and wellbeing. First Nations people's wellbeing simply cannot improve without an accompanying restoration, or healing, of their Country.

A more well known, equally destructive, pest is the cane toad. Originally introduced in the 1930s by sugar cane farmers as a biological agent to eat native beetles, the toad has decimated tropical Australia. There are estimated to be over 200 million across Queensland and northern New South Wales and they are toxic at all stages of their life cycle. Cane toads not only devastate insect populations and threaten the food sources of native animals, most reptiles and carnivorous mammals are fatally poisoned when they eat the toad, mistaking it for their usual prey. The toxic glands on the toad's back kill animals who eat it. This is occurring to such an extent in famous Kakadu National Park that pythons and lizards, once abundant, are now seldom sighted.

Biodiversity experts have recently publicly stated that wildlife in Kakadu has been annihilated by the cane toad. Biodiversity Watch's Graeme Sawyer described populations of thousands of toads along a 2.5 kilometre stretch of the Jim Jim Creek system, saying, "if you look at the water, in some of the remnant waterholes, it is a black soup of tadpoles."[121] The cane toad is spreading west and is a real threat to the biodiversity of the remote Kimberley region of north-western Australia. Fortunately, unlike in the Northern Territory where plans to combat the spread of the cane toad have been abandoned by government agencies, the Kimberley community is using some innovative methods.

In one pioneering example, local Balanggarra rangers in the Kimberley teamed up with university scientists to run a project teaching monitor lizards to avoid cane toads. Demonstrating innovative thinking and true cross-cultural collaboration, this initiative promises to minimize the toad's impact in the region. Called Conditioned Taste Aversion (CTA) training, the program teaches lizards to avoid cane toads. The process involves lizards first being exposed to small cane toads. These are not fatal, rather just large enough to induce vomiting. Lizards then give the full-size cane toads a miss when they arrive later in the season, thereby escaping being poisoned.

There was an interesting difference in temperament between the lizards caught by the Balanggarra rangers and the scientists. The rangers caught lizards who were shyer and more risk averse, while the scientists captured the more obvious, confident lizards. It was the ranger's subgroup of reptiles who responded to the aversion training and were able to survive the cane toad invasion when it came. The scientist's cockier, yet less clever, lizards didn't learn from eating the smaller toad.

Without the involvement of the Balanggarra rangers, the trial would not have found that lizards with certain personality traits could learn from the CTA training for only the bolder, poorer learners would have been caught. The scientists concluded, "our most exciting result, however, involves the scientific and conservation benefits of a cultural diversity within a research team. The responses of ranger-caught lizards to CTA training were critical to the main aim of our study: to test whether or not aversion training could enhance the survival of vulnerable native fauna. The success of that trial already has led to the rollout of CTA training on a landscape scale to reduce the ecosystem impacts of invasive cane toads across northern Australia. Indigenous collaboration is central to this conservation intervention".[122]

## Plants can be pests too

There have been over 28,000 exotic plants introduced into Australia since European arrival with 2,500 having naturalized. One famous example is the blackberry with Ferdinand von Mueller, the first director of Melbourne's Botanic Gardens, primarily responsible for its rampant spread. Wanting the bush to be more like Europe, in 1861 Mueller sowed blackberry seed wherever he rode in Victoria. The landscape, once carefully managed by First Nations people, was forever changed by Mueller's actions[123]. He also sent seeds interstate to be planted, ensuring blackberries a far-reaching and long lasting impact on the natural environment. Now a widely despised weed, the blackberry chokes creeks throughout the country and is extremely difficult to irradicate.

The blackberry infests over nine million hectares altogether and those endeavouring to rid the bush, or their property, from the plant try fire, mattock and herbicides. Sometimes, the treatment has caused further problems for ecological and human health. Herbicides like Triclopyr, currently recommended by government, are thought to have both short and long-term toxic effects[124]. Given blackberries cover great areas, large amounts of herbicide are required. These chemicals may disperse through the air, waterways or soil, and be inhaled or ingested by people and animals. Acute side-effects in people include eye and skin irritation, and dizziness. While animal studies have suggested chronic exposure may cause cancer or reproductive and developmental abnormalities[125]. Von Mueller's seemingly harmless actions have had disastrous ecological consequences for over 150 years and are a legacy of his seldom mentioned.

The loss of habitat and introduction of pests has meant possible solutions to various health problems have also been taken away. The gastric brooding frog, described earlier, is thought to have become extinct when fungus was introduced into its shrinking habitat. There was still more to learn from this species, especially how the stomach muscle was converted into uterine muscle. This knowledge may have helped us better understand human muscle diseases but is lost to us now.

# UNRAVELLING OF
# NATURAL SYSTEMS

While this exploration of threats to biodiversity is not fully comprehensive, it's clear the natural world is in dire straits. The fingerprints of humankind can be found on close examination of any single ecosystem. Some of Earth's most biologically abundant regions have endured multiple insults over more than a century and are now struggling to cope. It seems to be the proverbial 'death by a thousand cuts' as global forces marry ongoing local degradations. Australia's great river system, the Murray-Darling, is on the brink of collapse. Stretching over a million square kilometres, this aquatic complex includes the River Murray, the Darling and Murrumbidgee Rivers and all waterways which flow into them. It contains rich biodiversity with woodlands, mountain ranges, grasslands and over 30,000 wetlands and has supported the flourishing of many thousands of species and ecosystems. Over millennia, the waterways have been home to over forty First Nations. Under their stewardship, complex aquaculture networks thrived for tens of thousands of years, sustainably feeding many generations. The river system's demise is the inevitable consequence of many interconnecting factors. These all stem from the 'extraction at all costs' mindset which arrived with the first white people.

Since colonisation began, human activities in the rivers' catchments have triggered a cavalcade of insults to this once pristine and bountiful riverine ecosystem. Massive land clearing for agriculture over many decades saw over 15 billion trees removed from the Basin. This destabilised the earth, leading to erosion and secondary salinity as salty soil ran into waterways and floodplains. Ongoing sediment run-off periodically clouds river water, smothers plants and animals, and promotes algal blooms. These events involve dramatic shifts in the water's composition where a proliferation in algae de-oxygenates the water. When severe, fish and other aquatic life may suffocate. Excessive water extraction by farmers over the past 150 years has drastically reduced and slowed water flows and diminished seasonal inundation of flood plains. Slow-moving water carries less oxygen, further tipping the balance in favour of more frequent algal blooms. Additionally, the use of fertilisers and pesticides for crops has contaminated the waters contributing to the loss of once prolific animal life. Man-made climate change has added to this list of assaults by increasing the duration and intensity of droughts and heatwaves dropping water flows further. While introduced pests, like carp, have crowded out native fish compromising the river's ecological balance.

The culmination of these multiple harms was encapsulated by the shocking *fish kill* event in the summer of 2019. Graphic images of millions of dead fish in a forty-kilometre stretch of the Darling River and nearby Menindee Lakes depict the river system in its death throes. This natural disaster saw country towns endure the stench of rotting animals in their once healthy rivers for weeks on end. The human health consequences were dire. As well as the nauseating odour, affected communities suffered contamination of their water supply and the loss of a staple food source. There are less tangible impacts too. Watching the river's demise is devastating for local people because the waterway forms an integral part of their lives, physically, emotionally, and culturally. The psychological and spiritual distress of witnessing such an environmental catastrophe, solastalgia, may be more than some can bear. It is deeply sad yet unsurprising to see high rates of mental illness and suicide in rural communities, such is their lived experience of ecological disintegration.

## Ecocide, a Crime Against Humanity

The environmental tragedy unfolding in the Murray Darling Basin has taken place over some 150 years, with climate change and industrial agriculture amplifying the threat most recently. Even though the ruin of the river system is dramatic and confronting, for many people the pace and degree of change may be barely perceptible. In contrast, the havoc wrought on nature through chemical warfare during the Vietnam War was violent, sudden, and widespread. Employed by the American army to strip foliage off any trees the Viet Cong may have been sheltering under, herbicides were sprayed onto rainforests and crops. Called Rainbow Herbicides in reference to their colourful storage drums, the chemicals were systematically misted over the countryside for some nine years. The benign sounding Agents White, Purple, Blue, Pink, Green and Orange destroyed plants and animals and caused dreadful diseases in humans. This shocking act of war sparked community outrage and highlighted the need for the global community to curtail the use of such chemical weapons.

Galvanised by this planetary threat, some have sought to enshrine Earth's protection in international law. This required the creation of new terms, like *ecocide*. First coined by biologist Professor Arthur Galston in the 1970s, ecocide describes the deliberate killing of ecosystems by man. Galston wanted to convey the widespread devastation wrought on nature through Rainbow Herbicides. International discussions over the ensuing forty years by many governments explored the inclusion of ecocide as a Crime Against Humanity in times of both war and peace. However, while ecocide was in the founding document of these International Laws Against Peace, it was ultimately omitted following pressure from some wealthy nations.

Renowned Earth lawyer Polly Higgins worked tirelessly to mount the case for these international laws[126]. A barrister, writer, and advocate for the natural world, Higgins developed the Eradicating Ecocide campaign. This sought to have ecocide reinstated as an atrocity crime at the International Criminal Court alongside Genocide, War Crimes and Crimes Against Humanity. In Higgins' 2010 submission to the United Nations Law Commission, she defined ecocide as 'the loss, damage or destruction of ecosystem(s) of a given territory(ies) ... such that peaceful enjoyment by the inhabitants has been or will be severely diminished'[127]. She described the harm ecocide causes people as follows: "Ecocide adversely impacts on many levels, there can be harm both ecological and cultural. Our emotions and our senses are affected; we feel and see the adverse impact of ecocide. Communities most harmed by ecocide suffer what is known as *solastalgia*. At a collective level, communities feel a profound sense of isolation and intense desolation. This is compounded by the community's lack of power in the face of State and corporate might, the pain of being unable to console in times of great distress and the loss of homeland."[128]

Ecocide is embedded in the culture of rampant capitalism, the legacy of colonialism and patriarchy which forms the world view of 'developed' nations. Environmental philosopher, Glenn Albrecht created another word, *terracide*, to describe the extinction of all life on Earth, the deliberate desolation of the whole biosphere, an accumulation of multiple, regional, ecocides[128]. Could we be on the cusp of committing this gross, planetary crime? Much more than a crime against humanity, terracide is a crime against all life. Such catastrophic loss is difficult to contemplate, especially when the perpetrators are fellow citizens or international allies. Environmental, public health and social justice advocates, alongside First Nations people, have been pushing uphill, toiling against the inexorable forces of 'development'. Linking the interdependence of nature and humanity is essential to avert terracide through escalating climate and extinction crises. Yet it is only recently that this stance is being taken by those speaking from the wider health platform.

As the call from nature gets louder, and the threat posed to humanity by global environmental forces more graphic, the health/nature relationship is coming to the fore. As humans, we find ourselves in a precarious position as we enter the third decade of this 21st century. Facing a truly existential crisis, the decisions we make now will determine the future of all life on Earth. It is helpful to ponder how our attitudes and behaviours have gotten us to this point. Only once we understand our harmful patterns and destructive mindsets can we begin to make the pivot towards a regenerative and respectful relationship with nature. Canadian scientist and environmentalist David Suzuki calls for a change in the way we relate to the natural world. He asks, "is a river the veins of the land or simply potential energy and irrigation? Is a forest a sacred grove or just timber and pulp? Is soil alive or merely dirt? Is a house a home or just a piece of real estate? Is the planet a sacred creation or a world of opportunity?"

Such questions are timely and urgent, and cut to the heart of humanity's predicament. Let's turn towards this ugliness to explore how and why it is we have been Gaia's gold diggers rather than her gardeners.

# KEY POINTS

- Biodiversity underpins human health and wellbeing
- Keystone species support many others, their loss is profound
- Humans don't necessarily know which are keystone species
- Climate change is one of many human threats to biodiversity
- Other threats include pollution, pests, and land clearing
- Human pollution incorporates the use of chemicals and plastics
- Chemicals contaminate our bodies as well as the wider living world
- Endocrine-disruptor chemicals can lead to cancers and infertility
- Plastics accumulate in oceanic garbage patches and in the bodies of animals
- Pests kill native species and compete with them for food, water, and habitat
- Plant pests (weeds) invade and disrupt ecosystems
- Land clearing destroys forests and woodlands and kills native animals
- Loss of plants from land clearing destabilises soils and contaminates waterways
- Ancient cultural sites are destroyed as land is cleared
- *Ecocide* is the deliberate destruction of nature by man
- Ecocide is arguably a crime against humanity
- *Terracide* is global ecocide

# 6

# Today's Toxic Relationship With Nature

*"Our great boast is the possession of intelligence, but what intelligent creature, knowing the critical role of air for all life on Earth, would then proceed to deliberately pour toxic materials into it? We are air, so whatever we do to air, we do to ourselves. And this is true of the other sacred elements."*

~David Suzuki

## GAIA'S GOLD-DIGGERS

Nature, in all its beauty, complexity and variety, supports our health in ways big and small. It has inspired innovation and invention over thousands of years. So, why do we seem indifferent to its destruction? Encountering smart, kind, and well-meaning people who either don't notice the harm being done to the natural world, or don't seem to be especially bothered by it, is perplexing. Humans have an extraordinary ability to problem solve, learn from mistakes, and create clever solutions to complex challenges. Yet we seem to be unwilling, perhaps unable, to stop destroying the very planet on whose wellbeing we depend.

It's not as if nature's decline is hidden. We find ourselves amid the planet's sixth mass extinction event. Here, in Australia, we have a world-leading rate of mammalian extinctions, with twenty-eight extraordinary animals disappearing since colonisation began. In fact, Australia's official number of threatened species now stands at 1,775 – almost 50% more than eighteen years ago. This puts us amongst the world's worst performers in biodiversity protection[129].

Our record on climate change is equally disturbing. Despite massive reef systems bleaching year after year—a clear manifestation of climate change—our government has approved the largest coal mine on Earth. The public's response to this shocking decision has been a nonchalant shrug. There has been no widespread public outcry at this decision. No domination of news headlines or endless analysis by talk-show hosts. No preoccupation with it in general conversation for months on end. Rather, the environmental campaigners opposing the mine have been pilloried for jeopardising jobs.

Given Australia's unique biodiversity, we are especially vulnerable to climate disruption. There is a lot to lose. Iconic sites, like the Great Barrier Reef, Kakadu wetlands and Queensland Wet Tropics, are particularly at risk. But, as we saw in the summer of 2019/2020, nowhere is truly safe. Over a hellish few months, most of southern Australia coughed through smoke haze as endless tracts of forests burnt and billions of native animals perished. Australians hold the fate of a significant proportion of the world's plant and animal diversity in our hands. Yet, it seems we cannot be trusted with this role.

Collectively, despite the obvious urgency, we are failing to address the climate and extinction crises. Like many complex problems, multiple contributory forces come into play. First, we can't see, or perhaps don't notice, the loss of biodiversity around us. We seem to be so disconnected from our sense of place that we feel little care or responsibility towards the living world around us. When this loss is pointed out to us, we often minimise it, prioritising other issues. We reject the suggestion we live differently to minimise harm to nature because we don't want to experience discomfort or inconvenience, however temporary.

This lack of noticing and caring by many means those who gain financially by damaging nature, thrive (supported both overtly and covertly by governments). Globally, those in power have adopted measurements like Gross Domestic Product (GDP) to define the wellbeing of countries and economies. Thus, the ultimate determinant of whether something is valuable becomes its financial worth. Consequently, we see mining companies being given unfettered access to places of extraordinary natural beauty and cultural significance. Rights to unlimited amounts of precious ground water being granted despite increasingly frequent and severe droughts. Logging companies having freedom to clear fell forests to make woodchip for paper while the associated pollution of rivers, release of carbon and decimation of wildlife is ignored.

Governments seem to be complicit, even in democracies like Australia, and so legislation and regulation is minimal. In fact, proponents of small government neoliberalism deride checks on environmental compliance as 'green tape', something to be removed. The onus is on concerned members of the public and environmental advocates to check whether threatened species and ecosystems are to be harmed. These groups are often overwhelmed by the sheer number and scale of mining and other projects underway throughout the world. First Nations peoples are pushed aside and in the worst instances lose their homes and lives when the inevitable disasters unfold. This has been occurring for centuries with some standout Australian examples relating to nuclear weapon development.

## Bombing Country

The most awful is surely the British nuclear bomb testing at Maralinga in the 1950s and 1960s. This activity killed and injured many Anangu people and made their Country uninhabitable. Christobel Mattingley's 2016 book, *Maralinga's Long Shadow: Yvonne's Story*, provides a moving account of the devastation wreaked upon Yvonnne Edwards and her family during this time. Their Country was not only subject to years of nuclear bombing, the Anangu were also co-opted into the site clean-up which resulted in many dying from radiation sickness and cancer. As Yvonne recounted, "All Anangu mens who worked at Maralinga finished now. Lost a sister too from cancer. In her 20s. And an uncle in his 40s from cancer. And an auntie from cancer. Two of my sons died in their 40s from cancer. Sometimes I cry at night. Used to be a lot of old people. But not now... All our people end up in cemetery because of that bomb. It destroyed our old people. I cry at night – for my mother, grandmothers, aunties."[130]

Further displacement of Aboriginal people for the nuclear industry occurred in 1981 with the annexation of part of Kakadu National Park for uranium mining. This made a large part of the Mirrar people's Country inaccessible to them and has led to ongoing health and environmental problems. The UNESCO World Heritage-listed Kakadu contains extraordinary wetlands and experiences a deluge of rain during the wet season. This inundates vast floodplains. How it was thought tropical downpours would not lead to spills of contaminated water from the tailings site defies belief. Flying over Kakadu in a light plane reveals the scar of the mine to be an abomination in an otherwise glorious landscape. The tailings dam stores rock, rubble and contaminated water left after uranium extraction. A pond of poison sitting open to the air, it receives a high annual rainfall. With climate change, this is becoming increasingly unpredictable in its intensity, duration, and timing. There have been at least 150 leaks, spills and licence breaches at the Ranger uranium mine since it opened in 1981. Incredibly, as of March 2009, the mine has been leaking 100,000 litres per day of contaminated water into the ground underneath the national park.

The mine lease area contains wealth far beyond minerals. There are 171 places of Aboriginal cultural heritage significance and over 160 archaeological sites and artefacts, including some confirming Aboriginal habitation of up to 80,000 years[131]. Given the mine is scheduled to close in 2026, Traditional Owners and environmentalists are waiting to see the full rehabilitation plan. The land is supposed to be returned to pre-operation condition and to ensure radioactive mine tailings are physically isolated from the environment for at least 10,000 years. The criteria by which adequate rehabilitation is judged are set by the mining company itself, which highlights the poor regulation of this industry in Australia[132].

When we add to these especially horrific examples the rampant land clearing and destructive farming practices occurring widely across Australia, it's difficult not to feel a sense of outrage. Modern industrial farming and 'agri-business' act against natural systems. By employing chemicals and genetically-modified seeds, they grow crops in land that would be unfarmable if not for unsustainable irrigation. In all these ways, governments, extractive industries, and giant agricultural companies have pillaged the natural world while 'civil' society has stood quietly by.

Finally, climate change, has been unleashed. An unavoidable consequence of humanity's adulation of 'the market' and each nation's quest for a high GDP. Set in motion by unchecked global land clearing for mining, agriculture and logging, and the pollution from burning fossil fuels for transport and energy production, it is an almost unstoppable force. Climate change has disrupted all ecosystems services necessary for our health. We have overstepped the key planetary boundaries for ongoing human survival and urgent action is required to correct this imbalance.

What lies underneath society's indifference to the unravelling of natural systems? Perhaps it's the gradual disconnection from nature that's accompanied the industrial revolution as people have moved to the concrete jungle of ever-expanding cities. Or maybe it's the disruption of a sense of place, the inevitable consequence of migration, whether driven by economic need or conflict. Concomitant technological advances have seen a further retreat, as people move away from the physical into virtual worlds. Most likely it's a combination of multiple factors. This conundrum of complacency, carelessness and, often, sheer callousness is worthy of further exploration.

## BLINDNESS OR INDIFFERENCE?

Many people living in busy modern cities in the Western world seem to be suffering a type of heartache. Having lost our connection to the natural world, and our sense of place, it's as if our 'green' heart is broken. American author, Richard Louv uses the term *nature deficit disorder* to describe the hurt we feel because of this lack. While Australian academic, Mardie Townsend, describes it as *environmental deprivation*[133]. Either way, this want runs deep; our very spirit suffers without a meaningful link to nature. The damage this does to our bodies, minds and relationships is explored elsewhere in this book. Here, we'll contemplate how it is our heart has become so distant from nature.

Over the past few centuries, humanity has progressively moved from the countryside to live in cities where there is little green space amongst the urban sprawl. Still more than this, the stories we've been told have pushed the natural world from our hearts. These narratives have arisen from our cultural and religious beliefs. For those communities where Christianity dominates, the overarching story framework has been that nature is to be tamed and feared, controlled by mankind.

The rise of scientific knowledge and discipline has pushed us further from nature as we have become the dispassionate observer. Rational, scientific thought has seen us categorise, label, and dissect nature, dividing it up into smaller and smaller fragments to examine under the microscope. With the economic paradigm espousing the 'free market' and globalisation, pieces of nature have been commodified and are now bought and sold on the stock exchange. Economists tell us decisions about money are to be made without emotion, so this barter of nature's bounty is reduced to a heartless fiscal deal. Coinciding with these changes, the loss of the Commons and rise of individualism has seen us become self-focussed. In our rush to become the richest and the strongest we have pushed others aside and ignored values of community. We have forgotten the essential truth. The fundamentals our planet provides for us, life-giving elements like soil, water, and air, must be shared.

There are many reasons why most people living in modern cities don't see what's being lost in the natural world. Some of these are surely lifestyle related. Today, time is mostly spent indoors, in the home, car, or workplace. And recreational activities often take place within a huge shopping centre, exercise studio, or online. If you don't venture outside, you won't notice how dry the ground is or how the plants are wilting in the unseasonably warm autumn sun. Even if you do cross the threshold, chances are you'll be distracted by your device and, with headphones on, be oblivious to bird calls. One wonders, if all the birds went silent, how long would it take for people to notice?

Also, so many of us have *plant blindness* where we simply see green but don't truly know, or appreciate, the rich plant life around us. We also seem to have bird and animal blindness when it comes to our native species. Perhaps it is the loss of naturalists and field trips. In Australia, a much-loved past time was to go out and explore the bush, or beach, to look for new plants, insects, birds, and other animals. In fact, nature study was a key part of school education from the late-19th to mid-20th century. Teachers were encouraged to take their students outside to learn about plants and animals and get some healthy fresh air. Things are very different now. A 2002 study from the United Kingdom found children knew the names of more 'Pokemon' characters than local wildlife[134]. It's most likely a study of today's Australians, adults or children, would expose a similar dearth of knowledge given changes in education and recreational choices.

There seems to be such indifference to our flora and fauna it's no wonder that, despite leading the world in mammalian extinctions, most Australians would point the finger at other countries when asked to think about global hotspots for environmental harm. The loss of forests in Borneo seem to get more sympathy than the destruction of Victoria's old-growth forests. This is despite them being home to the largest flowering plants, and most carbon-dense forests on Earth. We are also understandably outraged by the threat to orangutans as rainforests are cleared to make way for palm oil plantations in Borneo. Yet, the industrial logging of Victorian forests, home to the Leadbeater's possum, our faunal emblem, is barely noticed by the average Australian.

Even our much-loved koala's plight is largely ignored. Outrageous rates of land clearing in New South Wales (NSW) have seen its population of koalas plummet from approximately 2 million at the time colonisation began to the current level of 20,000. Experts are deeply concerned this iconic animal will become extinct in NSW by 2050. The numbers are difficult to comprehend, with over two million hectares of native vegetation cleared between 1990-2016[135]. The devastating bushfires from the 2019/2020 summer wiped out a further one third of koala habitat. Koalas have evolved to eat only a few species of eucalyptus, so the loss of these gum trees, whether through fire or heavy machinery, is proving catastrophic.

## Ignoring our native species

There seems to be an entrenched disregard, often bordering on disdain, for native species. This may stem from the attitude of the first colonisers. Koalas were initially only valued for their soft fur and their numbers have never recovered from the decimation of the fur trade of the late-19th and early-20th centuries. Then, millions of pelts were exported to the United States and London for clothing manufacture. It is estimated 800,000 koalas may have died in 'Black August' 1927 when the Queensland government promoted hunting for the employment of rural workers. This followed some 2 million koala skins being exported from the east coast for the fur trade in 1924. After this savage and prolonged attack on koalas, remaining populations have continued to be vulnerable to ongoing habitat loss, disease, and threats posed by dogs and cars[136]. It seems we have a rather strange way of showing our love to this furry Australian mascot.

The shocking plight of koalas and Leadbeater's possums highlight how dire the situation is for Australia's unique wildlife. It seems as if, despite their vulnerability in the face of climate change and habitat loss, most people are untroubled by their predicament. This is hard to fathom and may be explained by the concept of *cognitive dissonance*. This psychological term describes the discomfort felt when conflict arises between our values, attitudes, or behaviours. To cope with this uneasy feeling, we may minimise the issue at hand, or attempt to rationalise our behaviour. We may see ourselves as loving animals and nature yet fail to act in environmentally sensitive ways. The awkwardness felt when faced with evidence of our own role in nature's destruction can be especially unpleasant. Experiencing shame and guilt for allowing this to occur is too difficult to cope with. So, we push it aside, preferring to criticise other countries on their environmental practices, or to distract ourselves with another issue.

The refusal to pay attention to death of native animals is especially apparent in the way most Australians simply walk past a dead possum on the nature strip of their street, barely giving it a glance. If it were a domestic pet, someone's 'fur baby', the response would be quite different. Efforts would be made to find its owner, or solemnly bury it in a special place. Similarly, driving along country roads in many places in Australia, the number of dead animals on the verge can be confronting. Yet we collectively dismiss it as roadkill, the price paid by our fauna for our need to rush from place to place as quickly as possible. Most people barely slow down, let alone stop to check for a baby joey in the pouch of an injured kangaroo. Perhaps we speed past to outrun our conscience, as much as to get to the destination on time.

## Attacking the land

Sometimes our disconnection from place can manifest more overtly in a harsh relationship to the land, and see us actively damage it. This behaviour may come at a personal cost. The fraught relationship between non-Aboriginal Australians and their land is encapsulated in the way farmers have often destroyed nature in their quest to live 'on' as opposed to 'with' the land. In his memoir, *The Nature of Survival*, third generation farmer Doug Lang writes about his efforts to repair the degraded farm he inherited. He recounts in vivid detail how various plants were wrenched from the ground when he was young. As an adult, Lang struggled with mental illness, including depression. Could some of this be a consequence of multi-generational, vicarious trauma from participating in, and bearing witness to, nature's destruction?

Lang recalls his involvement in ridding the farmland of native tree violet, called 'barrier bush' by his family. "I remember as a young teenager we were sent over to our barrier country to spend the afternoon pulling these bushes out by tractor and cable. We would then get the remaining roots of the bush out with a crowbar. I remember only too well just to break the monotony of crowbarring the roots... I would gingerly insert the detonator into the dynamite, place the plug of dynamite into a round hole I had crowbarred into the tree violet's root, light the fuse... and then run and take cover. The remaining root of the plant would be blown to smithereens as was the surrounding rock."[137]

The landscape was cleared with warlike aggression, literally blown apart. If this sanctioned destruction of nature is viewed as a war, a form of ecocide, these children were the child soldiers. It's not difficult to see how this activity could be traumatic on a psychological level and predispose to adult mental illness. One also wonders how Aboriginal people, witnessing this devastation, would have felt. Alongside the violence directed against them personally, was this decimation and violation of their homeland, of Country.

Our disconnection from nature may manifest through obliviousness, indifference, or outright aggression. Whichever way it arises, this dislocation makes it hard for us to truly know where we are. In either time or space. The upset may be more emotional than physical and colours our relationship with the natural world. The historical and cultural context of our lives is crucial in shaping this sensibility. Let's explore this further by reflecting on the colonisation of a small part of southern Australia.

## DISORIENTATION

In healthcare, one of the ways we assess a patient's thinking is to have them complete a Mini Mental State Examination, a series of questions to quickly ascertain overall brain function. The first question is to determine if they know where they are in time, place, and person. That is, who and where they are, both temporally and geographically. Most Australians don't truly know where they are – whose land they're on, or the full history of the place they live. Collectively, we are not fully oriented in time or place, or perhaps, even in person. In our ignorance of this history, we demonstrate our disorientation and a lack of deep connection to place.

This was certainly true for me. I didn't appreciate until my early forties where I was – on Wurundjeri Woi-wurrung Country, in the Kulin Nation. A land which for some 60,000 years had been occupied and cared for by generations of Aboriginal people. This place has a continuing, complex and ancient cultural history. Woi-wurrung, not

English, is the language of this place. I was ignorant of the correct name for the seasons or how to tell when they were changing. There are six seasons in the Wurundjeri calendar. Naturally, these are a much better fit for the flowering and fruiting changes in the bushland than the four seasons proscribed by English colonisers.

The nearby creek, named Gardiner's Creek in English, was known as KooyongKoot in the Woiwurrung language of the Wurundjeri people. Meaning 'haunt of the waterfowl', this descriptive term is much more suited to the land than the name of a man only here for a short time. Also new was information that Gardiner himself was a pastoralist whose behaviour towards the Wurundjeri was appalling. He forcefully stole their land, polluted their water sources with his cattle and had them shot at for stealing his potatoes when starving[138]. Gardiner's behaviour towards his own family was poor too. He left his house near KooyongKoot after only five years and moved further east before abandoning his wife and family to return to England, where he married his cousin[139]. Was this man an upstanding citizen, worthy of honouring? It's hard to think so. And yet Gardiner has many things named after him, streets, waterways, even a railway station.

More recently than Gardiner's invasion and occupation 190 years ago was the burying of a tributary of KooyongKoot with the soil discarded for a rail tunnel. The poorly named Back Creek was concealed underground for urban development. No more a briskly flowing waterway running along the floor of a deep gully, with habitat for birds and other animals. Rather grassy parkland with a flat pathway, amenable to dog walkers and joggers, sitting atop a huge, subterranean, concrete pipe. All over this city we have literally entombed natural and cultural treasures in the name of 'progress'.

## The blindness of the colonisers

Historically, we've not only submerged creeks, we've also ignored First Nations people's knowledge. Through our colonial lens we've missed seeing the whole picture, the richness and importance of what was already here. We've dismissed the extraordinary way First Nations people have lived on this dry continent for tens of thousands of years, developing a rich culture and way of living in harmony with the earth.

In his book *Dark Emu*, writer Bruce Pascoe provides numerous examples of how First Australians optimised the biological diversity of their country for medicines and food. In researching his book, Pascoe studied records of first contact as written down by white explorers and settlers. What he found is both fascinating and enraging because time and again Aboriginal innovation in agriculture, medicine, architecture, and culture is described in detail and recorded before being discounted as stupid or simply ignored. For example, the Brewarrina aquaculture system in north-western New South Wales is thought to be one of humankind's first constructions with archaeologists estimating it to be at least 40,000 years old[140]. It is comprised of stone ponds and races which channelled breeding stock up and down stream to create an enormous quantity of fish. Estimated to feed the 5,000 or more people who attended the annual harvest, it is truly phenomenal.

These types of aquaculture systems were noted by European arrivals over the entire continent near most inland rivers. The Lake Bolac system in western Victoria was used for trapping and harvesting eels and is only now beginning to receive the attention and protection it deserves. This is just in time because much was deliberately destroyed by farmers. Both in the first years of colonisation and then more recently, when anxiety about Native Title claims arose in the late-1990s. Sadly, appropriate recognition and celebration of Aboriginal innovation with aquaculture denoting intentional, careful land use ran counter to the preferred narrative. This was that Aboriginal people were nomadic, randomly wandering over a landscape of which they had no ownership.

The denial of the evidence of large Aboriginal communities living in stone dwellings with complex food systems enabled those taking the land to do so in the belief that Aboriginal people had no longstanding connection to it. The land, their Country, was free to be taken. The official term was *terra nullius*. Pascoe says, "Even at the time of writing, a massive roller is at work crushing volcanic stone in Western District pastures. On one level it is simple pasture improvement; on another it is heritage destruction. The operator of the roller is 'just doing what he is told' but he wouldn't be allowed to do it at Stonehenge or Easter Island."[140]

Recently, there has been criticism of Pascoe's description of Aboriginal people's land use as agriculture by some anthropologists and archaeologists. These academics argue about the terminology used, preferring the term *hunter-gatherer-plus* to describe First Australians, rather than farmers[141]. They also object to Pascoe's use of the word agriculture. As a non-Indigenous person seeking a fuller understanding of the history of the place I live, Pascoe's work has proved engaging and enlightening. Labels like farmers and hunter-gatherers come from English, the coloniser's language. As such, they are never going to adequately describe the complex relationship between Aboriginal and Torres Strait Islander people and Country. Most non-Indigenous Australians have been taught that farming and agricultural societies are more sophisticated and advanced than hunter-gatherers'. Perhaps Pascoe's advocacy for the use of these former terms was a way of appealing to this simplistic hierarchy. An attempt to positively shift regard for First Nations people's intellect and ingenuity. Whatever the response from academia, *Dark Emu* has shone a bright light onto the genius, complexity, and intricacy of First Nations peoples' stewardship of Country.

It's not only writers like Pascoe who are confronting us with evidence of our historical blindness. Historian Bill Gammage has also looked back at the pictorial and written descriptions of first contact to help portray the way the First Australians managed the entire landscape. Gammage uses the term *estate* to describe the way the whole country was tended to and looked after by the Aboriginal communities who lived here. Time and again explorers described parklands with large fields of grass edged by forest and the way fire was used to manage the country. We now know this was *fire-stick farming* where patches of grasslands are systematically burnt in a mosaic-like pattern. In this way, wildlife has time and space to move away from the area being burnt into adjacent country. Over time, the burnt section regenerates with new plants growing from seeds evolved to germinate through fire. Animals like kangaroos then return to feed on the newly growing grasslands so can be harvested for food as needed. It was the widespread use of firestick farming which led to this appearance of an estate at the time of first contact. The loss of this practice as the First Peoples' land-management skills were replaced by the coloniser's grazing techniques resulted in an extraordinary change to the landscape. What we now think of as forests, in many places, are in fact regrowth of scrub in areas which were firestick-managed grasslands before 1788.

Gammage's book, *The Biggest Estate on Earth*, reveals the enormous damage done to the Australian landscape as the First Australians who tended it were displaced and murdered and their practices disrupted. One quote from explorer Mitchell in 1848 seems especially prescient, "The omission of the annual periodical burning by natives, of the grass and young saplings, has already produced in the open forest lands nearest to Sydney, thick forests of young trees, where, formerly, a man might gallop without impediment, and see whole miles before him. Kangaroos are no longer to be seen there; the grass is choked by underwood; neither are there natives to burn the grass...These consequences, although so little considered by the intruders, must be obvious to the natives, with their usual acuteness, as soon as cattle enter on their territory."[142]

Aboriginal people were also observed working in concert with animals to get food. One extraordinary example, described by Pascoe, is the way in which the Yuin people worked with Killer whales to harvest larger whales[140]. The Yuin would light two fires on the beach and a man would walk up and down slowly between them. He would walk with a limp as they believed this made the Killer whale take pity on him. This whale would then shepherd the other, larger whales into the shallow waters of the bay. Here they were killed by the people who would throw the dead whale's tongue back for the Killer, thereby sharing their catch.

This is not the only example of co-operating with sea creatures. Gammage quotes the written observations of Tinker Campbell: "Here, for the first time, I saw the blacks fishing. There were many hundreds along the beach with their towrows (nets) in hand. As soon as the shoal of fish appeared in the offing some two or three of the blacks would advance to the water's edge, and striking the water with their spears as a signal to the porpoises to drive the fish into the bank—which signal the porpoises would instantly obey—the main body of blacks, some hundreds in number, would rush in with their towrows and dip up the fish...The blacks even pretend to own particular porpoise, and nothing will offend them more than to attempt to injure one of their porpoises."[142]. These stories clearly depict a people who were so attuned to the animals living with them they could communicate and collaborate with them. Surely, they are inspirational and worthy of celebration by our culture rather than being pushed aside, ignored or belittled.

As Gammage says in his conclusion: "If *terra nullius* exists anywhere in our country, it was made by Europeans. .... This book interrupts Law and country at the moment when *terra nullius* came, and an ancient philosophy was destroyed by the completely unexpected, an invasion of people and ideas. A majestic achievement ended. Only fragments remain. For the people of 1788 the loss was stupefying. For the newcomers it did not seem great. Until recently few noticed that they had lost anything at all. Knowledge of how to sustain Australia, of how to be Australian, vanished with barely a whisper of regret. ....We have a continent to learn. If we are to survive, let alone feel at home, we must begin to understand our country. If we succeed, one day we might become Australian."[142]

## First Nations people's insights

Fortunately, despite the horrors of colonial invasion, there are still many thriving First Nations communities and cultures to learn from and connect with. Contemporary Aboriginal and Torres Strait Islander academics, artists and authors continue to share with us their thoughts on the difference between their culture and this new, Western one. Tyson Yunkaporta is one example. Through his enlightening book, *Sand Talk*, this artist, poet, and lecturer shares the wisdom of Indigenous knowledge patterns and systems. Yunkaporta's view of our 'developed' lifestyle is incisive. He says, "I am often told that I should be grateful for the progress that Western civilisation has brought to these shores. I am not. This life of work-or-die is not an improvement on pre-invasion living, which involved only a few hours of work a day for shelter and sustenance, performing tasks that people do now for leisure activities on their yearly holidays – fishing, collecting plants, hunting, camping and so forth. The rest of the day was for fun, strengthening relationships, ritual and ceremony, cultural expression, intellectual pursuits and the expert crafting of exceptional objects. I know this is true because I have lived like this, even in this era when the land is only a pale shadow of the abundance that once was. We have been lied to about the 'harsh survival' lifestyles of the past. There was nothing harsh about it."[143]

Yunkaporta takes the reader on a journey through the patterns of complex knowledge systems and philosophies which provided guidance for Aboriginal people for millennia. Through his lens our society seems superficial, simple and damaging, especially to our young people, the natural world and our future. The focus we have on individuality and hierarchy comes with a cost. This is our loss of community and shared knowledge and erosion of the ancient intelligences we are born with. Yunkaporta leaves us with hope, and instructions on how to learn "patterns of knowledge and ways of thinking that will help trigger the ancestral knowledge hidden inside." He says, "The assistance people need is not in learning about Aboriginal Knowledge but in remembering their own." No doubt, this takes work and humility. But surely this project is worthy; to understand ourselves more fully, as we are, at this moment, in this place.

To truly orient ourselves we need to pause and make space, to look deeply with curiosity and openness at the true history of wherever we live. In this way we can nurture our connection to place, put down our roots and begin the work of restoration. If we are respectful and careful enough, we may also have the good fortune to establish meaningful relationships with our Aboriginal neighbours, colleagues, and friends. To learn from them how to live properly on Country, and with one another.

Apart from our historical and ongoing reluctance to listen to and learn from First Nations people, we also seem to be unwilling to hear scientists when it comes to the study of nature. This is a major obstacle when facing the global collapse of biodiversity. It seems incredible that while modern science undertakes exploration of distant planets, we remain almost clueless when it comes to a comprehensive inventory of life on Earth. This situation requires further discussion. Let's begin with the hierarchy of worthiness within science.

## Ignoring life scientists

Today, we are in an astonishing position. Life scientists, whose work involves species identification, are unable to keep up with biological losses from environmental degradation. So globally, we won't ever know the full complexity of life on Earth. There are simply not enough biologists, ecologists, and other life-based scientists to do the work to identify all species before many are wiped out. This work is not well funded privately or publicly. There seems to be more public and political interest in finding life on distant planets than understanding the myriad of life forms we are living with here.

There may also be an underlying gender issue feeding into the lack of funding and interest in these biological areas of science compared to mathematics, physics, and chemistry. The 'hard', or 'pure', sciences like physics and chemistry have historically been favoured by males, with the 'soft' sciences like biology the preserve of females. In Australia, most boys' schools didn't offer biology and girls' schools omitted physics and chemistry to fit in with social norms until the 1970s. The hangover of this persists today with scaling of final year school subjects seeing chemistry, physics and mathematics being weighted as most difficult, so worth more marks. Even admission to medical degrees reflects this bias with chemistry rather than biology (the study of life), being the only fixed requirement apart from English and maths for most universities. Currently, there's a push to encourage girls to study STEM (science, technology, engineering, and mathematics) due to the lack of gender equity in jobs like engineering and related research. It's a shame there's not a simultaneous will to build learning and career pathways in the study of life: plants, animals, soils, and ecosystems. An increase in people power would help address the huge need to restore Earth's ecological balance.

The lack of funding and prioritisation given to assessing biodiversity is a global phenomenon which is reflected in the incomplete tally recorded by leading agencies. The International Union for the Conservation of Nature (IUCN) is a worldwide body whose role is to monitor the status of nature. It is made up of government and civil society organisations and receives input from over 10,000 experts. The IUCN has developed its 'Red List' to keep track of the various species and ecosystems which are most vulnerable to extinction. It's the most up to date way to find information on global biodiversity. However, it has only been able to record a small proportion of species. So far, it's assessed 128,918 species and strives to increase this number to 160,000 as soon as possible.

The Red List aims to survey vulnerable species every three to five years and lists Australia in the top five countries for high rates of animal extinctions. We are also in the top ten countries for endangered and threatened species. According to the World-Wide Fund for Nature (WWF), about 1,700 plant and animal species are listed as threatened under the Australian Government's Environment Protection and Biodiversity Conservation Act (EPBC) with an additional 90 considered extinct. Australia has the highest rate of vertebrate mammal extinction in the world with invasive species, climate change and habitat destruction being key ongoing threats. Given this is not something to be proud of, governments haven't openly shared this fact with their citizens.

Another dubious first for Australia is being home to the first known extinction from climate change, the Bramble Cay Melomys. This small, brown, mouse-like marsupial was quietly declared extinct by Australia's environment Minister, Melissa Price in early 2019. In a media release misleadingly entitled 'Stronger Protection for threatened species' the recategorisation of the Melomys from endangered to extinct was buried in a table, rather than stated clearly in the Minister's text[144]. This example shows the level of government duplicity and cynicism as it works to keep extinction of species out of the public eye. The habitat of the Melomys, a Great Barrier Reef island, was swallowed up by sea level rise and storm surges, both due to climate change.

Also troubling is the fact our Australian figures are likely to be incomplete because the federal government has almost halved funding and jobs in the environment department over the past six years. So it's been unable to keep up with status of vulnerable species. And the classification of places like Tasmania's swamp gum woodlands has been postponed since 2016. During this time, bushfires and logging have continued, so it's highly likely the woodlands' critically endangered swift parrot has moved closer to extinction[145]. Given you can't protect what you haven't bothered to look for, species are sliding quietly towards extinction. This is disturbingly convenient for those keen to see habitat harmed in the pursuit of profit.

## The rise of citizen scientists

Despite these enormous challenges, the work of nature-based scientists is revealing the fascinating complexity and wonder of our world. Also uplifting is the rise of citizen scientists. These are members of the general population with an interest in nature, who are willing to step up and out into the field to assist research scientists. These ordinary people contribute to surveys of native animals helping those with the degrees and PhDs build their knowledge of the biodiversity of threatened ecosystems. The work of citizen scientists has been instrumental in protecting parts of southern Australia. They have gone into areas where logging or mining is proposed and identified vulnerable species. This provides a stay of execution while legal avenues can be pursued by larger environmental organisations to request habitat protection.

One example is the Bob Brown Foundation's (BBF) Tarkine Bioblitz. This annual event sees over a hundred citizen scientists go into the remote and threatened Tarkine/takayna region of north-western Tasmania where they survey flora and fauna. With the guidance of scientists, they have tallied over 1,000 records of species. In 2017 they made a world-first discovery, finding an enormous Tasmanian freshwater crayfish. Weighing over three kilograms, this species is Earth's largest freshwater invertebrate. Although currently listed as vulnerable because of logging and mining proposed for the area, it's not too late to protect their future. Scientists say putting aside 30,000 hectares would be enough. Without the volunteering of regular people as citizen scientists we may not even have known this blue giant existed.

As the scientist on site, Todd Walsh said, "You've got the Amazon, the Nile, the Mississippi, you've got all these magnificent river systems and this little pocket of northern Tasmania holds the world's biggest invertebrate in these systems."[146]

It is fair to wonder why the discovery of this special crayfish wasn't widely celebrated, and why its habitat wasn't rapidly protected. The most likely reason is because doing so would undermine industry proposals to mine and log the area. The wilful dismissal of the Tarkine/takayna's extraordinary natural and scientific values by successive governments highlights today's simplistic economic model. This sees the worth of a place defined by what can be extracted from it – timber or minerals in most cases. Prioritising dollar values above the intrinsic wealth of such places excludes their ecological, health-giving, and spiritual richness. The cost of this ignorance to humanity is profound and the sickness encapsulated in the capitalist model is exemplified.

## THE SYSTEM IS SICK

The pervasive disconnection from nature in Western societies manifests in a general apathy and reluctance to prioritise environmental protection. This allows commercial interests to corrupt democratic processes and participate in state-sanctioned destruction of biodiversity. We see this occurring in various ways. Sometimes the damage is an intentional and integral part of industry, as in hunting, mining, and logging. In other practices, it is regarded as a necessary consequence of 'development'. Like the flattening and fragmentation of natural areas, the draining and 're-alignment' of waterways, and when the atmosphere and oceans are polluted. Over centuries, ecosystems are progressively disrupted by the introduction of pests as plants and animals are translocated from their natural habitat in the service of agriculture, trade, and leisure.

In its most vulgar form, governments have placed a bounty on the head of native animals so millions have been killed for their fur. As described earlier, the impact this had on koala populations was devastating. More definitive though, and eventuating in complete extinction, was the attack on the Tasmanian Tiger. Sustained for more than a century, the politically motivated hunting of this quiet, nocturnal marsupial was brutally successful. Such ecocidal behaviour was akin to a national sport and occurred throughout the continent from the time of first colonisation until quite recently. Queensland had a Marsupial Destruction Act to enshrine this killing in legislation until 1994. Little wonder Australia leads the world in marsupial extinctions.

The financial institutions and markets in 'developed' countries are set up to take from nature and to place a monetary price on what is extracted. The damage caused to biodiversity and ecosystems, as well as to water and climate systems is not given a dollar value. So, it is unable to be measured by the current system. There is no price placed on the health-giving benefits of forests – their *ecosystem services*. These were outlined in detail earlier and are countless. They include purifying air, drawing down carbon, creating and cleansing water, providing shelter, cooling nearby lands, and offering food, healthy long-term jobs, and cultural and spiritual richness. This myriad of life-giving benefit is calculated as having absolutely no worth in the stock market or to governments. So damage to these things incurs no cost to the company, or individual, involved. These harmful consequences are simply written off as *externalities*.

## The suffering of local communities

Communities living at the intersection of nature and commerce, like those in logging towns, are caught between a rock and a hard place. Or, perhaps, a tree and a hard place. On one hand, they can earn money from logging and destroying the forest and all its creatures. Or they can preserve it and potentially suffer financial hardship. This is the false dichotomy embodied in the current system. Imagine the benefits to local communities if forests were instead valued for their ecosystem services. We could see a flourishing of jobs in ecotourism, nature conservation and scientific discovery. Also, the arising of new, nature-based health programs like forest bathing, bush-adventure therapy, and outdoor, nature-inspired counselling. This alternative scenario's benefits would extend beyond small rural communities to the wider living world.

Of course, governments who receive royalties from mining companies for resource extraction are fiscally glued to the extractive model, so reluctant to change what has been done for several hundred years. They are unwilling to recognise the harmful effects industries like mining and the associated fossil fuel and nuclear models of power generation cause to people's wellbeing. These adverse outcomes are benignly described as *health externalities* and include illness occurring both near extractive industries and further afield. One example are lung diseases from exposure to coal dust. These may affect people working or living near the mines themselves, or along the extracted coal's transport routes.

In the medical curriculum of the 1990s, *coal miner's lung* was portrayed as a historical illness suffered by those working in underground mines long ago, when conditions were poor. Coal dust was inhaled and accumulated in lung tissue causing it to blacken and scar and reducing its ability to transfer oxygen into the body, to breathe. Sufferers of this condition became increasingly breathless, eventually suffocating when their stiffened lungs could no longer expand to take in air. There has been a resurgence of this disease in Queensland and New South Wales' underground coal mines. Especially tragic is the plight of children who live near the mines, along the rail-route taken by the open coal trains, or close to the huge piles of coal waiting to be shipped overseas. Children's lungs are especially vulnerable to the air pollution generated by coal dust. So, we see high rates of asthma and other lung conditions in families living in areas of risk. Years of denial and obfuscation by local and state governments, and the companies involved, have only added to the suffering of these people.

Similarly heart-rending is the story of communities located near coal seam gas wells. Their water supply is at risk of contamination by chemicals used in the fracking process which extracts gas from deep in the earth. Hundreds of chemicals are involved, and privacy laws protect companies from fully disclosing details to health experts. Huge volumes of these compounds contaminate the water used in fracking. This often seeps into underground aquifers which animals and people depend on. Land and air near gas wells is also polluted and oversight of the industry is scant. The effects of exposure to these chemicals vary, depending on the compounds and processes themselves, the people or animals affected, and the duration and level of exposure. Reported symptoms in some communities include rashes, lung and gut issues, fatigue, and headaches. Hospitalisations for heart, lung, neurological and cancerous problems have been reported in communities living near fracking wells. Of great concern is the observation of effects on pregnancy and newborns. Some studies have found higher rates of extreme pre-term delivery, low birth weight and certain birth defects in pregnancies spent within three kilometres of gas mining[147].

## Putting profits above child health

It is not only fossil fuel extraction which harms human health. Other mining processes such as the extraction of toxic metals, contaminate soil and air and infiltrate children's bodies. In Queensland's Mt Isa, where lead has been mined for decades, local communities have been reassured by government health departments their children were not at significant risk of lead-related problems. This reassurance was provisional and required families to take measures to minimise the amount of contaminated soil ingested. These included hand washing, wet mopping of floors and trying to grow grass in their yards. The latter being an impossible task in an arid outback area which is prone to drought, especially for the Aboriginal community.

Eventually, rigorous independent analysis of soil and water lead levels in Mt Isa was undertaken. A tenacious and dedicated team of researchers led by Professor Mark Taylor from Macquarie University found approximately 40% of children under five years of age had blood lead levels greater than six micrograms per decilitre. Their report said, "such levels have been shown to result in significant and measurable impacts on socio-behavioural patterns including attention deficit hyperactivity disorders, learning difficulties, oppositional/conduct disorders and delinquency."[148] Ingestion and inhalation of lead from poisoned soil and air has increased risks to generations of local children potentially harming their learning and development. Aboriginal children are likely to have suffered the most, and to have this as an additional hardship to poverty and nutritional disadvantage.

What is especially shocking about this case is that children's health has become an index of environmental pollution. Surely best practice is thorough, transparent, and frequent measurements of soil, air, and water near the mine site. It was only following publication of this independent research that government and industry conceded such high lead levels were not a natural phenomenon. But were instead due to mining. As the researchers said, "the magnitude of the problem is demonstrated in our study where we showed that a child every nine days is lead poisoned, which is a situation that is entirely preventable with the correct remediation program."[148] There are many more examples of mining companies being allowed to create environmental pollution without adequate governmental oversight. Local communities have been let down time and again by the dismal failure of those in power to put people's health above profits.

## Shifting to a healthier society

A society that prioritises financial gains over the wellbeing of its children is surely sick itself. To also contaminate the earth and pollute the air and water upon which all life depends is both myopic and callous. A major shift in priorities is required. The systems we currently live under, especially economic, political, and legal paradigms, spell doom for the natural world. It is time to change the entire structure and its underlying philosophy. First Nations' culture and law, having supported Australia's First Peoples to live healthy, productive lives for some 80,000 years, provides a worthy template. As Pascoe says, "It's not the difference between capitalism and communism; it's the difference between capitalism and Aboriginalism. Capitalism provides a platform for decisions among fellow capitalists but shudders under the load of persuading communities over vast areas of the country. If that weren't so we would not have reached such impasse with our management of the Murray Darling basin, we would never consider leaving a state in our Federation without drinking water, we would not have laws which allow coal seam gas miners to ruin a farmer's land and threaten the very groundwater of the continent."[140]

There is so much for us to learn from the First Australians' way of managing the whole continent for the good of all, for the present and the future. It is in our collective interest to do so, urgently. To quote Pascoe again, "the start of that journey is to allow the knowledge that Aboriginals did build houses, did cultivate and irrigate crops, did sew clothes and were not hapless wanderers across the soil, mere hunter-gatherers. Aboriginals were intervening in the productivity of the country and what they learnt during that process over many thousands of years will be useful to us today. To deny Aboriginal agricultural and spiritual achievement is the single greatest impediment to inter-cultural understanding and, perhaps, Australian moral and economic prosperity."

First Nations' philosophies are embedded in nature and can provide us with ecologically sound guiding principles. Their concepts of health and wellbeing see humankind's interdependence with all other life on Earth and the flux of air, water, and soil. Their worldview places community of people, plants, and animals over individual wants, and seeks to care for future, as well as present, generations. They have been Gaia's gardeners, while those of us caught within capitalist, colonising structures have been her gold-diggers.

So, knowing how bad things are, what can we, as individuals do? Here's a list to start you off, but if you come back to the guiding question of 'is this choice beneficial or harmful to the natural world?', you can't go too far wrong.

# WHAT YOU CAN DO

- *Find out* the history of your home, its First Nations' story

- *Foster your curiosity* to better understand the indigenous plants and animals around you, think about their needs and develop an attitude of care towards them

- *Promote biodiversity locally* – plant indigenous and natives at home; advocate for these plantings in communities; join friends groups and others to replant and restore waterways and other degraded areas

- *Write to politicians* and join with others to campaign for programs to remove pests, increase control of chemical use and pollution by industry

- *Think about environmental outcomes* when you buy things; first, try not to buy new things – reuse, reduce and repurpose first, recycle as a last resort and purchase second-hand where possible. Give your time or experiences rather than objects. The most environmentally sustainable thing is the one you choose not to buy.

- *Eat less meat* and dairy and try to source organic, locally produced food

- *Avoid single-use plastics* and chemicals like fertilisers, pesticides, fragrances and other EDCs

- *Think about how you travel*; can you walk, cycle or use public transport to reduce transport emissions; do you have to travel so far for work or holidays? If you travel, consider giving back in some way to the environment where you go. Take a reusable cup, cutlery and napkin to avoid single-use plastics on the plane or when out exploring

- *Ask* whether the anaesthetist can avoid using nitrous oxide and other potent greenhouse gases for your elective surgery

- *Give* a proportion of your salary (if you can) to organisations working to protect nature and make sure your savings or superannuation aren't fuelling environmental damage

- *Consider joining a peaceful protest* – this is a powerful way to generate change

- *Talk about the problem*, give it the time and space it deserves and vote accordingly

*If not me, then who?*
*If not now, then when?*

The first half of this book has outlined the beauty and complexity of our world and the unfolding global threats of climate change and mass extinction. Understanding the importance of biodiversity and the ecological systems humankind depends on has encouraged a deeper appreciation of the dangers we face as these foundations are challenged. Also, the individual mindsets and societal systems that have led us to this time of climate chaos and biological collapse have been investigated. The ancient wisdom of First Nations' knowledge systems and philosophies has been touched on. This puts nature at the heart of wellness and sees we humans as part of the natural world rather than separate from it.

It may feel overwhelming to comprehend the plight of Earth today, as we stand here amid the Anthropocene and its unfolding mass extinction event. However, despite the seemingly desperate situation, all is not lost. We know where to look for help, and how to begin the repair. Addressing climate change and biodiversity loss together will improve human health. Acting to solve these problems on both planetary and local levels will see wellness outcomes realised for all people. And, simultaneously, actions to prevent and treat lifestyle related diseases have beneficial outcomes for Earth. If we embrace nature-based approaches, where people connect meaningfully with other living things, the gains multiply.

Let's move now to explore the domain of health, always remembering our place within the complex web of life and the interdependence of all living things.

# PART TWO

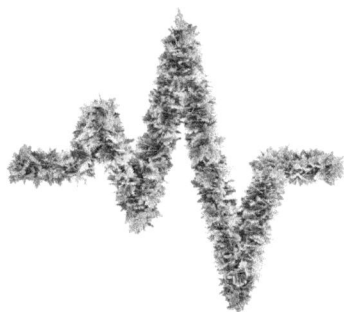

# Health & Wellbeing

Lifestyle changes over the past few decades have seen us move inside to sit down, away from other living things. At the same time, screen spaces have replaced green places in our lives and we have moved into virtual worlds. There has been an accompanying rise in illnesses like diabetes, heart disease and depression in increasingly younger people. The second section of this book will begin with an exploration of these lifestyle related health problems, particularly focussing on our youth, who are most at risk. Then we'll look at solutions, especially those found outside. For the simplest way to address these common ailments is to increase the amount of time people spend in, and with, nature.

Healthcare approaches which incorporate natural elements can be drawn together under the banner of *nature-based health interventions*. The possibilities and benefits of this new space are exciting. These approaches not only prevent and treat many common contemporary medical problems, they also foster a connection to the wider natural world which cultivates a sense of stewardship and care for Earth. This is key. Now, more than ever, our planet needs humankind to repair the damage we've done to her biosphere. Innovative, outdoor health programs see people restoring degraded ecosystems while simultaneously improving their own physical and mental health, forging new relationships and building community. Together, both people and planet heal. In becoming Gaia's gardeners, we help ourselves, our kith and our kin. And we return to an old way of being with the earth and other living things.

# 7

# Today's Health Challenges

*"When one is concerned with the mysterious and wonderful functioning of the human body, cause and effect are seldom simple and easily demonstrated relationships. They may be widely separated both in space and time. To discover the agent of disease and death depends on a patient piecing together of many seemingly distinct and unrelated facts developed through a vast amount of research in widely separated fields."*

~Rachel Carson

## LIVING INSIDE

Today, most of us live in cities, increasingly distant from the wider natural world. Despite the popular image of an outdoor lifestyle, Australia is one of the most urbanised countries on the planet. We tend to live in large houses with small backyards or apartments with very little outdoor green space. Most of us drive to work, going from inside our home to the interior of a car and then into the office. Even children are living this life, moving from one box to another, with less than 15% walking to school today compared to 55% in 1970[149]. We have essentially moved inside and sat in front of a computer. This has been especially so over the past few years as the COVID-19 pandemic has spread throughout the world. While staying home and working online has kept many of us safe from the deadly virus, this retreat into the virtual world has a cost. Many have become more sedentary and isolated than ever before.

Also, our working days have become longer and the line between work and home blurred. Being constantly accessible via email or social media sees the attrition of time free to spend in the 'real' world, with family, friends, or other living things. For many, even leisure time is spent inside with visits to multiplex shopping centres to watch movies and shop being preferred weekend activities. Those who are keen to keep fit will often drive to the gym to run on a treadmill while watching sitcoms on the attached screen. Children are ferried to parties at indoor play-centres to play laser force shooting games, drive go-karts or dress up as fairies. Of course, many are involved in organised sport on the weekend and this can be an outdoor activity. But it wouldn't really rate as nature time. Football, netball, or soccer are highly structured, goal orientated, adult supervised activities. Children seen gazing up at clouds or watching birds are generally not highly valued team members.

Weekdays are highly scheduled for most young people too. For many, the school day has lengthened, as before and after school care is tacked onto either end of the day. And they are often involved in an array of afterschool activities to 'enrich' their lives. The Australian Heart Foundation's Sitting Less for Children information sheet maps out the time today's young people spend sitting, often also looking at a screen[150]. It outlines the daily schedule for many children from breakfast in front of the television/ipad (or checking out social media for teenagers), sitting in the back of the car on the way to and from school, sitting in class (more screens here), afterschool study, computer games, or social media time. The cumulative total is a sobering seven hours a day of sitting for the average child. For those who experienced prolonged lockdowns with the pandemic and months of online learning, the tally may be even higher. This is far beyond the maximal amount of screen time advised by paediatricians. Given the emerging research on brain plasticity, the preponderance of sitting and computer-based activities in childhood clearly requires a rethink.

Neuroplasticity is the way our brain changes in response to the activities we engage in, both physically and mentally. Our brain is in a constant state of flux, reconfiguring itself from thought to thought, and action to action. If our children are spending a large part of their day sitting, to learn and socialise virtually, their brain's structure and activity will adjust accordingly. Changes in brain function and development ultimately manifest in new patterns of thoughts, emotions and behaviours[151]. We will dive more deeply into how our mind responds to natural environments later in this section. For now, let's look at some of the health problems that have arisen as we've moved to a more sedentary, indoor lifestyle. Taking a wide view to include environmental factors reveals how insidious exposure to pollution also plays a part.

## CONTEMPORARY ILLNESS

An extraordinary phenomenon over the past thirty years has been the rise of lifestyle related, or *non-communicable diseases* (NCDs). These include illnesses related to inactivity and excess weight, like diabetes, heart disease, mental health conditions and some cancers. The complex nature of these problems sees them often arise together. So, people who have a social situation and lifestyle which increases their risk of diabetes will also be set to have a heart attack, stroke, or kidney failure. The development of one of these conditions sets in motion a cascade of other changes in our bodies. This is much like tipping points that occur in other complex living systems. Once we have diabetes, our blood vessels are more likely to accumulate fatty deposits, reducing blood flow to important organs like our brain, liver, kidneys, and heart. In turn, this diminished circulation triggers a change in local chemical messengers. In our kidneys, this impairs blood purification and stimulates the production of certain compounds which increase blood pressure. In turn, elevated blood pressure places a strain on the heart as it must now pump against higher resistance. So diabetes, heart and kidney disease often develop together.

## Obesity – a marker of modern life

The tendency to accumulate increased body fat and to become overweight, or obese is a defining feature of modern Western societies. By disrupting the workings of key organs and upsetting hormonal balance, obesity is a major problem with many causes. Related foundations include a poor diet, reduced activity from increased screen time and exposure to environmental toxins. As touched on earlier, ingestion of endocrine-disruptor chemicals (EDCs), as found in plastics and industrial chemicals, is thought to predispose to obesity. Children born at low birth weights are also at higher risk of becoming overweight in later life. This is because their metabolism is primed to maximally take up calories. Those born in places with poor air quality from the burning of fossil fuels often fall into this category. Recalling the role of our gut's microbiome and its requirement for interaction with healthy microbes in soil sees the lack of green spaces in cities as a piece of the puzzle too.

The walkability of neighbourhoods is higher with more green space for recreation. Whereas obesogenic environments, with their lack of footpaths and cycleways, make active choices like bike riding, walking and public transport harder. Taking this broader view of obesity sees many intersecting environmental factors at play. Obesity is not simply the result of an individual's poor decisions. More exactly, it is a manifestation of modern societies' disruption of natural systems through an industrialised food supply, pollution, and urbanisation. And of our collective retreat from the wider natural world.

Like other Westernised nations, Australia's rates of overweight and obesity are growing all the time. We currently have some 60% of adults and 25% of children in these categories. Rather than a superficial, cosmetic concern, being overweight is extremely dangerous for our health. Not only does fat accumulate under our skin, it also builds up around internal organs and impairs their function. Fat accumulating inside the liver may eventually lead to changes in its architecture and the development of *fatty liver disease*. The liver purifies our blood, regulates circulating sugar levels and makes important proteins like clotting factors and hormones. It also manufactures bile, a special fluid which aids fat digestion. Damage to this vital organ has flow-on effects to the rest of our body.

Obesity may lead to the development of type 2 diabetes where regulation of blood sugar (glucose) levels is impaired. In a healthy body, the pancreas makes insulin, a hormone which stimulates cells to draw glucose from the bloodstream. When high blood glucose levels are sustained, cells become resistant to insulin, causing damage throughout the body. In the early stages, type 2 diabetes may respond to lifestyle interventions like a healthy diet and increased physical activity. But when more advanced, medication may be needed, perhaps even injections of insulin.

Also, obesity may affect seemingly unrelated body systems, like the lungs. In obstructive sleep apnoea an accumulation of fat narrows upper airways and impairs muscle function causing a temporary block to airflow. And breathing pauses or *apnoeic* episodes result. During these periods, blood oxygen levels drop and we rouse. When this occurs multiple times throughout the night normal sleep cycles are disrupted. The result is extreme fatigue and sometimes dangerous daytime sleepiness. Asthma is also more common in people who are overweight and in the children of overweight mothers, although the reasons for this remain unclear. Possible contributory factors to obese asthma include vitamin D deficiency, a poor microbiome, and diets low in fibre but high in dairy, sugar, and saturated fat.

Childhood obesity and related conditions are more common in the disadvantaged, with 33% affected compared to 19% for those more privileged. The suburbs these groups live in are said to be *obesogenic* because of their poor urban design. A preponderance of roads and paucity of footpaths and green space leaves residents overly reliant on cars with few active transport options. Without safely accessible footpaths and bike lanes few will walk or cycle, so people living in these poorer areas are exposed to high levels of air pollution from traffic. With fewer street trees and parkland there are less plants to draw pollutants out of the atmosphere to improve air quality. Also, limited access to fresh food markets and community gardens sees these communities consuming a less healthy diet. They are restricted to supermarkets and shopping malls where increased availability and marketing encourages the consumption of highly processed junk foods[152].

Children who are overweight are likely to grow into adults with obesity because most retain their excess body fat. This is a terrible burden to take into adolescence and young adult life. Not only does obesity increase the risk of NCDs developing, those afflicted are more likely to experience bullying, poor peer relationships and struggle with school[152]. Unsurprisingly, these difficulties may result in depression or anxiety, which make it harder still to eat well or move more.

Excess body fat may also harm future generations as it interferes with fertility by disrupting hormonal regulation. For overweight women, the challenges are not restricted to difficulties conceiving. Once pregnant, they are more likely to have a baby with an abnormality, a stillbirth or to develop diabetes. The birth itself is also riskier and more likely to require surgical intervention or be complicated by bleeding. Also, increased body fat manufactures the hormone oestrogen. Elevated levels of this are risk factors for breast and uterine cancer. They may also contribute to the increasing rate of prostate cancer we are seeing in men[153]. Once again, environmental pollutants, the endocrine-disruptor chemicals, may have a role to play.

It is simplistic to regard obesity as the consequence of irresponsible individual choices. Rather, this condition, and the constellation of diseases accompanying it, marks the failure of our society to take public health seriously. Comprehensively understanding people's need for healthy, fresh food, embedded daily physical activity and rich natural environments sees today's suburbs as a recipe for NCDs like obesity. Adopting the precautionary principle to reduce the pollution of air, water, and soils by eliminating the use of fossil fuels, pesticides and other endocrine-disruptor chemicals is an important public health action too. It is simply not possible to address human health problems without simultaneously repairing the damaged natural world. This principle is highlighted by contemplating the early stages of human development.

# THE FIRST ONE THOUSAND DAYS

Doctors and scientists are now learning that the first one thousand days of life are crucial in determining the risk of NCDs developing decades later, in adulthood. This critical time begins from conception, through a baby's growth in their mother's uterus, all the way through to about two years of age. How healthy a mother's environment and lifestyle is affects her child's risk of developing various conditions much later in life. These include obesity, diabetes, lung disease and behavioural problems. The father's health around the time of conception is also important.

Researchers have found low dietary levels of folate in men can impair gene expression in their sperm and predispose to autism in their children[154]. Folate is a vitamin found in green leafy vegetables and is now also added to bread flour in Australia[155]. So it is important to include at least five serves of fresh vegetables and two serves of fruit daily. Apart from folate, these foods are rich in antioxidants, other vitamins, minerals, and fibre. And organically grown vegetables also provide healthy microbes.

Dietary and environmental factors are important in the first one thousand days of life because they influence which of our genes are switched on via a process called *epigenetic change*. The new scientific field of epigenetics is expanding our understanding of which genes are expressed, and when and how, this takes place. Factors influencing epigenetic expression include our diet and general body condition and the health of our environment. Inhaling pollution from car exhaust, gas appliances or coal power plants when pregnant will influence how genes are expressed. This effects not just our own health, but that of our future children and grandchildren. Our grandchildren may be affected too, because the developing baby a pregnant woman is carrying contains the eggs which will, in turn, become her offspring.

Scientific understanding in this area is still in its early stages but it is reasonable to conclude that in addition to what we eat and how active we are, *where* we spend most of our time is important. Given we are now mostly inside sitting down our lifestyle is constrained and contained. Cutting off exposure to the world outside has coincided with the inextricable rise in NCDs. Despite major advances in modern healthcare, many people are chronically sick and unhappy.

## A WHOLISTIC APPROACH

The good news is that acting to reduce risk factors for one NCD, like obesity, will also help prevent others. And it's empowering to know we can stop the potential avalanche of health problems by simple lifestyle interventions early on. This thinking underpins preventative health strategies which might include encouraging people to be more physically active or to increase their fruit and vegetable intake. Many doctors also believe it should include helping them to move outside, into their nearest green space. By spending more time in a natural environment people are more likely to be physically active, have lower body weight, better fitness and improved heart health. The positives encompass how they feel emotionally too, with time spent in nature reducing feelings of stress and lifting mood.

In family practice we are privileged to look after people throughout their lifespan. Care begins before conception as pre-pregnancy counselling is provided to parents to optimise the very first days of their child's life. And it extends all the way through life's ups and downs, to the final breath. Family doctors are well placed to see health issues arising in childhood, manifesting in adulthood and possibly leading to an early death. It is gratifying to witness how supporting people to adopt healthy lifestyle behaviours leads to positive change and an avoidance of later illness. Helping a parent understand the value of healthy eating or spending time outside sees wellbeing benefits flow through to the entire family. In this way, the local clinic, with its doctors, nurses, and other health professionals, can have wide-reaching benefits in a community.

Doctors who take a big picture view of health see beyond lifestyle and social influences and incorporate environmental factors into their understanding. This means knowing that reducing exposure to industrial chemicals, plastics and fossil fuel pollution is a key part of combating NCDs. So too, is making it simple and easy for all people to spend more of their day outside, in nature-rich places. This involves advocating for improved urban design to increase the number of biodiverse, green spaces and to make active transport an accessible and attractive option.

We are now so used to living a contained, indoor lifestyle it can be difficult to grasp how essential it is for us to spend time in natural places. So, let's explore more deeply the various elements which make life outside, with other living things, so important for our wellbeing.

---

## KEY POINTS

- ❤ People living in Western societies spend most of their time inside, sitting down

- ❤ Screen spaces have replaced green places in our lives

- ❤ *Non-communicable* diseases are a modern phenomenon relating to inactivity and excess weight. ie. obesity, diabetes, heart disease and depression

- ❤ Obesity has multiple causes, including environmental factors like poorly designed, car dominated cities with little green space and pervasive exposure to pollution

- ❤ The first 1000 days of human life are crucial in determining risk of NCDs in adulthood

- ❤ *Epigenetic change* describes the process that determines which genes are expressed

- ❤ Dietary and environmental factors effect this gene expression

- ❤ Actions to reduce risk factors for one NCD, like obesity, helps prevent others

---

# 8

# Nature-based Solutions

*"I go to nature to be soothed and healed,*
*and to have my senses put in order."*

~John Burroughs

Stepping outside into a park or garden our orientation shifts subtly. We become aware of the day's temperature, brightness and soundscape. Inhaling fresh air encourages slightly deeper breaths and we may notice the scent of nearby flowers. We tend to look up and out towards the horizon, taking in our surroundings. It's often quite simply a relief to escape the confines of our mostly indoor life. Thanks to science we are now able to break down the beneficial elements to examine them more precisely, to understand better how nature sustains us and how we suffer when kept inside. Let's begin with the blazing star which determines the rhythms of our days, the sun.

# SUNLIGHT

Humans have a fundamental need to spend time in the sun. Most of our body's vitamin D is manufactured within the skin following exposure to sunlight. Only a small amount comes from dietary sources. Vitamin D acts like a hormone, working throughout the body to maintain good health. It is especially important for cell growth, bone development and strength, and for our immune, nervous, and muscular systems. Given our heart is a muscular pump, vitamin D's role includes maintaining the integrity of our entire circulation. Just as plants wilt without adequate natural light, human beings suffer when they are kept from the sun. Today, with our indoor lifestyle, it's unsurprising that one third of Victorians are vitamin D deficient[156]. This manifests in different ways, depending on age, and can cause significant suffering.

Vitamin D deficiency in children may result in a condition called rickets which, although rare, is on the rise in southern Australian cities like Melbourne. Rickets is more common in children with dark skin or those born to vitamin D deficient mothers[157]. Rickets causes developing bones to become weak, soft, and misshapen. Bony swelling results in painful deformity of the wrists, knees, and ankles. These children have delayed development because they are slower to walk and crawl than their peers. Beginning life with rickets is fraught with discomfort and frustration and requires early treatment to avoid permanent damage.

In adults, severe vitamin D deficiency may lead to osteomalacia where, like rickets, the bones are soft, and both bone and muscle aching occurs. If deficiency is more moderate, but protracted, osteoporosis may result. This condition sees bones become weak and brittle, and easily broken. Osteoporosis is a common condition, with many elderly people having the characteristic hunched posture from vertebral crush fractures in their upper back. While this is very uncomfortable, the most worrying complications of osteoporosis are hip fractures. These are often disastrous and culminate in death.

Vitamin D deficiency has also been implicated in the development of diabetes, depression, bowel cancer and heart and autoimmune diseases. It seems every system of the body requires this vitamin for optimal functioning, even tooth development. Given all this, ensuring we receive sufficient time in the sun is essential for wellbeing.

Paradoxically, while we have high rates of vitamin D deficiency in southern Australia, we also see large numbers of skin cancers. This most likely relates to how we spend time in the sun. Those who are seldom outside but then experience peeling sunburn on their annual holiday are especially at risk. So too, are those who spend prolonged time outdoors with minimal protection from high levels of ultraviolet (UV) light.

We need to be smart about sun exposure to ensure we don't overdo it while getting healthy doses of vitamin D. The risks of insufficient sunlight, as well as the risks of too much, need to be weighed together. Given sunscreen impairs our skin's ability to make vitamin D, it is reasonable to spend some time outside without applying sunscreen, providing the UV index is low. In Australia, the Cancer Council has a handy phone app to advise on how much sun time is safe on any given day. The data generated is location and skin-type specific, so provides an excellent, accessible guide[158]. Simple solutions like this help people make informed choices to get their sun-balance right.

## LOOKING INTO THE DISTANCE

A rise in certain visual problems has accompanied our move indoors and shift to screen-based work and recreation. When outside, we tend to adjust our gaze often, looking far into the distance and then back in closer. We are frequently changing our focus, exercising and strengthening our eye muscles. This eye movement also stimulates the visual cortex area of the brain, which processes what we see. Comparatively, looking at a computer screen or hand-held device sees our eyes focusing at a fixed distance for extended periods of time. This makes our eyes lazy, and the muscles lose tone. Much like sitting in a chair for hours at a time weakens our core and lower back.

This lack of focussing variation and eye exercise has accompanied our societal move inside to sit down and embrace technology. An increase in rates of myopia (short sightedness), is the unfortunate result[159]. This is especially so in young people. Also, staring at a screen for lengthy periods sees our eyelids blink less often. Consequently, reduced lubrication from tears causes eyes to dry out, feel gritty and sore, and be more prone to irritation. The combination of eye strain and inflammation may lead to tension headaches and difficulty concentrating.

Scheduling breaks throughout the day to step away from the screen and get outside can help ameliorate eye problems. Simply gazing at the horizon, or up into a tree's canopy, will provide necessary rest and respite from the demands of computer work. Even if unable to get outdoors, consciously looking out a window and into the distance at regular intervals will help eye health.

## EXERCISE OUTDOORS

While we can exercise inside, the benefits are greater out in a natural environment. There are a variety of reasons for this, but let's begin by considering air quality. As plants remove pollution and replenish oxygen levels, the atmosphere in a park or garden is optimal. Gyms or indoor stadiums are often poorly ventilated, and their air contaminated by various volatile chemicals. These are released from carpets, paint, and other indoor surfaces. Swapping to outdoor activities or classes reduces such exposure. So too, does switching to active transport options, like walking or cycling. The COVID-19 pandemic has highlighted the importance of ventilation and indoor air quality. Being largely airborne, the novel coronavirus is transmitted optimally where people gather inside in poorly ventilated spaces. So, avoiding exposure to this kind of disease is another benefit of choosing outdoor options for exercise, socialising or transport.

Stepping out of the car is especially good for children. As discussed earlier, because of their unique physiology, kids are particularly vulnerable to industrial toxins. And while many regard the back seat of a car to be a safe place for children, the air quality here is often poor. Small amounts of exhaust can enter the main body of the vehicle and combine with chemicals from synthetic interior surfaces to pollute the air. Ditching the car for active transport removes this risk and is especially beneficial if our route is through a natural space where we may encounter healthy, air-borne microbes.

Improving neighbourhood greenness makes walking or cycling for routine trips a more appealing option than driving. It also provides safe spaces for socialising and participating in outdoor exercise, either solo or with others. In this way, clever urban planning can address public health and social problems like obesity, inactivity, and loneliness. These steps also improve urban air quality by taking cars off the road and boosting the power of nature's air purifiers – trees, and other plants. Thereby better health outcomes companion greener suburbs and communities which are more pleasant to live in.

Outdoor exercise may involve a variety of activities from structured training sessions in a park through to simply tending plants in your own back yard. Gardening involves moving the whole body in a variety of ways and is good for strengthening bones and muscles and maintaining flexibility. It may be done at any age by anyone who has access to a garden. When done with others, gardening provides a means of social interaction and relationship building. This may occur in a school or community garden, or in residential settings like a retirement homes or prisons. Apart from fortifying the physical body, there are rich psychological benefits, which will be covered in more detail later.

Importantly, contact with the soil through gardening and other outdoor recreation may increase exposure to beneficial microscopic bacteria and other organisms. As discussed earlier, the complex interplay between our body's own microbiome, our inner garden, and that of the natural world around us, is becoming the new frontier of medical research. From this work, scientists are finding that regular contact with nature is essential for wellbeing as it supports the health of our microbiome.

When we are outside walking, running or simply enjoying the garden, we are more likely to encounter uneven surfaces. This stimulates our proprioceptive senses helping us gain better balance and stability. Proprioception is the awareness of our body's positioning, so strengthening this system helps us move safely. Improvements in balance prevent falls, which is particularly important as we age. One of the great things about being outside is that it encourages all our senses to work together in an integrated way.

Sometimes, it is difficult to tease out which is the most important element of outdoor exercise for wellbeing, especially for our emotional or mental health. Is it the physical activity, the clean air, the psychological relaxation from hearing melodic sounds and seeing beautiful sights, or the pleasant smells from plants and flowers? From a scientific perspective, it is almost impossible to analyse one aspect in isolation, which is why doctors have been slow to prescribe outdoor exercise as a health intervention.

As described earlier, doctors tend to look for randomized, double-blind, placebo-controlled trials (RCTs) when choosing a medication or intervention. These are the best scientific study, or *gold standard.* Here, the environment is so well controlled that only one or two very specific elements are assessed at a time. These experiments can be done quite readily in a laboratory but not so easily outside with the many variables found in nature. For example, the most well-known studies relating to exercise for psychological ailments look at group exercise sessions for people suffering from depression. This research revealed that such an exercise program, done three times a week, is as effective for moderate depression as medication. Most studies have been done in a gym environment rather than outside because this readily suits a reductive scientific approach[160].

This information is extremely useful for those of us seeing patients with depression as it supports exercise prescriptions as a treatment modality. However, it is not always accessible or affordable to attend a gym. Regular exercise outside in nature is likely to work as a preventative health measure by warding off mental illness before it develops. It could also form an affordable and effective therapeutic option, not only for depression but for physical problems too. For many, the cost of attending a gym for supervised sessions is prohibitive whereas a walk in the nearby park with a friend is easy and free.

# FOREST BATHING

When we are in nature, subtle shifts in our body's physiology occur. Stress hormones drop, as does our blood pressure. Even cellular activity alters, enhancing key elements of our immune system. Registering these changes, our body relaxes, and we feel less worried. Decades of research in Japan have measured these factors as scientists have taken people into forests and monitored their physical and psychological indices. Their findings have informed a drug-free health intervention called shinrin-yoku, or forest bathing.

Shinrin-yoku involves spending scheduled amounts of time in a forest environment as part of a health plan. It was first proposed in 1982 by the Forest Agency of Japan. It was initially thought being in a forest would provide a time and place for relaxation and inhalation of the woods' essential oils. Subsequent research has explored this idea further measuring chemical markers of stress and inflammation, blood pressure and heart rate, and mood. Early studies focussed on cardiovascular changes, especially blood pressure. However, recent analysis of decades of international data concluded forest bathing effected many cardiovascular parameters. Not only was blood pressure lowered, but heart rate also slowed, and heart rate variability (HRV) increased. HRV measures the heart's capacity to adjust to changing demands and correlates with overall vascular health. People with higher HRV tend to live longer with less illness. Spending time in a forest enhanced heart health with longer, more frequent visits having greater benefits.

Leading Japanese researcher, Dr Qing Li, studies the effect of shinrin-yoku on immune function and stress. He thinks the inhalation of minute particles released by trees is a key factor responsible for approximately half of forest bathing's benefits. Called *phytoncides*, these agents are a type of essential oil which protect trees from insects and decay. Japanese cypress, cedar, beech, and oak trees have all been shown to raise natural killer cell activity. They also all release phytoncides. Natural killer (NK) cells are a white blood cell which fights infection and prevents the development and progression of cancer. In one study, changes in immune function and levels of the stress hormone adrenalin were measured in participants of a three day, two-night forest trip[161]. This prolonged nature time increased NK cell activity and lowered blood adrenalin concentrations. The control group experienced none of these cellular and hormonal changes. They visited a city rather than a forest, while engaging in the same amount of physical exercise. Importantly, this research finding has been replicated by other studies showing maximal health benefit requires several days of forest bathing.

Much research has focussed on shinrin-yoku's effect on psychological wellbeing. Methods involved the use of questionnaires to assess stress levels and mood, and measurements of flight or fight hormones like adrenaline and cortisol, in the blood or saliva. Most studies found both physical and psychological stress marker levels fell, and vigour improved, following forest therapy sessions[162]. This nature-based intervention optimises health by simultaneously revitalising cellular activity, hormonal balance, and emotional state.

In Japan, forest bathing is now standard practice and certain forests are accredited as being a Forest Therapy Base or Forest Therapy Road. Criteria includes having certain tree species over more than a half hectare area with at least 10% tree canopy cover. There are sixty-two such places in Japan, with each having its own unique healing feature. Perhaps a particular variety of tree, a pristine stream, or tropical breeze. Some Forest Therapy Bases have doctors guiding participants mindfully through the forest, helping them slow down and connect with nature through all their senses. Health cabins provide stops where blood pressure and other indices may be checked[163].

When forest bathing, Dr Li says it's important to engage all senses and to refrain from heavy physical exercise[164]. Instead of rushing along a trail, as many in the West are prone to do, shinrin-yoku encourages slowing down. Participants may spend either a full day of four hours, or half a day of two hours, walking amongst the trees. Distances covered are low, just five kilometres for a full day, and the emphasis is on noticing the sights, smells and sounds of the woods. Gentle exercise, like Tai Chi, is considered appropriate, and it is also fine to simply sit and rest awhile.

Deep breathing facilitates inhalation of the phytoncide-rich forest air.

Li recommends a three-day, two-night trip to gain full immune benefits of increased natural killer cell activity. He has found the enhanced wellbeing from a full day of shinrin-yoku may last a month and surmises a daily walk in heavily canopied urban parkland would also be therapeutic. It is a simple practice to incorporate into daily life but requires a shift in approach to both activity and perspective. Rather than charging along a walking path through a forest, working up a sweat, the challenge is to slow down and pay attention to the plant and animal life around you. To notice the sights and sounds of nature instead of being distracted by the audio channelled through your ear buds. To soak it all in, to sensorily *bathe* in the forest.

The practice of shinrin-yoku has inspired similar programs in the West, with Forest Therapy guides and associations popping up in northern America, the United Kingdom and Australia. In the Japanese model, shinrin-yoku is embedded within the health system with strong connections to forest management and protection. However, in these other places, forest bathing generally sits apart from routine medical practice. Unfortunately, this means it is less accepted as a valid health intervention and regarded as 'alternative'. Thankfully, as the scientific legitimacy of shinrin-yoku becomes more widely known, perceptions are shifting. Many can see the health and environmental benefits of protecting forests for their therapeutic value and are calling for similar schemes. Optimists see a day when old-growth and other native forests are regarded as precious health resources. Where people go to restore their emotional balance and boost their immune function with guidance and encouragement from doctors and other health professionals.

## Dr Qing Li's tips for shinrin-yoku

- *Turn your phone/device off or leave it behind altogether*
- *Walk slowly and don't get tired, gentle exercise like Tai Chi is fine*
- *Focus on breathing in deeply, inhaling the air of the forest*
- *Pay attention to the sounds, sights and sensations you experience*
- *A full day would mean spending about four hours in the forest, walking about five kilometres, halve this for half a day*
- *You can rest or drink water or tea at any time*
- *Find a place to sit for a while to delight in the scenery or enjoy a snack*
- *To boost immunity via increasing natural killer cell activity a three-day and two-night trip is recommended*
- *The benefits from a full day forest bathing trip may last up to a month*
- *Walking every day in an urban parkland with lots of trees is also likely to be helpful if it's done slowly and mindfully*

## PRESCRIBING A TRIP TO THE PARK

While forest bathing is not yet a widely known health intervention outside Japan, other nature-based programs are gaining traction. The time-poor mindset of Western health systems has led to an emphasis on nature prescriptions. Through these, people are encouraged to spend time in nearby nature, rather than allocate half a day to 'bathe' in a forest. Unfortunately, as yet, there are no forests protected for their therapeutic properties with embedded health care practitioners in countries like Australia.

Nature prescriptions take various forms depending on the condition being addressed and the treating physician. In the United States, cardiologists are prescribing 'green exercise', like regular walks in nature reserves. Santa Fe's Prescription Trails program works to tackle diabetes with doctors giving their patients trail guides to encourage them out into parks[165]. The regular outdoor exercise improves blood sugar levels and heart health. Similarly, in Washington DC, the 'DC Park Prescription' program supports disadvantaged children to venture to nearby natural areas. Being at high risk of obesity and inactivity, they are especially vulnerable to lifestyle-related diseases from an early age.

Led by paediatrician Dr Robert Zarr, a team of researchers identified and rated all 342 parks in the city and linked this information to prescribing software. This enabled physicians to provide their patient's parents with their nearest park's location and accessibility. An accompanying prescription outlined visit frequency and suggested activities. This simple intervention resulted in more active children and families prioritising regular time outside together. Importantly, the prescribing tool was embraced by the busy doctors, who generally see some twenty patients per day[166].

Robert Zarr has recently been to Australia and shared his findings. Early adopters have been trialling his approach here, finding patients of all ages keen to embrace a non-pharmacological method. Understanding how time in nature reduces stress, improves mood, and benefits physical health is motivating for patient and doctor alike. So together, they choose the location, duration, and frequency of the nature experience to be prescribed. Through this shared decision making, a prescription is generated. Nature scripts may be printed, in the traditional manner, or sent electronically. Patients may also opt for a reminder prompt to help them stay motivated and on track[167].

To amplify this point, let's generate a prescription for someone who is inactive and overweight, so at risk of developing heart disease and diabetes. Or someone who is feeling stressed and sleeping poorly, perhaps struggling with sadness or anxiety.

We'll call this imaginary patient Alex. After identifying a nature prescription as an appropriate component of Alex's care, their doctor explains the benefits and process. Following this discussion, Alex suggests a nearby park as a place they enjoy visiting with their dog. The physician encourages leaving the phone at home to maximise Alex's engagement with nature – listening to bird sounds, delighting in the dog's antics, and noticing tree canopies and clouds. They also help structure the duration and frequency of the activity in a schedule which Alex feels is achievable. Alex opts to have the prescription printed so they can put it on their fridge as a daily reminder. A follow up appointment is scheduled in two weeks to check on Alex's progress and adjust the prescription as appropriate.

## ALEX'S NATURE PRESCRIPTION

PATIENT: Alex

LOCATION: nearby park

TAKE: activity - walk the dog without phone

FREQUENCY: every day

DURATION: 30 minutes

This method is a good first step, something motivated doctors are already adopting. However, the optimal outcome is for nature prescribing to become an integral approach, embedded within currently used medical software. Then, when it is time-equivalent to prescribe nature or a medication, nature prescriptions will be given regularly. This is currently the case for exercise prescriptions, which are focussed on physical activity. Interestingly, while movement alone can improve mental health, simply being nature, whether physically active or not, has huge emotional benefits.

Alex's nature prescription could just as easily have had them sitting under a large tree in the backyard without their phone, noticing nature.

The benefits for psychological rejuvenation would be equal to the walk, perhaps even greater. This is especially good news for those with physical limitations. How nature restores us mentally and emotionally was only briefly touched on in the discussion of forest bathing. This topic is important, so an entire section has been devoted to it, in Green Mind.

Nature prescribing varies depending on the level of encouragement and support people need. While some respond to a gentle reminder, others require a more structured approach. It's a matter of tailoring advice to the individual and having a range of options on offer. For many, a straightforward nature prescription will suffice. Others benefit from a single group session, perhaps a guided walk or forest bathing. Still others require a program organised over several months led by a skilled provider. The essential elements are flexibility, accessibility, and affordability.

Slowly, we are seeing a shift away from the quick consultation, rapid-fire medication prescribing by doctors. Instead, practitioners are moving towards a model where lifestyle behaviour change forms the keystone of care. This is certainly the case for diabetes management, where patients are linked to dieticians, exercise physiologists and diabetes educators at the time of diagnosis. We just need to broaden the scope a little, to incorporate nature-based health practitioners and programs.

There is certainly no need to reinvent the wheel as the evidence base for such work already exists. Various programs have been developed, shown their validity but then petered out as funding has dried up. One example is the Victorian Active in Parks (AIP) program from 2011. This collaboration between parks organisations, a community health clinic and private insurer generated a variety of health initiatives. Underpinned by sound public health policy, AIP saw parks as the setting for landscape health interventions. In the Bush Playgroup Program, young mothers struggling with poverty and single parenthood, were involved in regular nature play sessions with their children. Here, parents received general advice from early childhood professionals while enjoying time out in beautiful settings. Seeing firsthand how engaged children are by nature, new mothers learnt easy nature play activities for home. They also established new friendships and local connections. This simple program helped child development and socialisation while reducing parental isolation. This buffers against the loneliness and post-natal depression such women are vulnerable to.

Another initiative arising from Active in Parks was Green Referrals. This program saw those at risk of lifestyle related diseases referred to weekly supervised outdoor exercise sessions. Again, positive outcomes extended beyond the physical as emotional and social measures improved too[168]. Unfortunately, as funding diminished, Active in Parks evolved into an online platform rather than a driver of collaboration and program provider.

AIP demonstrated how a diversity of nature-based health interventions could address a suite of public health problems. Governments and community leaders can draw on these examples to devise preventative health pathways. This will help keep people away from expensive resources like medicines, tests and hospitals. With this approach, natural areas become places of healing, integral to our healthcare system. As such they are valued, protected and nurtured.

While nature prescribing and related programs see healthcare moving outside, there is a counter-current occurring too. A blurring between inside and out sees plants and animals embedded within hospitals and clinics. Whether through imagery, sounds, or indoor gardens, the therapeutic properties of nature are being utilised innovatively. Let's move on to explore how modern healthcare is embracing this philosophy.

## BRINGING NATURE IN

Most people prefer to looking onto a beautiful scene rather than a roadway or building. And a space flooded with natural light lifts our spirits much more than an internal room, no matter how large it may be. To work without seeing a glimpse of sky is deflating and constricting. This instinct for contact with the outside world is something we all share. It is reflected in both the price of real estate, and the coveted window office. Apart from aesthetics, there are great health benefits from having a natural view, or by bringing nature inside.

Researchers have shown that people recover more quickly from stressful events, like surgery, when they can see nature. One seminal study found patients with a park view recovered faster, required less medication and were discharged from hospital sooner, than those with an urban scene[169]. This has implications for medicine and the design of health centres and hospitals. Many now incorporate plants and gardens into their planning, aiming for natural light in most rooms[170]. Nature is most deeply embedded in hospitals who care for children, cancer sufferers or those requiring extended stays.

The new Royal Children's Hospital in Melbourne was built so inpatients look onto nearby parkland and enjoy a large inner garden. Likewise, the Victorian Comprehensive Cancer Centre has multiple gardens. Cancer sufferers, visitors and staff enjoy the tranquillity and relaxation offered by nearby nature. In these spaces, sunlight, fresh air, and plants provide a multi-sensory escape from the medical environment. At the Royal Talbot Rehabilitation Centre in Melbourne, nurse and horticultural therapist Steven Wells has developed gardens to provide respite, healing, and recovery. They are encountered by all who access the ward, providing a calming entrance point for relatives and staff. Most patients have severe brain or spinal injuries and are in hospital for many months. The garden gives them a vital connection to the outside world and to the plants and animals it holds.

As well as being places for quiet enjoyment, hospital gardens provide opportunities for specially designed rehabilitation programs. At the Royal Talbot, Steven runs both group and individual *horticultural therapy* sessions. Here, patients tend to plants and gardens in a purposeful and supported way. They strengthen muscles and improve co-ordination and balance while engaging in a variety of activities. Being outside in natural light, they receive healthy doses of vitamin D. Opportunities to look long distances, towards the horizon or up into treetops, are interspersed with closer, focussed tasks. This exercises the eyes, head, and neck spontaneously and functionally. Alongside physical benefits, horticultural therapy has huge psychological and social rewards. It enables patients to be a 'carer of gardens' rather than 'in care'. This is empowering for those who often feel helpless because of their illness.

While this approach is fairly new for Australia, in Europe and the United Kingdom, horticultural therapies are an important part of hospital care. The benefits are also being seen in a diverse range of residential settings, including aged care facilities, drug rehabilitation centres and prisons. In these places, gardening and nature-based activity provide opportunities for residents to be creative and grow self-confidence. Interpersonal skills strengthen through group projects and new friendships are forged. The development of these 'soft skills' is an essential part of rehabilitation and re-integration into wider society. Also, as many living in care experience mental health issues and these are soothed through contact with nature, such gardening programs are enormously beneficial. How simply being in contact with nature helps lift mood and reduce stress and anxiety will be explored further in Green Mind.

Designing hospitals and medical clinics with gardens and views of nature is best practice. However, simply bringing very small amounts of nature into a clinical setting, with the use of pot plants or fish tanks, is also beneficial. Scientists call this *indoor nature exposure*[171]. American researcher Virginia Lohr studies the interaction between people and plants. In one experiment, she found children immunised in a room with an indoor plant as a distraction rather than a colourful picture, cried less after their needle. Lohr surmised the plant's presence had a pain-reducing effect[172]. While more studies are needed to validate these findings, simply having a plant in the immunisation room could make necessary but painful experiences a little bit gentler. Also, recognising that just going to the doctors is an emotionally uncomfortable task for many adds to the case for indoor plants. Even if they reduce psychological distress by a fraction, it's worthwhile including them in waiting areas and other clinical settings.

Potted plants also have some very specific effects on air quality. Even the smallest work hard to clean the air around them, much like forests purify Earth's atmosphere. They do this by releasing oxygen and water vapour which increases humidity and freshness. Their foliage simultaneously absorbs pollutants like carbon dioxide ($CO_2$) and volatile organic chemicals (VOCs). These include benzene and formaldehyde and are released by synthetic hard surfaces and soft furnishings, like carpets, paints, computers, and furniture. It is thought VOCs, along with high levels of $CO_2$, can induce drowsiness and nasal congestion and impair concentration. This constellation of symptoms, called 'sick building syndrome', may also include eye and airway irritation. By increasing the humidity and oxygen level of an enclosed space, pot plants make the air inside fresher and less irritating to airways. This is beneficial for health care workers, patients, and families, especially those with breathing conditions like asthma. Even a small amount of greenery can make a difference. A plant just over twenty centimetres high significantly reduces both VOC and $CO_2$ levels[173].

With the advent of the COVID-19 pandemic, indoor air quality has become an object of interest. Many are now aware that high $CO_2$ levels indicate poor ventilation and are rightly reluctant to spend time in such places. While indoor plants don't remove virus particles, they do lower $CO_2$ concentration and freshen the atmosphere. So, the ideal indoor environment includes good ventilation, through open windows or air flow systems, in addition to pot plants. It is reasonable to expect healthcare settings provide information on their air quality, perhaps through live monitoring, and to see plants in most, as inexpensive, living, air fresheners.

People's reliance on clean air is not confined to hospitals and clinics. All places where prolonged time is spent indoors should be prioritising this foundational need. For office workers, there are great benefits in finding desk space for a plant and requesting greenery throughout the workplace. These extend beyond optimising air quality to include happiness. Research from the University of Technology Sydney found palms were best for reducing $CO_2$, but any variety will drop VOC levels. The same group reported a 40% reduction in stress and negative feelings in employees whose office had plants, compared to those without[174]. Other measures improved by plants include creativity, productivity, and satisfaction. Collaboration between colleagues lifts, along with mood, making the office environment a healthier and more pleasant place to be. Given we spend so much of our day at work, it's important our time there be happy and fulfilling, not just productive. A smart company would increase indoor greenery, plan for outdoor meetings, and ensure staff have regular opportunities to connect with nature during their day. These measures are not only common sense, they are also backed by science.

Just as society's adults spend most of their time at work, our young people are predominantly in school and early childcare. It's especially important these places have optimal indoor air quality. With their high vulnerability to environmental toxins and the large proportion of children who suffer from asthma, their need for clean air is critical. Also, the benefits of embedding nature within the school environment go far beyond air quality to support the health and development of the whole child. The importance of children growing up with nature will be explored fully later.

## WEAVING IT ALL TOGETHER

Once we understand and experience the benefits of weaving nature into our lives, we become motivated to prioritise giving ourselves and our loved ones the time and space to get outside. We will all have our own ways of doing this; I like to imagine sprinkling nature throughout my day, my week, and my year. I also aim to include different doses of nature in my life. From glimpsing the tree tops out my bedroom window and placing a plant in my office at work, through to time outside in my garden or local park. Deeper immersion through bushwalking or camping may take several days, or even weeks. These latter experiences may only occur a few times a year, but they are richly restorative, both at the time and after returning to the city. Memories of the beauty and grandeur of the landscape help buffer the inevitable ups and downs of modern life.

Envisioning various nature doses as analogous to ocean swimming is helpful. A natural view is akin to paddling in the shallows and time spent walking through parkland, or forest bathing, like wading into waist high water. The fully immersive wilderness experience mirrors diving into the depths. Whichever way nature comes into my day I know it is helping me be happy, calm, and strong.

As a mother and doctor, I try to provide a healthy example in how I live by eating well, exercising regularly, getting enough sleep, and ensuring I receive enough nature time. Aiming for a 'green hour' each day is an idea I find useful and it's a simple way of encouraging others to fit a dose of nature into their busy day too. The green hour may be one large chunk of time or many different pieces adding up to about an hour. But whichever way you get it, nature time is worth prioritising and scheduling into the diary.

With any new habit, aiming for a small change is more achievable. A good place to begin is by planning to sit outside for five minutes during a lunch break, or before the day begins. Most likely, you'll feel so good the minutes will stretch out and soon, you'll be scheduling longer and more frequent nature breaks. Just as important as the 'when' and 'where' of being in (and with) nature, the 'how' is key. Take care to really notice what's going on around you. This means putting the phone away and taking headphones off. Look at the clouds, listen for birds, smell the flowers, and maybe even put your cheek up against a tree trunk if no-one's looking! Later, in the Nature Play section, ways of deepening nature experiences will be explored. This involves taking a playful attitude, regardless of age, and sharing the joys with loved ones.

## SOME IDEAS FOR GETTING YOUR 'GREEN HOUR' OR 'DOSE OF NATURE'

| NATURE DOSE | EXPERIENCE |
|---|---|
| Looking at the water | • Having images of nature on the walls or computer screen<br>• Placing a vase of flowers or indoor plant on your desk<br>• Listening to sounds of nature<br>• Having an indoor fountain |
| Paddling in the shallows | • Looking out onto nature – a view, courtyard garden<br>• Having a walking meeting<br>• Being in nature but busy with other activities ie. jogging, fast cycling, power walking, group exercise program |
| Wading in up to your waist | • Spending time in your garden, surrounded by plants<br>• Having a regular 'sit-spot' to observe nearby nature<br>• Walking through or sitting in a park, without tech distractions<br>• Leisurely riding through a park, along a creek, by the beach<br>• Joining a relaxing, nature-focused community event outside; a playgroup, social gathering, environmental restoration |
| Diving in over your head | • Full or multi-day bushwalking, canoeing, rock climbing<br>• Camping in the bush, by the sea<br>• Surfing, sailing, snorkelling, diving – surrounded by water for hours at a time<br>• Birdwatching, sketching, deeply observing nature |

So far, the health and wellbeing benefits of optimising our time outside in the wider natural world, and of bringing natural elements inside, have been covered. From the sunlit synthesis of vitamin D through to horticulture therapy and nature prescriptions. The emphasis, to this point, has predominantly been on the physical effects time in nature has. Interestingly, simply being in natural settings influences our mind in profoundly positive ways. Let's turn towards this topic now, to see how nature can turn an upset, 'red' mind, into a calm and creative 'green' one.

# 9

# Green Mind

*"Those who contemplate the beauty of the earth find reserves of strength that will endure as long as life lasts. There is something infinitely healing in the repeated refrains of nature – the assurance that dawn comes after night, and spring after winter."*

~Rachel Carson

To understand how nature supports human happiness and mental wellbeing, it's useful to explore our brain's evolutionary path. The gradual shifts in structure and function of this mysterious organ over millennia have seen us evolve from simple organisms to highly functioning, creative beings. This slow process took place within the wider net of Earth's complex biosphere, in deep relationship with other lifeforms. The relatively sudden environmental changes over the past few centuries have seen our primitive brain grappling to adapt to modern life. This struggle has been especially pronounced more recently, with the advent of computer technology and virtual worlds. We are wired to live far more slowly and quietly than we currently are. Fortunately, we can use this knowledge to cultivate a sense of calmness and clarity, through mindful connection with nature.

## OUR BRAIN GREW UP IN NATURE

The human brain has evolved over millions of years as we progressed from basic lifeforms into the complex people we know and love today. Put simply, our brain developed in three stages, which correlate structure and function with each major evolutionary step. The consecutive formation of the vertebrate, mammalian, and then human sections of our brain occurred. Each structural part is governed by an 'operating system' which looks after one of our 'core needs'. These are to feel safe, content and loved. If any one of these primary wants are not being met, we feel distressed and unhappy.

The most primitive part of our brain, the brainstem, sits atop the spine. Along with our parasympathetic nervous system, and the oldest part of our Vagus nerve, the brainstem controls the basics. It monitors functions like breathing, digestion, and heart rate, and helps direct our behaviour to keep us safe. The Vagus nerve is one of twelve paired cranial nerves which connect the brain to the face, neck and torso. It is especially complex, arising in several areas of the brainstem, rather than a single site. It also has multiple branches, is asymmetrical and contains fibres which take information up to the brain as well as down from the brain to the body. It is often thought of as being *polyvagal*[b] due to its many features and functions[175]. The first part of the Vagus nerve to evolve was that originating in the dorsal motor nucleus, at the back of the vagal complex. Its formation correlated with the emergence of more complex life forms from the evolutionary swamp. It is a foundational part of primitive animal brains, like those of fish, birds, and reptiles. This old Vagus forms the most ancient component of vertebrate and mammalian brains, including that of humans.

The key operating system of the brainstem, parasympathetic nervous system and old Vagus grouping is *harm avoidance*. So, it looks for threats and starts the process of their avoidance or confrontation, via a flight, fight or freeze response. This ancient reflex to escape from threat occurs instinctively, with no thinking or cognition involved. Being subconscious, the urge to flee from harm is often difficult to describe

---

b   'Poly' from the Greek 'polys' meaning "much"

or explain. It often underlies feelings of anxiety or panic.

Next to evolve was the subcortex. Sitting above the brainstem, it occupies the brain's centre. The subcortex developed during the mammalian evolutionary stage and tends to our need to connect emotionally with others, to bond. This behaviour is essential for mammals, whose young require protection and nourishment via lactation[c] after birth. Along with the sympathetic nervous system, the subcortex looks after our core need to feel satisfaction. Its operating system is *approaching rewards*, or seeking, and it drives us to find food, shelter and a mate to reproduce with.

Finally, the outer layer of the brain, the cortex, developed. The cortex is important for reasoning, planning, remembering, and skills relating to being with, and bonding to, others. These include feeling empathy, developing language and the ability to co-operate. The cortex is thought to have evolved alongside the newest branch of the Vagus nerve which originates in the ventral (front) vagal complex. Unique to mammals, this part of the Vagus runs from the brain, down around the heart and back up, into the head. Its development coincided with our differentiation from other mammals as we evolved through the primate to human form. The new Vagus alters our facial expression and modulates our tone of voice allowing us to care for others[176]. Together with the cortex, this nerve is responsible for our core need to form relationships, to connect. Their operating system is *attaching to others*.

We are happiest when all three of our core needs are being met. When we feel safe, content and loved. As neuropsychologist Rick Hanson writes, "we meet our core needs for safety, satisfaction, and connection when we—metaphorically—pet the lizard, feed the mouse, and hug the monkey."[177] Modern society challenges our ability to feel this way as most media and many social systems often evoke feelings of loneliness, fear, or inadequacy. Thoughts or beliefs that we don't have as much money, possessions or friends as others can feed isolation and disconnection.

---

c   Lactation: the process where mammals secrete milk for feeding their young; breastfeeding in humans

Evolution has also seen our brain develop a *negativity bias*, meaning we notice threats and deficits more than positives in our world. Evolving on the savannah, it was essential to notice a predator so we could fight or flee, as need be. Parts of our brain constantly scan for threat so, when triggered, we can appropriately avoid danger. The *salience network* decides whether the things we are doing, or exposed to, are good or bad. Whether we should move towards, or away, from an object or situation. The main part of this network is our amygdala. This is comprised of small, paired, almond shaped structures, deep within the brain. If the amygdala is very active towards negative experiences, we are more likely to be anxious or sad. Whereas, if it's orientated more positively, we feel happier.

Another relevant feature of human minds is the capacity to imagine the future and remember the past. The *executive control network* manages our actions and thinking and is centred on the pre-frontal cortex, at the very front of the brain. It analyses what we think about a particular situation. Through this deep thought, we strategise solutions to problems, considering both short and long-term consequences, including impacts on others.

It's helpful to conceptualise the brain as having two key modes of activity. Rick Hanson encapsulates this beautifully, describing them as follows: "Each of your brain's operating systems has essentially two settings: *responsive and reactive*. As long as you experience that the core need a system handles is being met, then that system defaults to its responsive setting. When you feel safe, your avoiding harms system enters its responsive mode, which brings feelings of relaxation, calm, and peace. When you feel satisfied, your approaching rewards system shifts into its responsive setting, with feelings such as gratitude, gladness, accomplishment, and contentment. And when you feel connected, your attaching to others system goes responsive, evoking feelings of belonging, intimacy, compassion, kindness, worth, and love. For simplicity, I think of this as the "green" setting of your brain."[177]

When we are in the responsive setting, chemicals that relieve pain and inflammation and kill harmful bacteria are released. This allows for healing and a sense of calm. Conversely, when our core needs are not being met, we flip into reactive mode. Then, our sympathetic nervous system is triggered and chemicals like adrenaline and cortisol are released, readying the body to fight or flee. A cascade of changes in body function ensues. Our heart rate rises, and blood is diverted away from the gut, towards the large muscles of the limbs. Digestion shuts down, so our mouth becomes dry as saliva secretion is shut off. We may feel nauseated or as if there are butterflies in our stomach. Breathing becomes more rapid to increase oxygenation of the blood and if we don't move to utilise this, we may feel lightheaded. Our mind focuses on escape and thinking becomes preoccupied with the perceived threat. Emotionally, we feel unsafe, under attack, isolated and scared.

Over most evolutionary time, our brain was in responsive mode, flicking into reactive mode for brief spurts of activity. Threats were acted on immediately, via our flight/fight/freeze response, and we were primed to remember the threat to help us avoid a future danger. We then rested in responsive mode as our body and mind replenished. There was usually plenty of time to recover in this resting state before the next stressor. Importantly, this recuperation occurred when we were safely ensconced within our family group, and our tribe or small community. And within the wider nest of nature, companioned by other living things.

## OUR WORLD BEFORE

To appreciate the challenges modern life poses for the human brain, it's helpful to consider what life might have been like for our ancestors. During most of our evolutionary period, people lived in family groups within small communities. We were surrounded by a natural landscape rich with life and the night sky was pitch black, jewelled with stars. Compared to today, living was slow and our sensory input much less complex. Life was relatively quiet. The acoustic backdrop probably included gentle noises; bird calls, the wind in the trees, sounds of water and the voices of our companions. The smells of plants, soils, animals, and waterways were earthy and usually mild, diluted by fresh air. And the colours of nature were often soft – blues, browns, and greens. Splashes of vibrancy on birds and insects stood out from the gentler hues of the landscape. We walked over loose surfaces like leaf litter on the forest floor, grasses, and sands. Our feet were directly in contact with the earth, which we sensed as much as walked over.

Essentially, during this long time of human development, our ancestors lived in relative quiet, at walking pace. This evolution, in the presence of ecological abundance and few other people, is our origin story. It is what our brain was built for, and what soothes our troubled minds today.

Prolonged time spent peacefully in nature can reproduce similar conditions to this time of earlier humans. Such settings may help restore mental and emotional balance for those stressed by modern life. Meditation teacher Michael Taft's description of his time in a three-month silent retreat in rural America provides unique insights[178]. He found after several weeks that his brain was emptying out of thought content, "I would just sit, eyes and ears and nose and skin open to nature and let its silence and openness sort of soak into me". He describes it as being pretty boring, living in a low stimulus natural environment for several months. There was no television, music, or social media to entertain him when it got dark, and very few people to engage with. "All of this is not to disparage the Paleolithic, but instead to give you a sense of the environment your brain and nervous system were designed for. … There might be one or two exciting events in a whole month, and the rest of the time, it's just the sound of wind in the trees," he says.

Michael found that as his mind emptied of thought, it "was filling up with silence. I noticed that the woods, too, were silent and empty. There was a congruity there – silent mind, silent world – and I really, really liked it." He suggests this feeling was a return to how humans may have felt thousands of years ago. "Our brains would have been more than adequate to handle the few exciting things that came up and been perfectly content to sort of idle along the rest of the time. That idle mode feels really, really good, because it is probably the natural waking rest mode of the brain. Not caught in a seeking feedback loop. No stress, no anxiety or cortisol, and no overload of problems, problems, problems that our information overlords shovel into the gaping maw of our need for novelty." This idle mode is simply another way of describing the responsive state where our core needs are being met and our brain is not under any stress.

So, how has the world changed, and how has this affected our mind and the thoughts and emotions it generates? More specifically, how has our altered relationship with plants and other animals played out for our psyche, the way we think and feel?

## OUR WORLD TODAY

Just as the modern world sets us up to be overweight, it provides the perfect storm for generating unhappiness. The year 2007 saw a significant milestone passed as over half the world's population became urban, living in cities rather than villages. This collective move to the city, away from quieter rural locations, has upset our physical and mental wellbeing.

Contemporary urban life is characterised by feelings of busyness, pressure, and competition. We are surrounded by things our primitive brain sees as potential threats, so our stress response is heightened. The sensory overload may be overwhelming as we face a barrage of sounds, sights, and smells. The soundscape is often especially harsh. Outside, there's the beeping of trucks reversing, horns blasting, and the pervasive rumble of traffic. As phones are always with us, their ringtones, the ding of notifications and the endless chatter of social media is ever-present. Often, we are hearing this cocktail of city sounds well into the night. So, there may be no relief from this noisy bombardment, no truly quiet place.

Our eyes are accosted too, with the frenetic rush of traffic and concrete spreading from buildings, across shopping centres and carparks. Flashing advertising signs and billboards call out for our attention from almost any fixed surface. There is an almost constant stream of visual messages coming into our brains as we live our modern, urban lives. Even at night there are visual distractions, from our screen's blueish glow to the haze of light pollution obscuring the stars. This is very different to the often-pitch-black night sky our ancestors slept under.

The smells we are exposed to are also grating. City dwellers frequently inhale a toxic mixture of traffic fumes and industrial pollution when outside. While indoors, artificial perfumes are now everywhere. Recently, attention has focussed on the pervasive nature of fragrance in both personal hygiene and home products. Rather than scented products having naturally derived plant perfumes, as advertised, they usually contain a dazzling array of chemicals. And most compounds are present in much higher concentrations than found naturally. Manufacturers can put the word *fragrance*, or *parfum*, on the ingredient list of a product to represent any number of chemical agents. The exact composition remains a trade secret. But there are often over one hundred ingredients acting as the parfum. Almost three thousand chemicals are on the ingredient list published by the self-regulated International Fragrance Association. So, working out a product's contents is extremely difficult[179].

With the artificial nature of today's fragrances, it's unsurprising that many people experience headaches and other problems from them. The rates of headache are increasing and evidence suggests fragrance chemicals may be one contributor[180]. These poorly regulated agents are also thought to cause asthma and skin conditions in susceptible people[181]. Certainly, our physiology has not evolved with such concentrated, complex smells. The brain's olfactory system processes our response to smells. It is intimately connected to the amygdala and other regions associated with memory and emotion. Care should be taken with our exposure to fragrance as it may have subtle, yet important, effects on our thoughts and feelings.

City life is, literally, hard to the touch, with concrete, metal and glass surrounding those of us who live here. A proliferation of roads, skyscrapers and shopping complexes sees landscapes denuded and waterways buried. Underfoot are hard surfaces with bitumen roads, concrete footpaths and unforgiving tiled floors throughout office foyers and shopping centres. For school children, the softness of grass is rapidly being replaced by firm, fake turf, and sports courts. Rather than sense the gentle rebound of the earth under bare feet as our predecessors did, our footfall is jarring. We pad our feet against these rigid surfaces with thick-soled shoes. Or avoid walking altogether, preferring to drive instead.

There is also a toughness in the way we live with many families and communities being divided. City dwellers often live isolated lives with little meaningful social connection. So, despite there being millions of people in our cities, there is an epidemic of loneliness. The Australian Psychological Society's Australian Loneliness Report, released in 2018, describes one quarter of adults as being lonely[182]. A similar number experience social interaction anxiety, meaning they feel stressed when mixing with other people. Both these problems are associated with mental and physical health issues, like poor sleep, headaches, and gut upset. Feeling lonely, or worried about being around other people, is fuelled by a sense of isolation because our core need for connection is not being met. Physical elements contribute to this sense of unease as they remind us of our disconnection. We see this throughout urban environments in the form of barriers, like high fences and roadways.

Alongside these engineered elements, daily media reports on crime feed stranger danger. This often leaves us feeling afraid of others. Authorities react to this by expanding their presence, funding police and security services. This has progressed to such an extent that even in relatively peaceful democracies like Australia, railway stations are patrolled by groups of armed officials. Technology has fed this fervour for surveillance and now public places are constantly monitored through closed-circuit (CCTV) cameras. Rather than evoking feelings of safety, this level of scrutiny recalls George Orwell's novel *Nineteen Eighty-Four*. In it, Big Brother looks down on the people and all are watched. Such inanimate vigilance by the State contrasts to the care and concern reciprocated between members of a close, connected community.

We are not safe from machine generated threat within our homes either. Horrible scenes of terror and war from across the globe intrude into our personal space via 'smart' phones and other devices. It's as if modern society has conspired to constantly illicit a threat response from our brains. So, it's little wonder many people feel constantly unsafe and on edge, whether formally diagnosed with anxiety or not. And why many prefer to withdraw from others, retreating to the perceived safety of their homes and virtual worlds.

Understanding the processes which underlie our collective struggle to live in this often menacing, attention-demanding, urban setting is helpful. It enables us to see that it is not some individual weakness causing our distress, but rather, our environment. Let's explore the brain's processes a little further now. This will help us to reconfigure how we live.

## TODAY'S RED MIND

Our environment sets the stage for our lives, providing the sensory stimuli to which our brains respond. Remember, our primitive old brain is always looking out for threats, seeking resources and social connection. Meanwhile, our new brain (the pre-frontal cortex) has the capacity to plan, imagine the future and dwell on the past. Reflexive, subtle loops form between bodily sensations, external inputs and our thoughts and emotions. Meditation teachers, Paul Gilbert and Choden sum up the problems with this patterning for today's world beautifully, "Remember that the zebra will go back to eating soon after escaping from a lion, but a human may well ruminate about it for days and even be traumatised by the experience for their whole life"[183]. Distressing events can shape our brains and our experiences for many years as our minds get stuck in a loop of fear. This will come as no surprise to anyone who has suffered from Post-Traumatic Stress Disorder, or the complex trauma experienced through family or sexual violence.

Living in cities today we are bombarded by alarming sounds and images, particularly through television, social media, and news services. The visually overwhelming way news is presented to us on television is a good example. Designed to grab our attention, a band of writing streams across the base of the screen highlighting the latest information which is usually negative. Simultaneously, dramatic images flash up with alarming headlines and other visuals. Our brains perceive this as threatening and so trigger responses in our nervous system to put us on alert – flipping us into a 'red mind' state. Extended periods of time in this mode may result in mental fatigue and impair memory and judgement.

We are also more likely to experience panic. Or to try and calm ourselves by reaching for a beer, cigarette or chocolate. The tsunami of anxiety, attention problems and addictions flooding the health system is partly due to our brain's inability to cope with this sensory overload.

The harshness of urban life is also reflected in crime statistics, with women and children suffering most. For example, of Australian women over fifteen, one third have experienced physical abuse, one quarter emotional abuse and one fifth sexual abuse[184]. Soberingly, over 30 women annually are murdered by their current or ex-partner[185]. Social harms resulting from problematic men's behaviour, like family violence and sexual assault, culminate in relationship breakdown. Resultant homelessness, loneliness and isolation have repercussions for broader society. People self-medicate with alcohol and other drugs, while behavioural addictions, like gambling and pornography, are common. The consequences of these social issues manifest in the mental illnesses seen every day in general practice. Problems like anxiety, depression, poor sleep, eating disorders, self-harm, and drug abuse. Many people have a cluster of social, emotional, and physical issues all at once.

Those born in the city are especially vulnerable to psychological distress. Research has shown a dose response relationship between the degree of urbanisation at birth and mental disorders. The association occurs for a wide range of problems including schizophrenia, autism, substance use and mood, neurotic, eating and personality disorders[186]. There may be many contributing factors; these include exposure to pollution, stress, diet, lifestyle, family issues, infections, fear of crime and social difficulties. As discussed earlier, this may also be related to the loss of our microbial 'old friends' from nature.

Functional MRI scanning allows brain activity to be seen live. This is providing some answers as to why those with urban childhoods are wired to be more stressed. In one key study, researchers subjected healthy volunteers to social stress experiments while monitoring brain activity[187]. Measuring blood cortisol levels, heart rate and blood pressure, they could monitor participants' stress levels accurately. The more urban exposure the subjects had experienced during their lifetime, the greater their 'urbanicity' and the more their stress-muscle, the amygdala, responded. This means the subjects' stress sensitivity was heightened.

The scientists also noticed increased amygdala activity with current city living. So, those of us who had our childhoods in the city have brains which are primed to respond more to social stress. Given the inherently stressful city environment, it's little wonder we have high rates of unhappiness and anxiety in urban communities. Also, the cortisol stress response is exaggerated in adults whose mothers were distressed when pregnant. This may partly explain why mental illness can be found down the generations. Those born to stressed or traumatised women have a heightened response to life's difficulties.

Even for those not overtly suffering from mental health issues, our culture pressures us to consume. To buy more possessions, to use more social media, to drink more alcohol, seek more excitement and eat more food. As described earlier, this is our approaching rewards system when it's in the reactive mode. Meditation teacher, Michael Taft explains, "the drive to seek is deeply baked into the brains of mammals, and it is deeply baked into you. It was created for a world in which novelty was a rarity, a strange and wonderful newness in an enormous ocean of old sameness. The world of boring sameness is the world our brain expects, and it's why we get so addicted to the new, the exciting, the strange."[177]

Once we have consumed what we sought, we are but momentarily satisfied as our nervous system is skewed to push us to continue seeking. This constant drive to look for the next new and interesting idea sees us drowning in a world where novel messages and images are streamed into our consciousness via the ever-present digital device. To satisfy this need to be in touch and keep up with others, people constantly check their multiple social media accounts, emails, and messages. This multi-tasking impairs the brain's ability to think clearly and deeply.

## Our attention deficit

A newly recognised neurological phenomenon, *attention deficit trait* (ADT), describes this effect. ADT was first described in 1994 by Dr

Hallowell, an American physician and attention expert. It is thought this trait developed in response to the hyperkinetic environment of the modern, digital world. Hallowell says, "it is brought on by the incessant demands, temptations, and opportunities that hijack our attention, filling our heads with a cacophony of mental noise. As our minds fill with such noise – spasmodic synaptic snaps signifying nothing – the brain loses its ability to attend fully and thoughtfully to anything."[188] As it is elicited as an adaptive mechanism, the trait comes and goes depending on our device exposure.

When the brain tries to manage overwhelming input from digital technology, mental processing slows and thinking distorts. This manifests as disorganisation and difficulty prioritising tasks. There is also a tendency to think rigidly and to feel constantly on edge. The symptoms of ADT include heightened distractibility with an inability to sustain lengthy full attention. There's a tendency to jump from one task, or idea, to another. So, decisions are made impulsively, or avoided altogether. This elicits guilt about uncompleted tasks and feelings of impatience, restlessness, and tension. Given technology is ever-present, this group of symptoms is something many of us experience daily.

While it is hard for adults to identify and address problematic screen behaviour, the situation is even more difficult for children. They have little control over their environment, relying on their carers, and wider society, to look after their needs. When it comes to digital exposure, not enough attention is given to their vulnerability. The developing brain of infants and very young children is especially susceptible to being overloaded by visual and auditory stimulation. So, child behaviour experts are particularly worried about screen time in this age group. As technology advances so rapidly, it is impossible to gather long term data on the behavioural and developmental impact it has on children. Information on the effect of smart phones and social media on today's children, for example, won't be available for decades. Meanwhile, the nature of childhood is being transformed. An exploration of some currently available data is worrying as it points to disturbing trends in early development from exposure to television and computers.

## The impact of screen time

In Australia, children under the age of eighteen months are having an excessive amount of screen time. A Sydney research project found 40% of very young children are watching screens more than two hours per day[189]. This is associated with poor health outcomes because screen use correlates with sitting. If this behaviour continues for years, the effects on wellbeing are enormous. Some studies have found children over five who watched more than two hours of TV a day were more likely to be overweight, less fit, and have high cholesterol levels. Behavioural problems occurred too, alongside issues like poor sleep and musculoskeletal disorders[190].

Primary school children watching the same amount were also affected, being more likely to have behavioural withdrawal or trouble maintaining attention. The knock-on effects included poor mental health and struggles with learning[189]. Encouragingly, these effects may be reversible. One older study showed reducing TV viewing time over six weeks led to an improvement in both intelligence tests and attention[191].

Even having the TV on in the background may be harmful. In one study, fifty children between one and three years played with a variety of toys for an hour. For half of this time, the TV was left on in the background with a game show playing. The children only watched it for a few seconds at a time, and less than once per minute. Despite this apparently minimal distraction, their focussed attention during play was significantly reduced when the TV was on. They also played less with the toys[192]. This finding is important because play and concentration are crucial for early learning, yet children are rarely in a space without a screen. From doctors waiting rooms to petrol bowsers, public spaces are littered with the distraction of screens. Just as children's exposure to cigarette smoke is restricted for health reasons, we need to consider limits on digital displays.

Many new parents don't receive adequate information regarding safe technology use for children. Meanwhile, they are bombarded by messages from companies selling applications under the guise of 'early learning'. This can be confusing and frustrating. What's needed is clear advice from an early stage. Health professionals can communicate screen time guidelines sensitively and opportunistically. The current recommendation is that children under the age of two years have no screen time at all, and that those aged between two and five years have less than one hour per day[193]. It is best if this information is provided before birth, when it's easier to make behaviour changes. Setting good habits early helps lay the foundation for optimal communication. Making mealtimes a screen-free zone and putting phones away when having a conversation are good choices. This topic can be included in pre-pregnancy consultations when diet, exercise and other health measures are discussed.

## Our sleepless nights

Technology use in the evening, especially if it's in bed, impacts sleep. This is because the blue light and vivid imagery stimulate the brain, even if the content is not overtly stressful. Trying to stay off devices for at least an hour before hopping into bed is helpful, especially for young people. Also, leaving phones out of the bedroom altogether takes away the frequent interruptions of notifications throughout the night. If this is not possible, then adjusting settings onto 'aeroplane' or 'do not disturb' will minimise disruptions.

Traffic noise and light pollution affect sleep for city dwellers. Both require improved urban planning and environmental guidelines, so sit within the control of governments. The lightening of the night sky has been raised as a problem by astronomers. They are concerned that the Southern Cross, a four-star landmark for all Australians, is no longer fully visible from Sydney. Calling for a 'dark sky park' to be created, they want people to be able see the night sky more fully. "Sometimes we call it the Southern Triangle when only three stars are visible", says Sydney Observatory manager Marnie Ogg[194]. A dark sky park could be created by the adoption of LED lighting and other measures to reduce light pollution. Professor Fred Watson, the astronomer-in-charge at the Australian Astronomical Observatory at Siding Spring, says, "We are in danger of losing the night sky in cities. We've lost the intimacy with the sky that we all would have had one hundred years ago."

The connection with the night sky links to our overall relationship to place, to knowing where we are in time and space. For millennia we have used the stars to find our way and for many cultures the stars are imbued with spiritual meaning. We are losing this relationship to stars, galaxies, and constellations slowly so many are unaware of what's missing. Certainly, those living in the city are plagued by sleep problems. And no doubt the constant glow outside is a contributing factor, much like the ever-present grumble of traffic.

The relentless sensory input of urban life means a lack of deep rest, of night-time darkness, peace and quiet. Little wonder, despite modern medical advances, that so many people feel tired, stressed, and unhappy. Fortunately, there's a lot we can do change things. To make life better for ourselves, our families, and communities. Creating the time and space to bring nature back into our lives is the first step. At the core of this approach is restoring a meaningful connection to the natural world. This will help us to switch from an uptight 'red' mind, to a calm and steady 'green' one. Let's move on to look at how the mind responds to nature.

## GROWING A GREEN MIND

Scientists have been fascinated by the relationship between our minds and nature for decades. And the interest in this area is growing. Just as new technology has helped us better understand how modern life upsets our mind, science is also helping us figure out how to restore balance. By slowing down and planting nature back into people's lives we can help reduce their suffering. Time in nature helps cultivate peace, contentment, and connection to place. I like to call it 'growing a green mind'. As discussed earlier, others, like neuropsychologist, Rick Hanson, use the term *green mind* to refer to a calm state of mental activity. Scientist, Wallace Nichols, whose writing describes the ways water helps optimise our mind, calls it a *blue mind* [195]. Whichever calming colour you like to choose, a mind soothed by nature is able to function at its best and to be responsive, rather than reactive. There are various scientific theories as to why our minds function better in a more natural environment, here are the most common.

## Our inherent biophilia

First, there's the *biophilia hypothesis* which was described by Harvard biologist E.O Wilson in 1984. *Biophilia* is simply a love of nature and living things. So, this hypothesis describes humans as having an inherent love of nature due to our evolutionary story[196]. We evolved deeply immersed in nature. Our progressive separation from it over the past three hundred years is relatively recent in the multimillion-year timespan of our evolution. Over this long timeframe, our genes have been imprinted with an affinity for nature. In this theory, nature is not merely a resource for humans to exploit but is needed by us for our emotional, cognitive, aesthetic, and spiritual growth. We are thought to be genetically wired to love and need nature. This hypothesis suggests we've not had enough time to adapt to the progressive removal of nature from our lives and that this nature deprivation is harmful.

*Stress reduction theory* postulates that being in nature is less stressful because of the lower intensity of sensory stimulation in this environment. There is therefore less threat perceived by our brains and so less arousal of our nervous system and fewer associated negative thoughts and feelings.

*Attention restoration theory* describes how time in nature allows our brain to rest and recover from mental fatigue. It states that nature has four aspects of providing this recuperation. The first is simply *being away* from the source of our pain and stress. This might be physically away in a wild place, or simply allowing our attention to be swept away, looking at clouds moving past the window. The second aspect nature provides is points of *fascination*, like birds' singing and glorious sunsets. This sensory stimulation intrigues our attention and creates wonder. The third aspect is *extent*, which is the way nature helps put our worries into perspective. We notice how much smaller our concerns feel in the context of a majestic natural environment. Where we are just one person amongst thousands of other living creatures going about their day. The final aspect is that of *compatibility*, which describes the way nature feels comfortable to us because of our evolution in sync with it.

In all these ways nature holds our attention effortlessly compared to the demanding way the modern world shouts for it. As our attention is held easily by nature there is still sufficient capacity for our mind to think about other things, and so gain perspective on our problems. This theory may account for the way many people describe feeling back in balance emotionally after spending several days out walking in the wild.

These theories are not mutually exclusive. Instead, they provide different lenses through which to view the nature-mind connection. Often, several are used together to understand how nature restores our mind to a balanced state. It seems that a whole range of nature experiences can be beneficial. An American study found walking through a natural area reduced the amount of rumination, or worrying, a person did. It also lowered activity levels in the part of the brain related to behavioural withdrawal[(197)]. In the study, the authors compared walking for 90 minutes through parkland to walking alongside a busy road. They "suggest that accessible natural areas may be vital for mental health in our rapidly urbanising world".

A recent example of the importance of local parks and gardens for mental health was seen during the lock down period of Melbourne's COVID-19 pandemic. Then, parks and gardens were a place of respite for the crucial one hour per day when residents were allowed to exercise. People who would otherwise head to the gym found themselves getting acquainted with their neighbourhood green space. And children forbidden to play in playgrounds were seen climbing trees and riding bikes through puddles. Apart from physical exercise, the calming effect of this time in nature helped offset the stress associated with the pandemic.

Rumination is the tendency to go over bad memories and experiences in our minds, to dwell on the negative. In his book, *Hardwiring Happiness*, Rick Hansen explains, "since neurons that fire together wire together, staying with a negative experience past the point that's useful is like running laps in Hell: You dig the track a little deeper in your brain each time you go around it."[(177)] The more we ruminate, the more likely we are to suffer depression and other mental illness. So, perhaps it's the replacement of trees and parks with freeways and buildings that contributes to mental illness in city dwellers through its effect on increasing rumination.

## The three-day effect

The benefits of time in nature seem to be dose dependent. Extended time spent in wilderness areas having the greatest benefit for our minds. Researcher David Strayer describes 'the three-day effect' where clarity of thinking and creativity are improved after three days spent in the wilderness. He says the third day is when the "cleaning of the mental windshield" happens[198]. A cognitive neuroscientist at the University of Utah, Strayer thinks it takes several days of being in the moment, not distracted by technology, for the frontal cortex part of the brain to rest and recover. As discussed earlier, this region is responsible for complex thinking, like planning and problem solving. It gets exhausted by a pressurized, multi-tasking lifestyle.

In discussing their study, he and fellow researchers propose the benefits are due to twin factors: the rejuvenating ability of a wilderness environment and the removal of technology's sensory overload. "Exposure to nature may also engage what has been termed the 'default mode' networks of the brain, which an emerging literature suggests may be important for peak psychosocial health. The default mode network is a set of brain areas that are active during restful introspection and that have been implicated in efficient performance on tasks requiring frontal lobe function ... On a hike or during exposure to natural stimuli which produce soft-fascination, the mind may be more able to enter a state of introspection and mind wandering which can engage the default mode. Interestingly, engaging the default mode has been shown to be disrupted by multimedia use, which requires an external attentional focus, again pointing to the possibility that natural environments such as those experienced by the current participants may have both removed a cost (technology) and added a benefit (activation of brain systems that aid divergent thinking)".[199]

This experiment shows how several theories can be used to understand the findings of mental rejuvenation in nature. First, stress is reduced as screen-based distractions, the worry of work and home are removed temporarily. Attention is restored through the soft fascination of beautiful views and encounters with wildlife which provoke feelings of wonder and delight. The slow, steady pace of walking and awareness of a majestic natural landscape encapsulate perspective, putting problems into context with the wider world. Being with a small group of other people helps nurture our core needs to feel connected and safe.

When out in wilderness areas, we are far from light pollution and city noise. The night sky is dark, apart from stars, and there is only torchlight to see with. Our sleep-wake cycles sync with nature's rhythms. This allows our own diurnal patterns to be reset. We get to sleep more readily and have a less interrupted, more sound night's rest. Taken altogether, these elements make hiking with others for several days deeply restorative, mentally and emotionally.

A multi-day nature experience can be thought of as a sustained nature prescription or forest bathing activity by combining the elements of slowing down, removing screen-based distractions, and intentionally connecting with the wider natural world. All the benefits discussed earlier apply here too– lowered blood pressure and heart rate, reduced stress hormone levels and enhanced immune function. We can combine all of nature's stress-lowering features in a simple to read format, like a table:

## HOW NATURE LOWERS STRESS

| NATURE INCREASES | NATURE DECREASES |
|---|---|
| 1. Activity in the limbic system responsible for happiness – induced recall<br>2. Quality of sleep<br>3. Alpha wave activity in the brain, influencing relaxation and effortless alertness<br>4. Parasympathetic activity within the nervous system, which occurs when feeling relaxed | 1. Blood pressure and heart rate<br>2. Cortisol secretion and irregularity, which correlate to stress<br>3. Neural activity in the subgenual prefrontal cortex, active during rumination<br>4. Sympathetic activity within the nervous system which occurs when feeling stressed |

Graphic from *Planet Ark: Adding Trees Report.* 2016.[200]

Science is naturally reductive – we break down an experience or event into its various elements to better understand the how things work, to see how an experience like a bushwalk affects our physical body, thinking mind and emotions. Yet when asked to describe how we feel after such an outing we might simply describe ourselves as happy. There is a relationship between happiness and feeling connected to nature. So, let's see what research into this link has uncovered next.

## HAPPINESS

Happiness is something we all crave, and to be happy means something different to each of us. For me, happiness is feeling content and complete. I guess this is when my core needs are being met, when I'm feeling safe and peaceful, connected to loved ones and that my work is aligned with my values. The messaging we receive from much of modern society is that happiness is only achieved once we have all the things deemed desirable – good looks, a great job, a beautiful home, a loving partner, and gorgeous, happy children. Given it is pretty much impossible for any of us to have all these things simultaneously, many people are on a constant quest for the unattainable.

Surveys done by Planet Ark, an Australian environmental organisation, found people who have a closer nature connection are more likely to consider themselves happy[200]. The Planet Ark National Survey found that people who spent more time in nature had significantly higher self-reported happiness. Time spent in nature was associated with feelings of enjoyment, positive engagement and playfulness[201]. Their 2016 report, *Adding Trees- a Prescription for Health, Happiness and Fulfilment*, outlines how the increase in happiness is "linked to changes in the brain and hormone secretion, with nature quite literally creating a happier mind. These changes include activation of the dopamine reward system, structures in the limbic system that respond to happiness-induced recall and decreasing cortisol secretion and irregularity the more green space a person is exposed to."[200] As touched on earlier, the drop in stress hormone cortisol from time spent in nature reflects a calmer, happier mind state.

There is likely to be a long-term benefit from childhood nature experiences. Adults who described themselves as happier in Planet Ark's research survey were found to have engaged in a third more outdoor activities when growing up than people who rated themselves as low on a subjective happiness scale[201]. When I speak to groups on the benefits of nature time for children, I ask people to think back to their favourite place to play when they were a child. Almost every hand in the room goes up when I ask if this special place was outside, in nature. This aligns with a study of adults in which 97% identified the most significant place in their childhood as being the outdoors. The quality of the child's experience determines how it is engraved in memory. Experiences where children are actively involved with their body, senses and awareness are likely to be etched in memory for a long time[202]. As positive emotions are generated when children engage in nature play, these times outside become the cherished memories of childhood. Recollections of being happy and calm spring from natural experiences. This contrasts with playing video games and watching television, which do not tend to generate as many positive feelings to build memories of happy places.

Intimate relationships are an important contributor to our happiness. It seems time in nature can nurture them too. A survey of five hundred couples in the UK found a significant increase in sexual activity during and after a camping trip. Ninety-five percent said their love life improved dramatically when they were away and that the benefits continued once they returned home[203]. In another survey by Planet Ark, one quarter of couples reported tiredness and stress as being the top two reasons for their love life being less satisfying[200]. Perhaps, by addressing these problems, nature-based camping holidays can help a struggling love life and nourish intimate relationships.

Some relationship counsellors like George W. Burns, incorporate nature-based experiences into their work helping couples whose relationship is floundering. The rationale for this is that it helps rekindle the spark by evoking memories of the couple's earlier, exciting time of discovery. Often, as a relationship begins, time is spent together doing things out in nature – watching the sun set, going for picnics and walks by the sea or through a park. As time passes and couples get busy with the demands of family and work, these activities tend to get left off the calendar. To rekindle romance within a relationship, finding time for these things once again is important. Nature provides the backdrop, the beautiful, low stress setting for a time to just 'be' together. Unlike going to a movie or restaurant where there are many distractions and other people around, time together out in nature gives couples a relaxing place for reconnection. It is also generally free to go and do these types of things, so the barrier of cost is removed.

The relationships we share with our partners, children, other family members and those in the broader community, are the most important factor when it comes to our happiness. How connected we feel to others indicates how happy we are, with social isolation being a key contributor to depression. Studies have shown that more community green space is associated with improved social cohesion and relationships, with people feeling less lonely and isolated. There are also lower crime rates in neighbourhoods with more green space, making them safer. This is especially true in poorer suburbs. Residents of public housing, who have access to a common green area, have an increase in social activities, visitors, and more willingness to support each other compared to those without. Having more nature in our suburbs enhances human connection. This not only improves the physical environment and beautifies where we live, it also feeds our happiness.

Another rich human capacity is creativity. We all have an inner creative resource which is expressed in different ways throughout our lifetime. Nature supports this innate desire to use our imagination, to manifest our ideas, to create. Perhaps the truest representation of a green mind is some form of creativity – an artwork, a poem, a song, or a dance. Or it may be the solution to a tricky problem. Science has explored nature and creativity too, as we'll discuss next.

## CREATIVITY

The ultimate green mind is creative, and nature has been a backdrop to artists for thousands of years. Scientist and writer, Wallace Nichols, describes how the flow of water relates to the flow of creativity and reminds us that artists colonies often sprung up by water[195]. He says, "It is the layers of rhythmic structured symphony performed by waves and wavelets, stones and pebbles. It is the known shallows that taper into the mysterious abyss... It is the endless mutability the surprise and unexpectedness of its ever-changing colours and moods that stirs artists, film writers, and thinkers alike. Water unleashes the uninhibited child in all of us, unlocking our creativity and curiosity".

The curved shapes in nature contrast with the rigidly straight lines of man-made forms; think rulers, fences, and squares. Flying over outback Australia, it is striking to see the curves of waterways running through the landscape as hard lines of roads and fences cut across and through them. It seems human creativity may be sparked by interacting with natural curves. In one creativity experiment, participants were better able to solve maths problems and think of innovative solutions after drawing curved, as opposed to, straight lines[204]. Maybe our brain likes the flowing lines of nature and functions best when our body is looking at and creating these softer shapes? Certainly, many doodlers tend to make circular patterns.

Creating buildings in organic shapes rather than rigid squares or rectangles provides a nature-informed envelope for people to live and work in. This type of space feels completely different to the boxes predominating our cities. The Baya Gawiy Children and Parents Centre in the Fitzroy Valley in Western Australia shows how healing a building can be. Bunuba Elder June Oscar spoke to a group of us visiting in 2015, describing the genesis of the health centre. She recalled how the government wanted to build a rectangular box but she objected strongly. Instead, she had a building shaped in the form of the freshwater stingray (baya gawiy), designed and constructed. This animal is a Totem of her people. Generous curves flow throughout the centre and along one side are the 'healing rooms' where health practitioners see patients. It felt like such a nurturing building to be in compared to other hospitals and health centres around Australia. Almost as if you were being held gently by the space.

As touched on in Part 1, this use of nature to inspire architecture is called biophilic design and it is taking off around the world. It's not surprising that First Australians, an enormously creative and innovative people, are leading the way here. Their deep connection to nature, to Country, gives them unique insights and inspiration for creating healing spaces and programs.

We'll explore how nature play provides the foundation for creativity in childhood later in detail. But it's important to note here that when given opportunities to spend time in a natural environment, children can let their imaginations take flight, to weave stories into the landscape and to embed nature in their hearts. By prioritising time in nature for our young people, we are cultivating the artists of the future and growing new stories to feed the breadth of the arts. We are also enabling the creativity needed beyond the artistic sphere, in all domains of modern life, as we face the challenges of the 21st century.

## KEY POINTS

- ❤ Our mind has evolved within the quietness, spaciousness and tranquillity of nature
- ❤ Today's urban environment is overly stimulating and stressful for our mind
- ❤ Slowing down and mindfully engaging with the natural world soothes us
- ❤ The *Three-day effect* describes how prolonged time in nature improves creativity and mental clarity
- ❤ Spending time in nature can nurture connection within relationships
- ❤ Childhood nature experiences are linked to happiness
- ❤ Plentiful green spaces enrich community connection and harmony

# HOW TO GROW YOUR GREEN MIND

We can use research and ideas from the fields of evolutionary biology, positive psychology and nature-based health disciplines to work with and within nature to enhance our happiness and mental wellbeing. Whether life is going well for you or not, the more nature you bring into your world and the more time you spend getting out into beautiful, natural places, the healthier, happier and more content you'll feel.

## 3 key steps to nurturing yourself mentally and emotionally...

### 1.
### Orient to nature: turn towards nature and make space and time for it

- ❧ *Take off the tech:* switch off your device or, if that's too much, put it on silent mode and out of sight for a while.

- ❧ If possible *sit looking out* a window or at a natural object like a plant, picture of nature or fish tank, whether at your desk, in a café or when waiting for something.

- ❧ *Spend as much time as possible outside* in a natural place, whether it's a garden, a forest or the ocean.

- ❧ *Create a place* you can regularly spend time in which is peaceful and nature rich; this could be a garden, balcony or a room with lots of indoor plants or an aquarium.

- ❧ If you can't get outside, try meditating and *imagine* a natural place where you feel safe.

- ❧ Try to spend some time *outside at night* before bed, perhaps go for a night walk or just sit and stargaze.

# 2.
# Focus on the positive and the sensory when in nature

♥ *Use one sense at a time as a focus.* This can be done either sitting or standing in one place or when walking. For example, visually observe all around you, from the very smallest thing to the wide-open sky then close your eyes and listen to all the sounds around you before focussing on the felt sensations like the wind in your hair or sun on your face. Take some gentle, deep breaths and pay attention to the different smells outside and whether you can taste something different, like the salt spray when by the ocean. This can be a practice that takes only a few moments or one that extends over half an hour or so.

♥ *Do something novel and playful to maximise the benefit to your brain.* ie. put your cheek or belly against a tree trunk, take your shoes off and have a paddle or dig your toes into the sand or grass. Really pay attention to how these new sensations feel in your body.

♥ *Develop your sense of wonder.* Look at something you would otherwise pay little attention to. ie. Look under a rock or deep into the grass, really watch what the birds are doing, lie on your back and do some cloud spotting; 'put on some new glasses' to really see the world.

♥ *Breathe deeply* with your expiration taking longer than your inspiration and gently put your hand on your heart to stimulate the Vagus nerve's calming effect.

## 3.
## Engage in self-guided or facilitated deeper explorations in nature

- ♥ Go on a *guided forest bathing walk* or attend a meditation or gentle exercise session in a natural place (like yoga or tai chi).

- ♥ Try bushwalking, camping or kayaking taking care to *spend some time reflecting* on the beauty of the place you are in rather than rushing through it. Ideally, this would be for at least 3 days but even a few hours bushwalking once per week is beneficial.

- ♥ You could participate in these activities on your own, with your family or maybe *find a nature-buddy* to commit to regular green mind times.

We know connecting to nature helps grow our green mind, fostering happiness and creativity. And lacing nature through our day is something we can all do to enrich our lives. Developing greater awareness of the present moment through mindfulness meditation practices can help us do this. Let's explore how this might work next.

## MEDITATION – NATURALLY...

Over many years, I have developed a regular mindfulness meditation practise and have done various courses and lots of study and exploration of different types of meditation. Through this I have come to understand that being in nature provides an opportunity for the mind to rest and reset, like the meditation experience. Combining the two enriches both. This may mean meditating out in a natural environment, using natural elements as a point of focus, or nature as a background soundscape.

Mindfulness meditation has its roots in Buddhism – essentially being a secular form of the mind training practised by Buddhist monks and teachers. Buddhism is a philosophy espoused by Gautama Buddha, a man who lived in 6th century BC in northern India. His teachings are focussed on reducing the suffering of humans and other sentient animals. A major cause of our emotional pain is accepting the inevitability of change and difficult experiences – loss, sickness, ageing and death. Mental training to improve concentration and awareness is a core practise of Buddhism. It helps people see things more clearly and to cope with the ups and downs of life.

In mindfulness meditation, you learn how to pay attention to the present moment by noticing your thoughts, feelings and the sensations felt both inside your body and coming in through your senses. The practice cultivates a sense of curiosity and self-kindness towards experience. It is a state of heightened awareness of the present and can be quite restful. This contrasts with the state of restless thinking where the untrained mind worries about the future or ruminates on the past. As past and future are largely beyond our control, spending a lot of time thinking about them is reliably anxiety provoking. Long-time meditation teacher and author, Eric Harrison ruefully states, "we don't have to live permanently in the present and never think of other things. Just to spend 5 to 10 minutes of each hour consciously on Planet Earth would be a huge improvement!"[205]

Initially, many people become aware of the chaotic nature of their minds with thoughts and images chasing one another seemingly at random. With regular practise, it becomes easier to simply notice the nature of the mind without becoming caught up in thinking. Just as with learning any new skill, mindfulness meditation takes time, patience and perseverance. It can help to remember how challenging it was to master other abilities, like playing an instrument or a sport. The first attempts, or first few hundred, are often humbling.

## Mindfulness basics

Mindfulness practise usually begins with consciously becoming aware of your body. The points of contact between you and the floor, chair, or ground, your breathing, and the sounds and sights around you. There is often a point of focus. This might be sounds or bodily sensations, like breathing. What many don't realise is that mindfulness meditation can be done anywhere. You don't have to be sitting crossed legged on a cushion in front of a candle. Often, it's good to be moving in some way, especially if you are feeling unable to sit still. This is why slow walking or stretching can be restorative. The key is to be paying attention to whatever is happening in the present moment rather than distracted by thinking.

It can be good to practise in different ways throughout the day. Craig Hassed, a medical doctor and mindfulness meditation teacher, speaks of punctuating your day with *full stops* and *commas* of meditation[206]. A comma might be an episode of a few minutes where a full stop may be longer, say 15-30 minutes of a more formal practise. In this way, there is an increase in overall awareness of the present moment throughout the day and you learn to come out of your head and into your body. This takes you away from worrying about the future or ruminating on the past, and brings you more fully into the present moment. Doing this helps to switch off underlying tension from the sympathetic nervous system and turns on the restful vagal response described earlier. As a result, the overall tone of the day is less pressured and, because of the intentional focus on the full experience, you become better at noticing the good things. For example, rather than rushing around mentally ticking off your 'to do list', a mindfulness comma encourages you to stop, feel the earth under your feet, the warmth of the sun on your face and the breeze on your skin. Pausing to notice a few slow breaths helps the tension run off your shoulders and you can continue with your day more focussed and less stressed. It only takes a few moments but, when done often throughout the day, the impact may be profound.

## *Sparking the relaxation response*

Including these moments of mindfulness is a way of intentionally inducing what has been called the relaxation response by scientists. This term was first used by Dr Herbert Benson in the 1960s and describes the ability we all have to encourage our body to slow down and relax. A cardiologist, professor and founder of Harvard's Mind/Body Medical Institute, Benson's work helped demystify meditation and make it more mainstream. The relaxation response is essentially the opposite of the flight or fight response. It helps bring the body back from a stressful state into a relaxed, responsive state. He describes it as "an inducible, physiologic state of quietude".[207] In his book *The Relaxation Response*, Dr Benson outlines a structured way to create this response, but many other practices can initiate it. These include sitting practices like prayer and meditation, moving mindfully through yoga, tai chi and qi gong and hands-on therapies like massage and acupuncture. Spending quiet time in nature, while not specifically mentioned by Benson, is also likely to elicit this state. Incorporating nature into the mindful moments, or as the backdrop to a formal meditation practice, enriches the experience, deepening the relaxation response. Helping turn the red mind green.

In the decades since Benson first published his work, the research on mindfulness meditation has grown exponentially. Thousands of scientific papers have been published exploring how this ancient practice affects our mind and body. This has especially influenced practitioners in the fields of neuropsychology and positive psychology. The paradigm shift that occurred with the discovery of *neuroplasticity* underpins much of this work. Neuroplasticity describes how the connections within our brain and nervous system change according to our experience. The adage 'neurons which fire together, wire together' encapsulates how recurrent thoughts are laid down into brain structure. So, if we are frequently thinking negatively, criticising ourselves and others, we are laying down the hardware for hurt. Alternatively, we can actively practise positivity. We are not stuck with a fixed mindset. Neuroplasticity enables us to change our brain to increase feelings of safety, connection and satisfaction. And if we incorporate nature into this approach, we can turn our brain from red to green.

## *Turning a red mind green*

Presenting at the Australian Meditation Conference in 2018, neuropsychologist Rick Hansen described how we can use mindfulness practice to rewire our brain to increase happiness. Hansen described the mind as being like a garden and outlined three key steps to creating greater happiness. The process involves embedding positive experiences into our brain by focussing on them. He calls this 'taking in the good'. It begins by fully engaging with what is present by noticing all elements of the current experience, a simple mindfulness practise. The second step is to reduce the negative or 'pull the weeds' by letting unpleasant elements be. The last step, increasing the positive, is 'planting flowers', or paying attention to the enjoyable things around you.

We can use the everyday experience of standing on a suburban street to unpack this further. Mindfully noticing all the information coming in through the senses helps you become aware of the soft breeze in your hair and the fragrance of nearby flowers, as well as the busy traffic. These pleasant sensations can be thought of as the 'flowers' of your experience. Focussing on them, while simply letting the sight of the traffic be, will help increase feelings of happiness and rewire the brain accordingly. It's important the negative is not actively suppressed because this would require mental effort. Instead, unpleasant elements are just noticed and then left alone.

In his writings, Hanson emphasises the need to really stay with a positive experience by focussing on it intentionally to truly embed or *install* these changes in the brain. He dives into deeper detail explaining how internalizing experiences of our core needs being met "builds up a sense of fullness and balance so we can meet the next moment and its challenges feeling already strong, already happy, loving, and at peace."[208] Remember our core needs are to feel safe, content and connected. So, to stay with the same example, after noticing the flower's fragrance, you can enhance the experience by taking a few deep breaths to deeply inhale the perfume. Consciously evoking feelings of gratitude that someone has grown flowers for you to enjoy reassures your old brain. It relaxes, knowing your core needs for satisfaction and connection are being met. Happiness and contentment flow from this. The simple experience of smelling a flower has then been embedded into your brain as an expression of gratitude. As Hanson says, "we become more grateful by repeatedly installing experiences of gratitude. We become more mindful by repeatedly installing experiences of mindfulness."[208]

Slowing down and practising mindfulness is the first step because it gives us the mental space to notice the flower's fragrance, the birdsong, or the drifting of clouds overhead. When we step outside, there is always an element of the natural world we can appreciate in this way. Understanding the principles of various meditation teachings and using them in combination with the delights found in nature, helps develop a deeper mindfulness experience throughout the day. The work of Rick Hansen and others tells us that doing these brief practices regularly will change the structure of our brain, so we feel happier more often. Just as repeatedly lifting weights will bulk up our muscles and increase their strength.

## How meditation protects our genes

Researchers have also discovered that as well as reducing feelings of stress and unhappiness meditation helps protect our genetic material. In 2009, Australian scientist Dr Elizabeth Blackburn and her colleagues won the Nobel Prize for discovering the link between ill health and short *telomeres*. Located on the ends of our chromosomes, the iconic double helix shaped chain of our DNA, telomeres behave a little like the end on a shoelace. They protect the chromosome from damage as a lace-end stops the lace from unravelling. The shorter telomeres are, the less healthy you are. In this way telomere length is a marker of the age of our DNA, our biological age, if you like. This research helps explain why some people look much older than their chronological age, and vice versa.

Regular meditation increases the length and strength of the telomeres so protects the chromosomes they bookend. It is thought meditation does this by reducing anxious rumination and inducing the relaxation response. The increase in telomere length is thought to improve immune function and reduce harmful inflammation in the body by ensuring the correct genes are switched on and off[209]. So when you're meditating, or achieving a meditation-like mind state, you are doing some personal genetic engineering. Studies haven't yet confirmed that time in nature confers the same benefit but given the evidence to date that forest bathing reduces the stress response in a similar way to meditation, this is highly likely. Slowing down and mindfully connecting with the natural world allows us to combine the benefits of these two medicines – nature and meditation. The effect of this is powerful and goes to the core of our being as the relaxation response is switched on, our brain is rewired, and our telomeres are lengthened.

## KEY POINTS

- ❤ Mindfulness meditation is a secular form of the mind training practised by Buddhist monks
- ❤ During mindfulness practise you cultivate awareness of the present moment
- ❤ The *relaxation response* describes our body's shift into a calm state
- ❤ Meditation and mindful time in nature both elicit the relaxation response
- ❤ We can use mindfulness practises to rewire our brains to increase happiness
- ❤ Meditation has been linked to the health of our chromosomes

While knowing the science and keeping up to date with current research is satisfying, there's nothing quite like personal experience for learning. The ups and downs of life provide plenty of fodder for self-understanding, and for working out how best to cope when difficulties arise. Nature can be our friend, therapist and teacher in dark times. Let's move on to explore how, beginning with my story as a case study.

# 10

# A Green Mind Approach To Mental Illness, Stress, And Suffering

*"Climb the mountains and get their good tidings. Nature's peace will flow into you as sunshine flows into the trees. The winds will blow their own freshness into you, and the storms their energy, while cares will drop away from you like the leaves of Autumn."*

~John Muir

## GRIEVING WITH A GREEN MIND

While writing this chapter, I was blindsided by the sudden death of my mother. This followed close behind several other hugely stressful events. These emotional shockwaves pushed me to expand the practices I was already using to keep myself well – mindfulness and nature. I started reading and investigating different approaches to meditation and went on a mindfulness retreat set deep in the wilderness. I spent as much time outside as possible and used all I'd learnt about gratitude and focussing on the positive and applied it, especially when in nature.

This meant that when I woke each morning, I would lie in bed and really pay attention to the chorus of birdsong. I can see into nearby treetops from bed, so I would listen to the birds and watch the leaves moving, notice the sky and feel the breeze from the open window move across my face. I consciously went through how safe I felt, nestled in bed, and how grateful I was that I awoke this way each day – with birdsong! I also allowed myself to feel a deep love for where I was, for my family asleep in their beds, our dog resting on his blanket and the beautiful part of the city I lived in. In this way I was deliberately evoking feelings of safety, gratitude, and love to remind my brain that my core needs to feel safe, satisfied and connected were being met. This calming ritual began before I stepped out of bed.

Then I would take my breakfast outside to eat, mindfully savouring each mouthful. Using all my senses to soak in the nature around me, I'd appreciate all the delights, from the play of light in the gumtree's canopy to the feel of cool air on my face. There is almost always a constant state of motion outside, leaves rustling on some tree or plant, a bird going about its day or an ant marching purposefully somewhere. This movement is a reminder of the inevitability of change. While the other animals' activity offers the perspective that I am but a small part of a much larger world. Noticing the canopy of gumtrees overhead I'd take time to appreciate the shade and shelter they provide, the oxygen they generate for me to breathe and the carbon dioxide they take in from my exhalation. This exchange of breath between me and the trees helped me feel connected to the world around me and grateful for simply being able to breathe in fresh air. I'd consciously allow feelings of gratitude to flood me as I inhaled deeply.

Depending on the day, I might then take the dog for a walk through the park or ride to work. Whatever I did I would pay attention to the details of nature, both large and small, through as many senses as I could. Making these simple activities mindful and nature focussed, literally stopping to smell the roses.

I committed to spending two to three hours every week in deeper nature immersion to really calm my stress and lift my mood. I found a great book with day walks in Melbourne and went to as many different places as I could. This was a silver lining because I discovered many beautiful remnants of bushland and wetlands within a city of five million people. Each time I went, I found a spot to sit and mindfully take in where I was, again using my senses to really pay attention and 'be'. To embed the beauty and gratitude and learn from nature.

One remarkable experience was being surrounded by kangaroos. I was walking through an expansive nature reserve with a large, central lake in the middle of the big homes and fat roads of sprawling suburbia. Around the lake are two paths. The outer gravel path is preferred by most. Couples or groups power walk or ride this way, seemingly oblivious to the nature they pass. A second trail, a meandering nature walk, veers from the busy path through grassland and bush to the water's edge. As I emerged from the paperbark forest, I found myself interrupting a mob of wallabies and kangaroos relaxing in the sun. Being outnumbered by another species, observed as an outsider, and treated with careful indifference was heart stopping. It was also very grounding. It's simply impossible to be away in your head worrying with a mob of kangaroos watching. Once again, the landscape provided a lesson on perspective. I was just one person amid many other animals, all sharing the same air and sunshine.

I have had to prioritise nature experiences and commit to them, putting time aside and not allowing other things to get in the way. This is a part of my therapy, like going to a counsellor. I treat it with the same respect, writing a time in my diary and making sure I get there on time to be with myself, in nature.

Mum died just before our annual family camping trip. As we had to wait for a coroner to investigate the cause of her death, we were in limbo, not quite knowing what to do. We decided to go away, but for a shorter time than usual. The bush camp site we visit is remote, out of phone reception and without power. The few days we spent there allowed me to really feel the loss of my mother and to place it within the wider landscape of my emotions and my life. She was my first nature mentor, the person who developed my curiosity and love of the natural world. As I watched the sea, clouds, and birds I could feel her presence and hear her voice in my head pointing out the beauty around me. It felt right to be immersed in a beautiful natural place to feel my grief.

As part of my grieving process, I decided to go away for a four-day meditation retreat to a remote part of Tasmania, overlooking the ocean. Part of the retreat was in silence. Admittedly, had I known this before leaving, I probably wouldn't have gone. The thought of being with others and not speaking to them was foreign. Surprisingly, I enjoyed the silent time. It removed the need to engage in social chat with strangers, which was quite restful. As someone who works with people, being around others, meditating, walking and eating together without having to speak felt good. There was the feeling of being with fellow travellers but not responsible for attending to their needs. Also, the comparing, judging, criticising, and social engineering that often goes on when a group of people get together, disappears. This is such a relief.

This nature-rich approach helped hold me through my pain. Others suffering with grief, burn-out or mental illness could also consider a method which incorporates nature. Perhaps in its setting or within the therapeutic process itself. There are a whole range of practices to help us rebuild ourselves and our relationships where nature forms a central role. Let's step through a few now to see how beautifully natural elements can be woven into treatment programs, both inside and outside healthcare environments.

## NATURE GUIDED THERAPY

Nature-guided therapy is a type of counselling which draws on the philosophies of positive psychology and ecopsychology. Ecopsychology aims to enhance both individual and environmental wellbeing and the relationship between them. A person's thoughts and feelings are understood within the broader context of their natural environment, and nature is seen as an intrinsic part of human emotional wellbeing rather than separate from it.

This contrasts with the model of psychotherapy founded by Sigmund Freud where the inner workings of the individual, the 'psyche', take centre stage. When thinking about psychotherapy, the image of a patient lying on a couch in an austere room while the learned psychiatrist listens intently, springs to mind. There is no nature in the room, no flowers, no view out the window. Perhaps this was intentional. Freud is reported to have said "nature is eternally remote. She destroys us – coldly, cruelly, and relentlessly."[210]

Nature is also absent from today's hospital-based psychiatry. Often patients are admitted involuntarily for the safety of themselves and others. Those suffering from severe mental illnesses like psychosis, have lost contact with reality. So, they're no longer safe to live in the community. In the process of receiving inpatient care, they are shut away from the natural world, often only able to go outside into very small courtyards to get fresh air. Having very unwell and often quite traumatised people kept inside, away from other living things, seems harsh. Might there be a gentler way to ease their suffering and help them recover while also keeping them safe?

Thankfully, some health professionals are now moving to a different way of thinking about the workings of our mind and what therapy might look like. Either by stepping outside the traditional consulting room into the open air, or by encouraging their patients to purposefully engage with nature. As nature holds an enormous variety of positive sensory stimuli, it provides a terrific resource for this new type of therapy. As described above, the positive nature-encounters we gloss over every day can be thought of as delights, precious and special. Rushing through our busy lives we barely notice them. Our baked-in negativity bias makes sure we notice the potential risks and harms, but not these beauties. Yet, nature is full of them, we just need to be on the lookout. The melodic birdsong, the tree's patterned bark and the softness of grass underfoot – sensory pleasures are everywhere.

George W. Burns is a psychologist who uses a nature-guided approach to help individuals and couples improve their relationships. He writes, "If you want to enhance self-concept, self-esteem, and self-confidence, facilitate treatment of the mentally ill or improve family relationships, then the research is clear: assist your clients to engage in more nature-based interactions."[211] As a therapist who focusses on helping couples achieve happiness, he uses nature-based experiences as a way of increasing the frequency of positive feelings in his clients. Research has found stable, happy, and lasting partnerships are characterised by a five-to-one ratio of positive to negative emotions[212]. Many couples, busy with work and family, find themselves struggling to achieve this ratio and nature can be a way to tip the balance back in the right direction.

In his writings, Burns uses case studies to outline the process. Let's break it down further and explore how it works in practise. First, Burns asks couples to recall when they met and how they spent their first times together, looking for positive, nature-based resources within their experience. Perhaps walking by the ocean watching the sun set or going on a picnic together. They then reflect on whether perhaps these activities have been brushed aside as the busyness of life has taken over. Couples are also asked to complete a Sensory Awareness Index (SAI). In this questionnaire, the requirement is to list twenty enjoyable experiences under each of the five sensory headings. For example, under sight – flowers; ocean; laughing children; in touch – sun on skin; wind in hair; feet in sand etc.

Each person is then asked to increase the amount of positive sensory experiences in their life by deliberately scheduling them into their diary, so they are not forgotten. The next step involves the couple deciding how to increase time spent with one another having these enjoyable encounters. To help build engagement and connection to the pleasurable nature-based activity they are taken through a nature-guided mindfulness exercise using each sensory modality. This can then be practised individually and together to enrich the experience and deepen the impact it has on them as a couple.

To move towards meaning, Burns facilitates a reflection and discussion to help the partners understand how to enhance their relationship. He uses simple questions like: 'what did you discover in doing that?' Burns describes one married couple who spend time together watching a glorious sunset. The wife says the view of the sunset is ruined by the presence of power lines, while her husband doesn't understand why she would let these small things diminish her enjoyment of the sunset. Upon reflection, she understands her tendency to focus on negative aspects of their marriage, rather than positive. Through this introspection, she begins the process of valuing the good in their relationship. In turn, this reinforces positive interactions with her partner, helping heal the rift between them.

As you can see from this example, nature-guided therapy is a simple way to repair strained relationships. And nature-based interactions are readily available and free. Every day there is a sunset and sunrise, a morning bird chorus and the night sky almost always has a star to spot.

There are also many therapeutic approaches which take place far from a consulting room. Bush Adventure Therapy is an Australian version of Wilderness Adventure Therapy and has programs for families, adults and teenagers where participants are taken out into the bush for physical adventures. This builds on personal strengths and helps those involved gain valuable insights into the path their life is taking. There are programs for those with cancer and other chronic illness, those living with a disability and for families going through a tough time. Programs range from day trips to multi-day hikes.

With a similar approach to Nature Guided Therapy, Bush Counselling is offered by some therapists and may suit those who want to talk but need more than the hour usually offered by clinic-based mental health professionals. It will appeal to people who want to talk outside four walls and who like to be doing things when they're outside. This innovative approach can include bush walking, fishing, kayaking or walking a labyrinth with the metaphors to be found in these activities used to help solve emotional problems. For example, the flow of a river can help ease a situation and help a dilemma move towards resolution, while the rhythm of bush walking punctuates a conversation with silence yet keeps the conversation moving[213].

One of the most healing natural elements is water. Simply looking at the sea, listening to a river running or immersing ourselves in a bath, we are soothed by it. Let's dip our toes in to uncover how water can help us address health problems.

# THE COMFORT OF WATER

Water can be therapeutic in all sorts of places, both inside and outside. It is a great way to bring the relaxing effect of nature inside, into our homes, hospitals and other health settings. Whether submerging our bodies in a deep bath, looking at an aquarium or indoor fountain, or listening to the gentle patter of rain, the calming effect of water is profound.

Immersion in water can be very soothing, especially for a distressed infant or elderly dementia sufferer, with a deep, warm, relaxation bath. Many women also find water helps them cope with the pains of labour. The warmth of the water relaxes muscular tension and supports body weight. Perhaps there's a primitive reflex involved which helps calm both mother and baby in this often-stressful time around birth.

Aboriginal Elder and musician, Archie Roach, sung about sacred waterholes where Aboriginal women gave birth. Afterwards, the placenta (afterbirth) was buried under a nearby tree. This tree would belong to the infant's Dreaming. In his song 'A Child Was Born Here', Roach described this beautiful, sacred practice[26]. He used his music to educate audiences about the care needed when walking near waterways. Many were special birthing places.

Perhaps this ancient ritual accounts for the sense of sacredness felt when near billabongs and other waterholes in the Australian bush. Maybe there's an ingrained memory of this connection between water and childbirth in all of us. Most likely, throughout all our evolutionary stories we gave birth near rivers, pools and ponds. It's just that most non-First Nations people have lost this consciousness. The remaining fragments being the pull many labouring women feel to be in, or near, water.

In the days before Aged Care facilities were businesses run by corporations, elderly people who could not be cared for at home were often looked after in Nursing Homes by trained nurses. Distressed dementia sufferers, who would often wander about at night, were given a relaxation bath to calm them. The warm water soothed, and they would then settle and return to bed. This was a much kinder and more natural approach than sedating them with medication, although was more demanding from a staffing perspective. Might we hope to shift back towards these watery methods in the future?

Interaction with water doesn't have to be passive and relaxing. Sometimes the healing process requires the vigorous engagement and activity of the surf.

## Catching waves

Outdoor experiences in water can help a variety of health problems. Apart from the enjoyment and physical exercise, getting out into and onto the water can calm the mind. Here in Australia, we have a strong surf culture. So, it's not surprising that catching waves is proving to be a great way to help those struggling with emotional difficulties. Surfing programs can form part of a treatment plan for those with drug dependency, social isolation and mental health issues. Participants range from children living with autism through to returned service men and women. For those with drug dependency problems it seems the thrill of catching a wave can match the high of drug use and, combined with the mindfulness of surfing, may reduce drug cravings and agitation.

Surfing for Autism is an innovative approach where kids are taken into the water to learn skills like balancing on a surfboard or body surfing. They are guided by experienced surfers and so can do something that might otherwise be thought impossible for them. The need to be completely focussed on the body in this way can help reduce the anxiety experienced by many people with autism. These children are often distressed by sensory triggers, like the feel of clothing or footwear. The steady, hydrostatic pressure of the ocean, along with being supported by someone they trust, can help alleviate this distress. They are held physically by the water and emotionally by their mentor.

Surfers Healing is an American non-profit organisation which has come to Australia to run annual events with like-minded groups here. They are motivated by the positive responses from children with autism and their families and say, "when we help kids get up on a board, we're challenging preconceived notions of capability. When we encourage participants to dive in, we're supporting them to engage with the world. And when we go out and ride waves together, we're empowering families to believe their kids 'can'."[214]

Another program aimed at children, but those experiencing social isolation or mental health challenges rather than autism, is Open Mind. Based on the Victorian Surf Coast, it began as a pilot project for the UK based surf therapy model created by The Wave Project. The initial pilot was a success, with most participants reporting an improvement in their wellbeing indicators, the biggest improvement was in the measure 'I've been having fun'![215] Open Mind has gone on to provide surf therapy programs to many children, offering the combination of group surfing and mentoring to improve participant's confidence and happiness[216].

Soldier On Surf Therapy is a program created by a collaboration between Surfing Australia and Soldier On, an organisation which supports returned veterans. It aims to help men and women struggling with mental health issues like Post Traumatic Stress Disorder and depression. It involves both two-day surf camps and learn to surf programs to get participants confident about being out on the water surfing. Underpinning this program is the knowledge that surfing provides not only physical exercise, but also a mentally restful and restorative experience.

When learning to surf you need to be completely focussed on where your body is in relation to the board and where the board sits on the wave. You need to be alert to everything around you. All your senses are engaged as you feel the water on your skin and in your hair, get bobbed up and down by the swell, hear the swish of the waves, see the movement of each wave as it comes towards you and taste the salt as you go under water. Surfing is literally an immersive experience, forcing you to be completely in your body and in tune with your senses, and this drowns out the 'mind chatter' of worry or sadness.

Australian world champion surfer Layne Beachley says, "the ocean especially has helped me through some of the most dramatic and dark periods of my life, from the deepest depths of depression, pain and suffering. The one place I always resort to is the ocean because it's free of judgement, free of criticism and it's a place where I can leave my troubles on the beach and dive into the water, which rinses my mind, body and soul. I use the visualisation to cleanse me of the torment, pain and suffering that I may be experiencing at the time. It allows me to be present in the moment and enjoy the environment that I'm in. My time in the water is when I can do a lot of my own healing, thinking and I just feel free and liberated. I commit to immersing myself in nature every single day, whether it's in the ocean, walking barefoot on the grass, going for a bushwalk or a bike ride – it's an important part of my life and it's something that I prioritise every day."[201]

You can see from Layne's description how healing surfing is for her. While she engages in hours of time in the surf, just a short swim in the ocean gives many of the same benefits for everyday people. The way plunging into the waves stimulates all the senses, shifts our focus from the thinking mind into our body. We are grounded as we float, held by the ocean and rocked by the swell. The sound of the ocean can be soothing all on its own. And we can be far from the shoreline to benefit from it. Water soundscapes can be used in the most sterile places, like hospital wards. Let's see how we might bring the seaside into the bedside.

## THE SOUNDS OF NATURE

The sounds we would have heard when in utero, like the rhythmic whoosh of our mother's circulation and breathing, accompanied us throughout our early development. Natural sounds arising through the movement of water are also rhythmic and quiet, like the ocean, falling rain or a waterfall. Perhaps this explains how studies have found that listening to these natural sounds can improve sleep for patients after surgery and in critical care wards. In these specialised medical units, there is often a lot of background noise. The hum of various machinery, alarms going off intermittently and staff talking as they monitor the condition of their patients.

This noisy environment can impair sleep, interrupt rest and slow a patient's recovery. In a 2013 study in Tehran, patients were played sounds of water—the sea or rain falling—for one hour during the night.

A control group did not have these nature sounds. The results showed that sleep was improved for those patients hearing water during the night, even if only for one hour. The authors concluded, using natural water sounds is "recommended as a method for masking environmental noises, sleep induction, improving sleep, and maintaining sleep in the coronary care unit."[217]

Listening to nature sounds, including water sounds, has also been found to help recovery after psychological stress. In a Swedish study, participants were stressed by having to do an arithmetic question under timed conditions. They were then exposed to either nature sounds, road traffic noise or to the ambient noise of ventilation systems in nearby buildings. The group who listened to nature sounds recovered more quickly as measured through their heart rate and other bodily signs of stress[218]. Playing ambient water sounds seems to be such a simple and effective way to reduce stress and improve sleep, yet this is not something currently part of most health care settings. A way to combine the positive benefits of both the sounds and sights of water would be to have an indoor fountain or perhaps play sounds of water and have pictures of the ocean, a river or a waterfall on the walls.

## HEALING NATURE WHILE HEALING YOURSELF

The *ecopsychological* approach sees benefits to both people and the wider natural environment. Healing of troubled minds occurs alongside regeneration of the landscape. A great example of a community project incorporating this approach was Feel Blue, Touch Green[219]. In this program people experiencing social isolation and chronic mental illness were involved in environmental rehabilitation work in coastal Victoria. They would come each week and participate in various nature-based activities including tree planting and plant propagation. This provided time with others and so increased their social interactions, and there was also the healthy physical activity out in the fresh air. For many of these people in their daily life, most of their time was spent inside on their own. Getting out into nature with others and working on an environmental project which had benefits for the broader community had immense value. There is also a powerful metaphor of healing the land as they were healing themselves.

In his memoir, *The Nature of Survival*, Victorian farmer Doug Lang captures the benefits of this approach for people like him who have struggled for years with mental health issues[137]. Lang has chronic depression and obsessive-compulsive disorder and has also experienced the ups and downs of alcohol and drug dependency and personal loss. He has a compelling story to tell about resilience and how nature has been a part of his therapeutic tool kit. Lang writes about how small things add up to make a positive impact in his day. He calls these things the "one percenters".

Doug Lang worked over many years to rehabilitate the degraded landscape on his family farm by planting trees and wildflowers and he refers to the Feel Blue, Touch Green approach saying, "it is the basics of this program I personally try to build into my lifestyle on a daily basis". [137] Seeing trees and flowers he has planted survive drought and weeds gives him a sense of satisfaction and purpose. Doug writes, "When I witness a plant survive like this, I feel a sense of achievement. I feel good about myself and my spirit is lifted immediately no matter how I am feeling beforehand. For me, it's like taking one of Mother Nature's natural uppers. In fact, that is what is happening. I am actually doing just that. I am getting a natural lift from one of the millions of Mother Nature's gifts. The great thing about this gift is that it is there for us all on any given day at any given time. We just need to stand still or walk quietly within the nature that surrounds us, look and listen and this little upper is there for the taking and it's free, but a little addictive. I know only too well that some days this works better than others. I am not silly enough to think that this little miracle will lift a grey depressive mood, but it will help. With depressive illnesses we need to look at the 1%. If we can rake in a few 1%ers during a depressive episode they will add up. I know if I go down the paddock feeling low and flat and do a bit of work amongst our trees, I never come back feeling worse. It is this little 1% that we can grab hold of and work with to improve our own wellbeing and to help us through another challenging time."

# GARDENING AS THERAPY

Therapeutic horticulture programs are a more structured approach with a particular rehabilitation or therapeutic outcome in mind. Officially, Horticulture Therapy is defined as 'a process of using plants and garden related activities to promote wellbeing of mind, body and spirit' (Horticultural Therapy Association of Victoria). These programs can be run in hospitals or in the community. As discussed earlier, the horticultural therapy approach is used in many different types of hospital settings with rehabilitation facilities often leading the way. There are also some community programs which are targeted at those who are living at home with their families. At Kevin Heinze Grow, a charity in Victoria, some 300 people a week engage in therapeutic horticulture sessions in sprawling gardens. There are 70 volunteers who come along to help, supervising gardening for program participants. Many people who participate in the programs have some sort of disability or are recovering from an acute brain injury (ABI). They are often in their teens or early adulthood, having been injured in car accidents and, as well as the garden activities providing them with physical rehabilitation, they get the social interaction of being with others. Importantly, they also learn skills like plant propagation and may gain retail experience as the centre has a small nursery where plants are sold.

Sitting within a busy suburb, this garden-community centre has a ramshackle quality, yet is a true jewel in the way it supports its community. Like many community-based organisations, the staff do transformative work on a tiny budget, providing vulnerable people with essential rehabilitation. Simply replanting a seedling into a larger pot engages the body's fine and gross movement systems as well as proprioception. This is the ability to know where parts of the body are in space and in relation to one another. It also strengthens eye muscles as the plant's tiny roots and leaves are focussed on. All sorts of gardening activities provide great physical therapy, and rather than being a boring set of repetitive exercises, participants are creating something, working with living things and helping plants grow. They engage in purposeful and helpful ways and give back to the community by creating potted plants that can be sold to raise much needed funds. When this activity is done with others in a small group, an additional therapeutic goal is met as participants engage in low demand social interactions. In this way the whole person is involved – physically, mentally and emotionally. This entire process takes place in the fresh air within a rambling garden rather than in the sterile environment of a health clinic.

The centre provides professional development for practitioners who facilitate horticulture therapy sessions for residents in nursing homes or, for those living independently, in community centres where elderly locals come and garden together. Some innovative nursing homes have garden spaces specifically designed for their residents with dementia. They have features like clothes lines, post boxes and bus stops. Patients will go to sit and wait for a bus, post their letter and hang 'washing' on the line. People suffering from dementia have impaired short term memory but are often able to recall experiences from long ago. These simple activities provide them with something to do that's easy and non-stressful and, because they are out in the garden, they are getting much needed sunshine and exercise. Trained staff also engage residents in gardening, a pastime they often fondly remember from their earlier life. Tending shrubs and flowers is relaxing, and being out in the garden provides opportunities for these elderly people to have serendipitous encounters with nature, from feeding birds to noticing new growth on plants. These are welcome distractions to the unpleasantness of being in a nursing home. As old-fashioned varieties such as roses and geraniums are chosen, pleasant memories are evoked, and feelings of reassurance arise for those who may feel stressed and lonely.

Some people are more likely to develop mental health issues than others. Those exposed to traumatic experiences, perhaps during their childhood, or through natural disaster and other calamities. Some have a strong family history of these health issues and others have a social background increasing their risk, maybe living with poverty, exposure to substance abuse or social isolation. Getting your green hour can be seen as a preventative health strategy for those at risk of developing stress-related mental health issues. Most city dwellers may fit into this category given the inherently stressful nature of urban life. This knowledge adds weight to the case for protecting the green spaces within and on the fringe of our cities, especially forests which meet criteria for forest bathing. Researcher Mardie Townsend says, "the need for therapeutic landscapes is greater than ever but most approaches to address health fail to recognise the therapeutic benefits of nature contact."

## SOOTHING TEENAGE ANGUISH WITH NATURE

Given that some quarter of Australians will have experienced an episode of depression before they turn eighteen, adolescents are a high-risk group for mental illness. Supportive relationships with family and friends are protective and it's important for parents to find time to be with and talk to their teenagers. Many health experts suggest using time in the car to talk to your children but time out in nature is a much better opportunity for a rich, quality interaction to occur.

When walking together by the sea or in the local park, the mind is resting and relaxed, in its 'green' responsive mode. Whereas in the car our minds are busy looking for potential threats and much more likely to be in 'red' reactive mode. Some health professionals promote the 'car chat' as optimal because eye contact is avoided, and the teenager is confined in the car, unable to get out of the conversation. However, the idea of a simple walk through a park is much kinder. It provides the soft visual distractions and calming sounds of nature, and gentle exercise helps to release any physical tension that's present. There is also the opportunity for the young person to move away if that's what they need to feel safe.

It might be fun and novel to go on a night walk with your teenager. This can be a time to chat about life in general and any worries they may be having. Spending this time outside at night is especially beneficial because the darkness and time away from a screen helps ready the brain for sleep, allowing the melatonin levels to start to rise. Melatonin is the hormone released by our brain which signals to the body it's time for sleep. Our melatonin level rises in the evening and drop towards dawn. Disruption to melatonin production affects sleep quality and duration. Sleep is enormously important for keeping our emotions and mind happy, and most teenagers don't get enough. If unable to go out for a walk, try sitting in the yard for a while. Simply noticing the stars and any wildlife moving about is relaxing. There's nothing quite like seeing an owl silently swooping through the night sky or watching a possum making its way through the trees. Doing this with the young people in your life is a simple, calm way of being together and enriching your relationship.

## Bush Adventure Therapy

Sometimes teenagers have huge struggles and need specialist help. We often hear about connecting with mental health professionals in a clinic, but there are unique opportunities to be had outdoors. An example of a structured, nature-based approach to help unhappy young people are the Bush Adventure Therapy (BAT) programs. These help adolescents experiencing mental health issues, isolation, and disengagement from school. Or those with family tension or drug and alcohol addictions. Participants are taken out into areas of wilderness and provided with carefully planned challenges and scenarios to help work through life difficulties. These programs provide time away from the stressful negative influences of the young person's usual life and a time to disconnect from the demands of social media.

The BAT guides create challenges like multi-day walks, caving, rafting, and climbing. During these activities things may go wrong and risks are taken. It can, of course, be quite stressful for teenagers in these situations to work out how to navigate the next step. They may feel hungry, tired, and sometimes scared. But they have the support of mentors who encourage them to look deep within themselves and keep going. Participants might not think they can complete a fifteen-kilometre hike and yet, with encouragement, they do. The teenagers learn they are stronger than they believed, have capacities they didn't know they had and feel proud of their achievements. In this way, these young people are developing their inner resources. So, when they go home and things are going wrong, instead of reaching for a drug, or doing some other harmful activity, they make a better choice.

There is great strength in doing this with others, watching how they navigate the difficulties and sharing both success and failure. A skilful mentor uses metaphor to relate these wilderness challenges to situations back home. This helps the teenager explore their internal emotional landscape within the broader natural landscape. Opportunities for solo time provide a space where boredom may be felt. Teens are used to being almost constantly entertained by technology, so they learn how to sit with the discomfort of little stimulation, of nature's quietness. This time alone allows for inner reflection. During conversations with mentors afterwards, the experience is unpacked, and the teenager has the chance to explore the meaning of it more fully.

Bush Adventure Therapy is different to outdoor education, where teaching experiences are offered to school students in the outdoors. There can be significant overlap between these two approaches, but BAT is generally more individualised. A survey of the evidence by Adventure Works found that BAT helps healing, restoration, growth, learning and development[220]. The survey's authors break the outcomes into three main facets; being socially connected with peers and mentors, spending time in nature and experiencing a sense of adventure. The social connection benefits help to reduce stress, promote feelings of value and support recovery from mental illness. Spending time in nature promotes restoration of mind and body and inspiration for change as well as improving concentration and clear thinking. The component of adventure builds self-esteem and confidence, strengthens independence and assertiveness, and increases internal control and motivation.

Some young people need regular engagement over a period of months rather than a single multi-day adventure. One example of a weekly, community-based project is the Active in Parks' Youth Ambassadors Program. Here, teenagers experiencing lack of engagement at school or other issues become 'park ambassadors'[221]. They go on surfing, canoeing, sailing, hiking, and beachcombing to get to know their local parks and beaches. Apart from learning these outdoor adventure skills, they develop communication, team building and leadership capacities. They then go on to share their knowledge about national parks with peers. Having the opportunity to teach others builds self-confidence and a sense of agency. Getting out of the school environment and into the 'real' world can help break patterns feeding disengagement from education. This rich experiential learning, or 'learning by doing' is powerful and can be transformative in a young person's life.

Another high-risk group for mental and emotional suffering are Aboriginal and Torres Strait Islander people. Many innovative programs to address these issues have been developed from within their communities. Connecting to Country forms a key part of the healing process. This involves relating to nature in meaningful and spiritual ways and is often led by Elders. We can learn from First Nations people about how to heal through being with nature in a deep way. Let's explore some of their ideas a little.

## YARNING AND GANMA

Aboriginal and Torres Strait Islander people have endured over two hundred years of dispossession, displacement, and trauma through the process of colonisation. Like other First Peoples, they may experience feelings of helplessness as their Country suffers environmental degradation from extractive industries, poor farming practices and land clearing for the building of roads and cities. Being uprooted from Country and often also torn away from family through a series of government-sanctioned interventions is profoundly damaging. This trauma may manifest in drug dependency, homelessness, incarceration, or domestic violence occurring down through generations. Such deep pain is reflected in high suicide rates, especially for young people, and the impact this has on communities is devastating.

As the legacy of colonisation lies at the root of their suffering, it can be difficult for First Nations people to engage in Western-style counselling for their mental health issues. The framing of a white 'expert' and black 'patient' can evoke colonial connotations of a master/servant relationship. A more culturally sensitive, and therefore effective, approach incorporates the Aboriginal practice of yarning, which involves storytelling, sharing history and exploring common ground.

A slow process, sometimes taking weeks or months, yarning gradually builds a trusting relationship through which problems are shared and worked through collaboratively. This contrasts to the much quicker, more direct Western-style where the doctor or therapist may interrupt and ask sensitive questions with little preamble.

Another Aboriginal practice and philosophy being incorporated into counselling approaches is ganma. The word is used by language groups of the Northern Territory to describe a place where salt and freshwater meet. Ganma is used metaphorically to describe the coming together of two different tribes and may be interpreted as 'if you'll listen to us, we'll listen to you'. Some are working to shift the field of psychology in Australia to increase the number of First Nations psychologists and have Indigenous concepts like cultural continuity, yarning and ganma brought into university psychology courses. One key initiative shaping this is the Australian Indigenous Psychology Education Project (AIPEP) led by Pat Dudgeon. A collaboration between university educators and students, Indigenous psychologists and support staff, AIPEP has developed a clear curriculum framework and advocated strongly for structural change to make mental health care more culturally sensitive and appropriate[222].

Specifically developed for suicide prevention in rural Aboriginal communities, 'We-Yarn' workshops facilitated by retired footballer Nathan Blacklock and mental health worker Fiona Livingstone encourage sharing of lived experience. While often given in an indoor venue, the outcomes seem to be best when held outdoors, on Country. Blacklock says, "That's where the healing can take place. For something personal to you, something that needs healing, it's best to be in a circle outdoors. Mother Earth looks after us."[223]

Sometimes these workshops bring together people from both Aboriginal and non-Aboriginal rural communities who are experiencing distress from witnessing the degradation of their Country or land through climate change-induced drought. These may involve facilitation from both Aboriginal and non-Aboriginal mental health workers. Such sessions provide space for personal experiences of ecological suffering to be shared. Ultimately, depressed farmers may come to understand the suffering Aboriginal people have endured through their displacement from Country, and this may shift and soften their attitudes.

Through such workshops, non-Aboriginal Australians are the beneficiaries of Indigenous wisdom of caring for Country. One farmer experiencing depression says, "Some of the Aboriginal people spoke about feelings of shame, like not seeing enough of their family or not providing enough. I sat there thinking it's an emotion Westerners should feel more of until we start helping fix the land we are helping to destroy. Now it's affecting our livelihoods." She goes on to describe an evolving sense of stewardship for the land, "At the end of the day I felt I came away with ideas about responsibility to not just our farm but to the river nearby, the birds and kangaroos too that live on our farm. We spoke of family and land ties during the day, too. If nothing more, I feel now like a custodian of the land I live on and that gives me pride. I am responsible for the living things that depend on the farm. ...I feel taller, as a result."[224]

We would all benefit from taking a more considered, thoughtful approach to helping those with mental health issues and if we could adapt our health system so that ganma and yarning underpin all consultations in which we seek to ease emotional suffering. Now, in general practice, the process is rushed. Doctors push to gather a history and make a diagnosis using a tool comprised of direct questions. They then generate a management plan and referral to a psychologist. This is all usually done in thirty minutes or less. And that's if the doctor involved doesn't take the quicker option of prescribing medication.

Taking the time needed for a person's story to unfold and providing a calming space for the interaction is so important. This time and space and gentle, open attention are part of the healing process. Shifting the location outside into nature adds another therapeutic element. The restorative powers of the natural world work their magic to soothe the nervous system. This eases the path for discussing difficult thoughts and feelings. It's not surprising the outcomes for We-Yarn, and similar programs, are better when sessions take place on Country.

# HEALING EMOTIONAL WOUNDS WITH NATURE

❤ *Nature guided therapy* sees the natural world as the place of healing

❤ Surfing programs help those experiencing trauma and those with autism

❤ Yarning and ganma are First Nations approaches

❤ Gentle immersion in water can soothe distress, emotional or physical pain

❤ *Bush Adventure Therapy* is a mode of outdoor therapy especially helpful for young people

❤ *Horticultural therapy* can be done individually or in groups

❤ Landscape restoration sees personal healing occur alongside repair of the Earth

❤ Nature sounds can soothe, even in critical care units within hospitals

# 11

# Growing Up With Nature

*"A child's world is fresh and new and beautiful, full of wonder and excitement. It is our misfortune that for most of us that clear-eyed vision, that true instinct for what is beautiful and awe-inspiring, is dimmed and even lost before we reach adulthood. If I had influence with the good fairy who is supposed to preside over the christening of all children, I should ask that her gift to each child in the world be a sense of wonder so indestructible that it would last throughout life, as an unfailing antidote against the boredom and disenchantments of later years, the sterile preoccupation with things that are artificial, the alienation from the sources of our strength.*
*If a child is to keep alive [their] inborn sense of wonder without any such gift from the fairies, [they] need the companionship of at least one adult who can share it, rediscovering with [them] the joy, excitement and mystery of the world we live in."*

~Rachel Carson, A Sense of Wonder [225]

A few years ago, when out walking, I came across a scene reminiscent of my childhood. Playing in an enormous puddle alongside the dirt road were three children around six to eight years of age. They had crafted old plastic milk bottles into boats. The little boy proudly explained how he had built a berth for his boat at the edge of the puddle. His sister had decorated several dirt mounds within the puddle with flowers and these were islands in their game. A misty rain fell but the children were oblivious, engaged in their story and the creation of another world known only to them.

Growing up in the suburbs of Melbourne in the 1970s, before computer games, the internet and smart phones, outdoor play was the norm. At the end of our street an area of bushland traversed by a creek was where neighbourhood children would gather to play. We spent hours 'down at the creek', after school or on the weekend, returning home for meals or when it got dark. Children of all ages would play together and there was never an adult in sight. I recall feeling safe, happy and free. The play we engaged in varied from making houses in the bushes and calling one another on our 'stick phones' through to more daring adventure. Sometimes we climbed into trees and once we had a challenge to jump from the high bank of the creek to the low bank. I hesitated on the edge just a moment too long, miscalculated the jump and landed in the water, twisting my ankle on the way. My friends dragged me out, helped me onto my bike and back up the street to home.

These types of exploratory nature play experiences shaped my early life, and that of my friends and many other children at that time. In his landscape memoir, Australian author and nature lover Tim Winton lyrically describes his childhood on the outskirts of Perth and the special way children explore nature[226]. "Being short and powerless, kids see the world low down and close up. On hands and knees, on their naked bellies, they feel it with an immediacy we can scarcely recall as adults. Remember all that wandering and dithering as you crossed the same ground again and again? It wouldn't have seemed so at the time but with all that apparently aimless mooching you were weaving a tapestry of arcane lore- where the chewy gum bulges best from the tree, where the yellow sand makes a warm pad to lie on beneath the rattling banksias – that didn't just make the world more comprehensible, but rendered it intimate, even sacred."

Our childhoods were characterised by the freedom to explore local natural areas without adult supervision for extended periods of time, either alone or with others. By groups of different aged children playing together, a variety of both adventurous and contemplative experiences emerged. The lack of an adult presence allowed for self-determination and problem solving.

Today's parents struggle with the worry of kids being out on their own in car-dominated suburbs. And the quiet judgement of others for granting their children this freedom. It is a battle to provide opportunities for children to develop their resilience and sense of confidence in navigating their neighbourhood, by just letting them cycle, walk or catch public transport without an adult. The social and physical constraints can be difficult to overcome.

Apart from developing self-agency, time alone travelling their home turf provides children with the opportunity for serendipitous encounters with nature. Watching as a bird gathers sticks for its nest, scuffing through autumn leaves, brushing up against a neighbour's cat, and wondering at the coolness of a tree's bark on a hot day can never happen in the back seat of a car. The windscreen view of your suburb will not help you feel connected to *your* place and confident to find the way home. You won't get to know the smell of rain, or to note the changes in the natural world occurring as the seasons shift.

As a mother myself, I lament the lack of this freedom for my own children and worry they have missed out on developing their independence, problem solving and social skills within the natural world. For young people today, there is less freedom, less space and less nature left for them to explore. This nature deprivation is stifling children's inherent sense of wonder. And it risks snuffing out the joy and creativity wonder fuels.

In light of this, it's deeply gratifying to see the counter-current arising as parents and communities push for the right of children to simply play in nature. Interest in bush kinder, kitchen garden programs and nature play philosophies continues to grow. The social movement that prioritises giving children the time and the space to be in nature is exciting and community driven. Early childhood environmental educators are strong advocates for child-centred nature play. Christine Joy led the education program at the Royal Botanic Gardens in Melbourne for many years. To hear her speak about nature play, what it is and how to facilitate it, is a delight. It is a great honour to have her contribute to this book by sharing her insights.

## NATURE PLAY

Chris Joy was part of the team at the Royal Botanic Gardens in Melbourne who developed the Ian Potter Children's Garden – a ground-breaking natural play space for children designed specifically to facilitate their connection to nature. She is especially interested in how nature play can nurture the development of creativity and empathy in children.

She believes nature play is innate, a centuries old way of learning and behaving that is the way children react to the world around them. Nature play is 'just what children do' rather than an outcome focussed program. When children are involved in nature play their imagination is powerfully engaged and they are connecting to the world around them in a very physical and sensory way. This is a rich, intense learning experience which has an important role in building culture as children are able to act out things they've observed in the world around them.

Although children have been playing in nature for millennia, lifestyle changes over the past few decades have disrupted this. As Chris Joy says, "the culture of play has been lost from our society". So, we may now need to use some 'play invitations' to get children started in nature play. Ideas include placing bundles of branches on the ground for children to perhaps build a cubby with. It is essential children do not have the outcome dictated to them by an adult. But instead, be encouraged to explore the natural materials themselves and play with them using their own unique imagination.

Nature play can be engaged in from the very beginning, with babies gazing up into dancing leaves overhead. But it begins in earnest when children can be left alone outside. Once able to walk around independently, they can be playing, and from the age of three or four a parent can be some distance away, so the child is unaware of being watched. The urge to play remains even through adolescence when social networks are stronger. Of course, adults still want to play too! They can model playful behaviour when outside providing subtle prompts for children.

For parents who are unfamiliar with nature, a simple way to begin is to walk through the backyard or park with your child in an exploratory way. Engage all your senses. For example, take the time to feel things like the texture of bark or leaves, not only with your hands, but perhaps with your cheek. Some children delight in putting their bare belly against the smoothness of a tree trunk. Pick up 'treasures', like leaves or flowers, noticing how they smell, or perhaps look at them in a different way, maybe peering through holes in leaves so the sunlight is dispersed. Perhaps lie on your back and gaze at the clouds, finding animals in their shapes and then roll over to peer into the jungle that is the grass. Close your eyes to feel the warmth of the sun on your face, or the breeze on your skin, and listen carefully to the different bird calls or the crunch of a leaf under your weight.

A range of approaches can be used, from providing no prompts – just the time and space for children to freely to engage in nature play, through to giving invitations, like natural materials, which the children can use as they wish. Finally, for those who may need a little more structure, an idea for play might be introduced. This could be something like the creation of a mandala where children are asked to make a shape on the ground from leaves and other treasures. They usually work with others to do this and come up with their own design. The main risk to nature play is over-engagement of adults who often want an 'outcome'. It is important parents and teachers try to hold back from this outcome focus as it can squash creativity and imagination.

The 'delight factor' is what Chris Joy calls the intense emotional and joyous response children have when playing in nature. She describes children's faces being lit up, eyes wide and them saying things like 'I love you so much' and 'this is the best day of my life'. These children are learning through the delight factor and Chris Joy believes that learning should be a joyous part of daily school life. Given the whole child is so engaged in this approach, their learning encompasses the physical, the emotional and the sensory.

It is also important children playing out in nature are not 'protected' from physical discomfort. Learning how to manage this is essential for the development of resilience. In her nature play sessions, Chris Joy encouraged children to walk through the flax 'jungle' where they needed to move through cobwebs and lie on the ground even when it was wet. In our modern lives, we have weeded out much of the physical discomfort for children. But learning how to keep going and not miss out on great things, just because we might be experiencing a degree of unpleasantness is important. Developing a tolerance of these little grievances in childhood helps lay the foundation for coping with discomfort as we grow up.

## A nature play approach

Another way of thinking about structuring a nature play experience is to consider it as consisting of three components. These being adult directed, adult initiated and child initiated. Most nature-based educators tend to utilise a blend of these. An introductory technique might involve roaming across a landscape together before coming to a more static phase around a tree and considering the macro and micro parts of the space. Incorporating large and small play materials supports both gross and fine motor development. Gross motor skills are acquired when large muscle groups and balance are used, as in climbing a tree, walking across an uneven surface or balancing along a fallen tree trunk. Fine motor skills use precision finger movements like carefully picking up and manipulating a delicate flower or seed pod.

The rich outdoor environment of a bush kinder provides a wonderful example of the *ecology of learning* which occurs in a nature play setting. To illustrate this point, Chris Joy described a bushland session. Here, one boy was peering down wombat holes while another climbed on a fallen trunk. Nearby a group of children were focussing on a small area of dirt. Within the soil was an ant's nest. When the children realised they'd hurt some insects they were fascinated by watching the ants die. They then became worried about the ants and so built a fence around them. As they were doing this, they discovered some tiny mites which were only just visible to the naked eye. The boy who had found the wombat hole then called the others over to share what he'd found. All this took place within the one play session and exemplifies the 'biodiverse experiences' found in nature play. The children were learning about life, death, complex ecosystems, biology and geology as well as developing their gross and fine motor skills, problem solving, teamwork and empathy.

The nature play session described above contrasts greatly with an indoor, regular kinder session. Here children are much more restricted in what they do because they're limited by the materials provided, time pressures and often also given a specified outcome to achieve. In their 2013 film, 'School's Out', lessons from a Forest Kindergarten, Lisa Molomot and Rona Richter compare a forest kindergarten's nature play approach with that of an American kindergarten[227]. The film beautifully demonstrates the rich learning that occurs with prolonged time in nature and the role educators have in facilitating this. It is also thought provoking in its comparison to the more rigid, indoors American kinder which is akin to many learning environments here in Australia.

## Sparking imagination through nature play

"Fact and fantasy shimmer together – the thing about nature is that it blends and mixes the two things. The two are intertwined and children find this exquisitely delightful", is Chris Joy's way of describing the powerful need children have to integrate nature and culture. One way they do this is to see story characters in nature. To wonder if Moonface really is up the enormous tree, or if Snugglepot and Cuddlepie are hiding in the gum nut blossoms. Stories, traditionally from books but in First Nations communities shared orally and in our modern, Pokémon-driven societies through devices, are a deeply ingrained way in which we develop and share our culture. I recall spending an afternoon with my young nephews and teenage son in some local bushland where enormous old red gums draped in bark were alive with birdsong and the ground was littered with sticks and leaves. Almost immediately my thirteen-year-old grabbed a huge stick and proclaimed himself Gandalf with magical powers, and Chris Joy's words came to mind.

Books can be a way to link the young people in our lives to nature. We can take story time outside and choose books which feature the natural world. There are many to choose from with old fashioned favourites being *The Magic Faraway Tree* and *Wind in the Willows* and Australian stories like *Snugglepot and Cuddlepie*, *Diary of a Wombat* and *Wombat Stew*. The children's book, *You and Me, Murrawee*[228], is a lovely picture book introduction both to the natural world, and to Aboriginal ways of understanding nature. It serves to build cultural knowledge as well as provide nature play ideas.

Simply telling a story outside while sitting on the ground, using animation in voice and posture, is a wonderful way to teach children. Especially if you can mix fact and fantasy and use strong archetypal images. The story can even be scary, so children learn how to deal with a low level of anger or violence. Chris Joy uses the example of sharing with children a story about a tree being struck by lightning. What it might have been thinking when it was struck and split in two and having the children go away and play out the story afterwards themselves. Art, music and drama teachers and librarians are all especially skilled at telling stories in creative ways. They can bring nature into their repertoire or take their teaching out into nature for inspiration and context. Of course, grandparents, parents and others in a community also have a wonderful capacity to tell stories. There's nothing a young child likes much more than being held safely, in a warm embrace and listening to a tale.

The Ian Potter Children's Garden at the Royal Botanic Gardens Melbourne is a tangible example of combining the skills of those from the fields of horticulture, education, landscape design, art and interpretation to produce a delightful place of nature play for children[229]. The success of the garden to inspire nature play stems from the cross disciplinary approach of its planning. Chris Joy's understanding of how children develop and learn informed the design of the space and plants were chosen so it would be conducive to free nature play for children of all ages. Entering this garden as an adult is wondrous as you are drawn to crouch and walk through the plant tunnel, wind through the bamboo forest's smooth trunks, clamber over rocks around an ancient tree trunk or paddle in the small waterway. Many elements of this garden could be incorporated into a home, community or school's garden design and would serve to bring this type of nature play to all children (and adults!). Similar gardens are springing up all over Australia as the value of natural play experiences are appreciated and the hard, brightly-coloured plastic playgrounds of old are slowly replaced.

## Growing a sense of wonder

Rachel Carson's *A Sense of Wonder* was written many decades ago yet still rings true today. In it, she provides a lyrical manual on how we can be the important adult guiding the children in our care as they begin their journey with the natural world. How we can help foster their love of nature through play, and grow their sense of wonder which provides the foundation for a thirst to understand, to know. Although she never had children of her own, Carson delighted in taking her grand-nephew Roger out to the tidepools and woods of her rural property. These adventures formed the basis for her book. Like Chris Joy, she urges adults to be child-like in their approach to exploring nature with children. To use all our senses, be curious and refrain from explaining by taking the view that nature is a place for shared adventure and enjoyment. A place where children can form "a sense of wonder so indestructible that it would last throughout life."

It is now over half a century since my mother first introduced me to nature by putting my pram out under the waving leaves in a suburban backyard. She would recount how settled I became when put outside. So as an infant I had plenty of time in the garden. In northern Europe this is the norm for infants, as it's felt that they should be in fresh air as much as possible. In modern Australia most babies are tucked up inside for their rest. Recently, a Melbourne childcare centre started putting infants outside to sleep and has found they are more settled as a result. It seems my mother was ahead of her time, or perhaps we have moved away from what has been natural and instinctive for many parents[230].

My mother would also stop the pram so I could get close to flowers. As far back as I can remember, she would point out the daily wonders in nature, the clouds in the sky or the birds coming into the yard. Rachel Carlson describes the importance of children having at least one 'Elder' to guide them in their nature journey. At key moments in my early life, my mother and nature were there for me. I especially remember her taking me to Tasmania's Cradle Mountain National Park after my final school exams. We walked through the extraordinary landscape and marked my move from school to adulthood in nature. Just a few years ago, after she turned eighty-four, we visited Victoria's Wilson's Promontory National Park, a glorious, rugged expanse of coastal bush. She was determined to explore as much as possible. One day we walked for about seven hours! Even when her arthritis was clearly uncomfortable, she continued to point out the birds and flowers. Her sense of wonder as strong as ever.

It is my greatest wish that my children have the same enduring fascination for, and love of, the natural world and that their grandmother's legacy lives on in this. Like Rachel Carson, I hope all children can receive this guidance from the nature mentors in their lives, so they can draw strength from nature and that the fascination and sense of wonder provides inspiration for a meaningful life.

## NATURE PLAY

- Can start as soon as children can play on their own outside, around the age of three

- Has no predetermined outcome

- Uses *loose materials* like sticks, leaves and stones

- Brings nature and culture together

- Take stories outside into nature and tell stories about nature

- Often means getting wet, dirty, cold, hot or a little bit uncomfortable but it's worth it!

- Is fun, fascinating and exciting

- Nature experiences foster imagination and wonder

- Adults can be nature mentors, sharing the exploration without teaching or explaining

## LEARNING IN GREEN

In 1915 a unique school was opened in bushland on the outskirts of Melbourne. Set underneath the shade of gum trees, amongst wildflowers and fragrant wattles, the Blackburn Open-Air School was modelled on similar schools in Europe and America. Its students were the poor and malnourished children of the inner city. They would take the train out into the fresh air of the bush to be educated in an open-air pavilion. Alongside lessons in spelling and maths, the students enjoyed nature walks and had their afternoon naps in canvas deck chairs[231]. Students attended this school right through until the 1960s when improved health and social services deemed it was no longer required. In the early 1970s I attended primary school near the site of this open-air school and was also lucky to spend time between lessons playing in bushland.

The ensuing decades have seen the green space around most schools diminish and children's opportunities for nature play during the school day almost vanish altogether. The time of an afternoon nap under the shade of a tree, or any daytime rest, has well and truly passed. Instead, the pendulum has swung the other way. The school day has been extended to encompass before and after school programs and lunch time is now often spent on a device of some kind rather than stretched out on the grass or climbing a tree. There is little time for either the minds or bodies of today's children to rest and, in most urban schools, nowhere natural to go.

Given our children spend most of their childhood in a school, its teachers, programs, philosophy and grounds are all important considerations for parents and care givers. Many parents have little choice about which school their child attends. So it's important all provide an optimal learning experience and that the buildings and grounds are healthy places to be.

## Nature-rich school grounds

The school environment plays a crucial role in the wellbeing of its students and staff, and the more nature in its design, the healthier the environment becomes. This section outlines how greening a school makes it a place where children's learning, happiness and development are best supported. As well as looking to the past for inspiration, today's policy makers, planners and teachers can look to research both overseas and here, in Australia.

Simply having a view of nature from the classroom helps restore attention and lift mood for students and teachers. Understanding this can inform decisions on how best to orientate learning spaces both in the broader school design and within the classroom itself. The more nature-rich a schoolground, the better students can focus on return to class. This knowledge should see a prioritising of trees, gardens and plants in school planning and budgets.

As part of her PhD, Australian researcher Kathleen Bagot undertook a detailed analysis of some twenty primary schools[232]. She measured what's called 'perceived restorativeness', which is what makes an environment experienced as restorative by the child. As discussed in the Green Mind section, Attention Restoration Theory (ART) was first proposed by Kaplan in 1995 and is 'the theory that exposure to nature reduces directed attention fatigue, restoring the ability to concentrate at will'.[233] Directed attention includes activities like learning to read and write or watching a video. Kaplan found natural environments are especially rich in the characteristics needed for restorative experiences. We all need nature to help our brain recover from the exhaustion of living in a modern world that's constantly demanding our attention.

The purpose of Dr Bagot's study was to try to understand whether school playgrounds could become a psychological resource for students by maximising their perceived restorativeness. They did this by asking the children how they felt when they were in the playground using the ART framework. The study included 550 students across a broad range of social groups with an even number of boys and girls. The school playgrounds were scrutinised deeply to look at the amount of nature they contained. They counted the number and size of all shrubs and trees to come up with a figure in cubic metres. They also measured the percentage of grass covering and used photo ratings of perceived naturalness to ask adults how natural they considered a space to be. Apart from the amount of nature in the playgrounds, the number of play areas, play resources like climbing frames, sand pits, sports ovals and overall percentage of school grounds given over to play was measured. It was a truly comprehensive look at the composition of these schools' outdoor play spaces.

The types of play experiences were also analysed by measuring the amount of physical activity and social interaction enjoyed by the children. Positive and negative mood states and their 'perceived affordance' was also checked. Perceived affordance is whether the children felt they could do the sorts of things they wanted. For example, whether they could run around, sit to play quietly or spend time alone if desired. Essentially, Dr Bagot's team looked at how much nature and other play spaces and equipment were in the schools, the types of activities the kids engaged in and how they felt about being able to do what they wished. And whether they felt happier after being out in the playground.

Dr Bagot and her team found the more plants and shrubs there were, the more the children experienced the playground as restorative. They felt better after spending time there. Compared to the amount of nature, other physical playground characteristics did not provide psychological restoration. This fits with other research that concludes natural rather than built environments are mentally restorative. Importantly, positive mood states were associated with this psychological restoration. The children were happier on return to class after being in a more nature-rich playground. Interestingly, physical activity did not contribute to perceived restorativeness in this study. Play experiences were important however, with the opportunity to socialise, and a wide variety of possible play activities, being notable positive factors.

Another interesting finding was that the amount of nature present was perceived differently by adults who tended to find areas of grass more natural than lots of different trees and shrubs. Given that the best psychological outcomes for children were associated with vegetation volume, it is important that their health requirements are understood when planning playground composition. Otherwise, we end up with school yards that parents and teachers think look nice, but which aren't supporting optimal child wellbeing. This might explain both the current preponderance of flat lawns in our schools and parklands and the increasing rates of anxiety and attentional problems suffered by young people.

To sum up findings from this detailed study, the ideal school ground for children should have lots of different trees and plants and a variety of natural play areas. There should be opportunities for them to play alone or with others. It's also better if an emphasis is placed on enriching the natural areas in school grounds in preference to constructing play equipment, sports fields and courts.

Looking out onto a natural view is also likely to support academic achievement and positive behaviour in the classroom. An American study from 2010 looked at 101 public high schools and measured student performance and nature exposure[234]. Children who looked out from class or the cafeteria onto rich natural spaces with lots of trees and shrubs were more likely to perform better on academic tests, to graduate, and be less likely to engage in criminal behaviour. Interestingly, if the views included featureless landscapes like large areas of lawn, sports fields or car parks, the reverse was true. The greater the volume of nature, the richer in trees and shrubs it is, the more mental fatigue is restored. It makes sense that if you are better able to focus and feeling happier as a student then you will engage more with learning, perform well in tests and go on to complete school.

Not surprisingly, taking this further by getting kids outside to learn in outdoor classrooms has been found to improve academic outcomes. Another American study found that year six primary school students who attended an outdoor school program had a 27% improvement in their science scores after participating, and this improvement lasted for 10 weeks. Interestingly, and sadly, of this group of over two hundred and fifty at-risk children, 56% reported that this outdoor school experience was the first time they had been out in a natural setting. Teachers were also asked to rate the students, and the study found children who attended the outdoor science school had higher ratings in self-esteem, conflict resolution, relationship with peers, problem solving, motivation to learn, and behaviour in class[235].

Embedding nature within the curriculum sees young people learning outdoors with the natural world providing a living canvas for teachers. A paradigm shift in the underlying philosophy of how children are taught has seen the evolution of nature pedagogy.

## NATURE PEDAGOGY

Pedagogy is the art and science of teaching. The guiding principles for opening children to the joys of learning.

More recently, some educators have developed the field of 'nature pedagogy' which is how teaching can be done with nature[236]. One of the thought leaders in this field is Claire Warden, a Scottish teacher and family support worker who has focussed on teaching *with* nature, rather than just *about* or *in* nature. Warden talks about a learning journey and calls for teaching in nature to be implanted in the curriculum, so all children can benefit. The learning journey she espouses covers the whole life span. Just as it's beneficial to understand wellbeing from cradle to grave, it makes sense to think about nature pedagogy all through life too.

Learning with nature can begin in early childhood, where kinder can take place partly, or even entirely, outside. Primary and secondary school children's teaching can emphasise time outdoors for learning across the whole curriculum, for example using maths and science to understand different species within the school landscape. And residential facilities for the elderly can include gardens, which stimulate happy memories for their occupants.

Warden also has a *child-centred* approach where adults are with children but careful not to be dominating of them. This echoes the nature play philosophy espoused by Chris Joy as discussed earlier. Warden urges us to consider what's natural for us as humans to help guide the learning journey. This includes having children of different ages together, keeping groups to a relatively small size of under thirty, encouraging preparing and sharing a meal, and keeping the design of a school or kinder as home-like as possible. At the Nature Kinder she runs in Scotland, the house-like atmosphere means that children move at their own pace from inside, through a garden area, into a forest. This child-led and centred approach contrasts sharply to the mostly indoors, highly-structured formal approach seen in many childcare centres elsewhere.

In her exploration of the nature of childhood and how it has changed over time, English author Jay Griffiths gives a scathing critique of schools[237]. She describes today's schooling system as being a *denatured*, sterile environment. Griffiths charts the history of European schooling, upon which our Australian system is based. She writes "in the history of European schooling, certain concerns echo down the centuries: hierarchy, obedience, violence and class control (pun intended). A school system was established, half factory and half prison, in order to create a passive and disciplined workforce where schooled, uniform obedience was demanded." Griffiths mounts a sustained attack on the regimented curriculum of today where everything is measured and compared.

Having recently had my children complete their final years of schooling, where their entire education is crystallised by the system into a single score for university entrance, Griffiths' arguments give pause for thought. "Children, strangled by ties and regimented by soldiers, are learning a covert curriculum of power relations and normalised militarism. They are learning a right-wing political ethos that hierarchy is inevitable, that obedience, discipline and control are all-important. They are being taught that competition is the basis of education and that test results indicate superiority. In age-based classes and measured by numerical marks, they are learning that classification and measurement are the most important tools of thought."

Perhaps it is in response to this highly ordered and competitive system that we are seeing some nature getting through the cracks with a new wave of educators diversifying the experience of the children in their care. In a variety of settings, from the early years through to the end of schooling, nature pedagogy is finding its place.

## *Inspiration from across the globe*

In the United Kingdom, an exciting project called Natural Connections worked with one hundred and twenty-five primary, secondary and special schools to embed use of local green spaces for learning across the curriculum. The program was huge, with some five thousand teachers and assistants involved over the four years of its duration. The impetus for this far-reaching program was a government policy outlined in the 'Natural Environment White Paper' of 2011 that aimed for 'every child to (should) experience and learn about the natural environment' and committed to 'remove barriers to learning outdoors and increase schools' abilities to teach outdoors when they wish to do so'.[238]

The Natural Connections project was evaluated and findings confirmed that learning in natural environments resulted in 'greater pupil engagement, enjoyment of lessons and environmental awareness, and improved social skills, health, wellbeing and behaviour'[239, 240]. Importantly, the impetus for this project was the understanding within the department of education in the United Kingdom that learning in outdoor spaces supported academic achievement across all subject areas and was to be encouraged and promoted. This runs counter to the common perception here in Australia that outdoor learning is 'just' about sustainability and the natural environment and developing 'soft' skills like flexibility, motivation and the ability to collaborate and work in a team. One example of this from the Natural Connections project was when a primary school ran a series of maths intervention groups, with one of these being held outdoors. The intervention was designed to learn maths for space, shape, time and measurement. The outdoor learning group made more progress than the other group. Not only were they outdoors in a healthier environment, but they came to better learn the maths concepts[241].

Denmark, a leader in education, introduced its new curriculum in 2014. This has an emphasis on increased physical activity and 'uderskole' or learning outside the classroom. Uderskole involves teachers taking children out into the local community for learning on a regular basis and may include visits to museums or galleries as well as trips to natural places. The frequency of uderskole is generally on a weekly or fortnightly basis and the idea is to provide a motivating school setting to teach 'often abstract academic concepts in a more concrete and illustrative way.'[242] With 18% of all schools in Denmark relocating some of their subject-related teaching to places outside on a regular basis, the concept of uderskole is becoming embedded in the curriculum having initially begun as a grassroots movement[243].

Singapore, which is regarded as having a highly academic and disciplined educational ethos, has also moved to embrace the value of outdoor learning for students. In their 2014 Framework for learning, the Singapore Ministry of Education describes desired outcomes for 21st century learners as stretching beyond the purely academic to include creativity, innovation, cross-cultural understanding and resilience. Learning outdoors is understood to be a way for students to develop these skills, which are thought to increase the likelihood of success in a globalised economy. This shift away from a simple academic focus was outlined in a speech by Acting Minister for Education Ng Chee Meng in 2016, "We need a better balance in our students' education journey.

This means dialling back an excessive focus on academics. We need to free up time and space to nurture other dimensions that are just as important for our children's development. Let them not just study the flowers, but also stop to smell the flowers, and wonder at their beauty. We want to cultivate a generation of young people who grow up with a sense of curiosity and a love for learning, asking both the 'whys' and sometimes even the 'why-nots'."[244]

To support this move, their government is investing in more frequent, diverse and longer outdoor educational experiences for students. In this speech, the Acting Minister also outlines plans to move away from competitive reporting of academic results and a lessening of homework demands. All good news for children and parents alike given the knowledge we now have about the importance of free time, sleep and play for development.

Importantly, learning out in nature nurtures creativity which, according to the late education guru Sir Ken Robinson, is the 'ability to have original ideas of value'. In his wonderful TED Talk from 2006, Do schools kill creativity?, Sir Robinson espouses why "creativity is as important as literacy and we should treat it with the same respect"[245]. He complains that today "we get educated out of creativity" by a school system that places the arts at the bottom of subject hierarchy where literacy and maths are over emphasised. Even within the arts, dance and theatre studies sit below music and fine art, and yet these subjects are instinctively important for children with dance movement and self-expression through acting being wonderful vehicles for creativity. In the grading of final marks in the school system here in Victoria, students are discouraged from taking these so-called 'easier' subjects as they attract a lower score. Sir Robinson's talk has had over forty-five million views, so it has clearly resonated throughout the world with those of us wondering how best to support the growth of creativity in our children. No doubt 'original ideas of value' will be extraordinarily important in a rapidly changing world.

More recently, Sir Robinson put his support behind the push to promote outdoor classrooms. He described the key reasons being that nature stimulates creativity, is a powerful resource for learning, provides hands on, active learning and is both fun and social[246]. "Education takes up a great deal of children's time," Sir Ken said, "this is their childhood, the only one they get and learning outdoors, working together, playing together is fun. It's about the quality of our lives and experiences." He endorsed the value of The Outdoor Classroom Day in the UK and Ireland. This began in 2011 as a small initiative and has grown to see over 400,000 children taking part in 2016 with the idea spreading to 51 countries around the world[247]. Put simply, it is one day a year in which schools are supported and encouraged to take classes outside to inspire ongoing outdoor learning and play.

Looking around the world at education systems in Europe, the United Kingdom, America and Singapore it is apparent that the value of nature for learning and development is becoming more deeply appreciated globally. This is backed by research and, in some lucky countries, supported by government policy. There is no need to reinvent the wheel but rather to be inspired by programs like Natural Connections which can be adapted to suit any school community. A simple aim is to have school grounds full of nature, where kids can look out the window onto nature if they're inside and where they can have as many lessons as possible outside, either in the school's own green space or in nearby nature. This may mean rethinking the design of the classroom, the school yard and the curriculum but the benefits are truly great. As a teacher from the Natural Connections project says, "We try to look at learning as something pupils enjoy, and they absolutely love outdoor learning and enjoy it. And when you get enjoyment, you get enthusiasm and you get raised results. So it's a win-win!"[241]

Surrounding young people with nature during their journey through learning not only helps them discover, create and enjoy. It also ensures they are spending time in a healthy environment. Let's turn now to consider how plants, especially trees, can provide the clean air, shade and shelter essential for growth and development.

# BREATHING IN

We are understanding more and more about how important air quality is for health, especially since the COVID-19 pandemic. It's simple, the cleaner the air, the healthier we are. Areas with high levels of pollution, from the burning of fossil fuels like coal and gas for energy, or fuel for cars, are unhealthy for our bodies in many ways. Apart from the obvious respiratory effects like lung cancer and asthma, poor air quality can increase the rate of heart disease and stroke.

It may seem incredible that substances in the air we inhale can hurt our brain and heart, but because of their tiny size, these particles are a significant cause of illness. Called fine particles (PM2.5), these smallest pollutants, once breathed in, can pass through the exquisitely thin membrane between the air in our lungs and our bloodstream. They can therefore move throughout the body to cause harm[248]. Poor air quality has been recognised as a modifiable risk factor by the American Heart Association along with cigarette smoking, diabetes and inactivity[249]. In Australia, more people die prematurely each year from air pollution than from accidents on our roads. In 2021, the road toll was 1,127 while the Australian Institute of Health and Welfare has estimated some 3,000 deaths from urban air pollution[250].

Pollution from car exhaust contains a mixture of chemicals and these interact with each other, especially when the weather is very hot. So, on a warm summer's day when a school is surrounded by cars idling with their air conditioners on, the air quality is likely to be extremely poor. Unfortunately, there is no current practice of measuring air quality around schools, and most school communities are unaware a problem may even exist. For schools sited in industrial zones, near coal-fired power stations or near major roadways there is an even greater likelihood that children are being exposed to damaging chemicals in the air they are breathing.

Indoor air quality can also be a problem with aerosol sprays, fabrics, paints and carpets releasing chemicals called *volatile organic compounds* (VOCs) into the air. These compounds can settle onto the floor and other surfaces and make their way into our bodies by either being inhaled or unknowingly swallowed. They are present within cars too, and so the air quality in the back seat can be as poor as that outside, near the car exhaust pipe. The problem with these sorts of chemicals is that they are readily absorbed by the body and tend to accumulate in our tissues. There is concern amongst researchers and doctors that early life exposure to these chemicals may be associated with an increased range of problems including obesity and cancers.

Children are particularly vulnerable to these sorts of environmental exposures for several reasons. First, despite their small size, they take up toxins from the environment more than adults. This is because they are growing and so breathe, eat and drink more per kilogram of body weight compared to adults. They also have a proportionately larger body surface area. The smaller the person, the greater the ratio of surface area (skin) to size. Consequently, children absorb toxins through their skin more readily. Children have more active gut absorption than adults, for example they absorb four times more lead than adults for the same exposure. Lead is a heavy metal released into our environment through industries like mining and from the widespread use of lead-containing petrol in the past. Even today, exposure to lead is a significant risk factor for brain damage in Australian children, particularly in mining towns and for children exposed to lead containing paints in old homes[251].

Second, children's behaviour puts them at greater risk of environmental exposures than adults. Infants and toddlers love to put objects in their mouth, exploring the world by using all their senses thus increasing their risk of accidentally swallowing toxins. They also play on or near the ground. Their breathing zone is just above the floor where some indoor environmental toxins tend to settle and concentrate. The way toxins move through the body is also different in children. For example, the barrier between the blood and the brain is more porous in children and so these harmful chemicals can more easily cross from their blood stream into their brain to cause harm.

When it comes to air pollution, children are especially susceptible because their lungs are growing until well into late childhood. Exposure to air pollution can begin from before birth, when toxins from a mother's cigarette smoking or other air contamination passes through the placenta to impact on the developing baby's lungs. When they are infants or toddlers, children can be exposed to smoking, indoor or outdoor air pollution or allergy-causing substances. These may all cause lung problems and affect lung growth. Breathing problems may occur in childhood, with the development of asthma, or have a delayed presentation where lung disease surfaces later in life. It is now thought some adult-onset lung disease may have its origins in early life exposures to various environmental toxins.

## MAKING A CASE FOR TREES

How can we take this information and use it to better care for children? After learning about these environmental risk factors, I spoke to leading child lung specialist, Professor Peter Sly from the University of Queensland. I asked if there were any measures that would protect children from developing lung problems apart from the obvious, like not smoking around children or when pregnant and avoiding traffic fumes. Sly said a diet rich in nutrients and antioxidants could help and having plenty of green space in a child's life is also probably beneficial.

This makes sense because plants, apart from producing oxygen and absorbing carbon dioxide, take up environmental pollutants and so clean the air. Ensuring school grounds and suburbs are rich in green space, with a variety of trees and shrubs, is an important way to improve air quality and the health of young people[252]. Schools can also use pot plants as a way of making indoor air cleaner. Bringing greenery inside has the additional benefit of increasing the humidity, or moisture, in a room and this may help those with lung and skin problems.

As anyone who has sought shelter in the shade on a hot summer's day will appreciate, trees cool our gardens, streets and public spaces. This is important when we appreciate the accelerating effect heat has on the formation of certain gases in polluted air. Through the effect of climate change, the duration and intensity of heatwaves in Australian cities has risen over the past few decades and this trend is expected to continue. Melbourne is predicted to experience a tripling of the number of days over 35 degrees Celsius by 2100[253]. Children are markedly at risk of heat-related illness during a heatwave and so maximising the cooling effect of trees in their environment is a protective health measure[254].

In the built environment, surfaces like concrete, bitumen and brick absorb heat. This leads to the *urban heat island effect* where cities are hotter than the surrounding countryside. This can be countered by increasing the number of trees and other vegetation present because plants help reduce both day and night-time temperatures. They do this by shading footpaths and buildings and by reflecting more sunlight and absorbing less heat than man-made materials. Trees also use a cooling process called transpiration where they release moisture into the air through their leaves having drawn it up through their trunks and branches from the ground[255].

To make the air in our school grounds as healthy as possible for children we need to ensure they are well shaded by trees. Trees provide a pleasant respite from the heat for both children and staff, as well as wonderful places to play and relax. This goes against the current trend to remove trees from school grounds because of a fear of injury from falling branches. Following on from the tragic death of a schoolgirl in a New South Wales primary school in 2014, authorities removed more than five thousand trees in schools across the state. An arborist commenting on the decision to remove such a large number of trees said that the mortality rate of children dying from falling tree branches was one in every 30 million student years, so the tree removal was an extraordinary over-reaction to a devastating but rare event[256].

The benefits to children of improved air quality, shading during hot weather and the positive psychological effects of a rich natural school yard far outweigh the small risk of harm from falling trees. When speaking to educators about the benefits of nature for child health and development I am invariably asked about risk. It seems there is an excessive focus on some risk and not others, and a refusal by decision makers to fully consider all risks and all benefits. Of course, it is challenging to think about long term or non-physical factors, but this is what needs to happen. Some are beginning to think of risk: benefit ratios rather than just 'risk management'. This is a welcome step, but there needs to be a broadening of our understanding on this issue. It is essential advice be sought from those in the health sector, as well as the actuaries and lawyers from insurance companies before decisions on tree removal are made.

Yes, there is some risk for children playing in a natural space. They may fall from a tree, trip over a log, get sunburnt or have a branch fall on them. These events are usually accidental and can be minimised by reasonable protocols. Serious injuries are thankfully rare. On the other hand, the benefits of outside activity in a natural school ground are enormous and provide for optimal physical, mental and emotional development. A lack of time outside predisposes children to the delayed, long lasting, lifestyle-related health problems resulting from inactivity, excessive body weight, vitamin D deficiency, poor sleep, low mood and increased stress.

## GREEN UNDERFOOT

Unsurprisingly, natural surfaces like grass are better for wellbeing than the artificial turf gradually taking over many schools' outdoor spaces in Australia. Not only used for soccer pitches, this 'astro turf' is also incorporated into playgrounds and general landscaping. Like trees, grasses use transpiration and so are cool to sit on when it's hot. This contrasts to sitting on fake grass on a warm day. Apart from finding the surface surprisingly hot despite its cool green colour, it is unsettling to notice the petrol-like fumes it releases. It is also disconcerting when your children have countless black tar balls drop out of their shoes and socks after playing on such a surface. And alongside the annoyance factor of having to clean up the mess, there are health concerns relating to these grains of tar. Tar balls are made from ground up car tyres and are referred to as 'crumb rubber' by industry. This term is quite misleading because unlike natural rubber, which is derived from tree sap, these black balls are an industrial product.

In the United States, there has been some concern amongst the soccer community over the long-term health effects of these artificial turf surfaces. This is because a group of goalkeepers have developed a type of blood cancer called lymphoma. They are wondering if their illness could be related to their exposure to the fake grass from a young age. Goalkeepers are more exposed than other players as they are often diving to the ground, getting the tar balls into their clothes, hair and sometimes even their mouth and eyes[257]. Given the reasons outlined above, which make children more vulnerable to environmental toxins, these concerns need to be taken very seriously. It is known that car tyres, from which these tar balls are made, contain many different chemicals including hydrocarbons and even small amounts of heavy metals like lead[258,259].

There is little long-term safety data on the use of these artificial surfaces in school grounds where growing children are playing. Decision makers should apply the precautionary principle when deciding how to landscape their schools. This overarching philosophy of public health states that, if the current science is unclear and there's potential for harm to the environment or human health, the path of least risk is best chosen. So, if it is unknown whether exposing children to a new, chemically-based surface like artificial turf, is safe, then their exposure should be minimised. It is about being 'better safe than sorry'[260]. In the United States in 2016, President Obama announced an inquiry to investigate the safety of artificial turf more fully for players. It will be sometime before this information is available to the public and at the time of writing, clear guidelines for caregivers seem many years off. So for now, it is best for children to avoid playing on these surfaces for a long time, or in very hot weather, and to wash their hands after playing[261,262].

As outlined earlier, because of the exposure to beneficial micro-organisms found in soil, the presence of plants and dirt in a playground aids the development of a healthy immune system. So, even though synthetic turf might seem like a 'clean' option for a schoolyard, it is not as healthy for kids as old-fashioned dirt and grass. Grass stains on the knees of children are a sign of healthy contact with nature, of exploration, play and probably exertion. They can be regarded with satisfaction by educators and parents alike.

Some new approaches inspired by nature pedagogy involve children spending a large amount of time outside. In Australia, for the preschool years, this has taken the form of bush kinder.

# BUSH KINDER

The bush kinder idea is inspired by the nature or forest kindergartens seen in Europe and the United Kingdom. Essentially, these involve young children spending long periods engaged in unstructured play in a forest or beach setting. Duration may range from several hours to entire days at a time over the course of one or more years. Children engage in the natural place, observing the seasonal and daily changes in the weather, plants and animals and explore at their own pace, gently guided by parents and teachers. The approach is child-centred and led, and allows children to develop self-management skills and take some risks. Activities might include tree climbing, water play and experimenting with the varied loose materials found in nature like sticks, stones and dirt.

In the northern hemisphere this method has been researched and evaluated and findings include multiple benefits for children and educators. Children in these kinders were found to be physically fitter and stronger and to have increased social and imaginative play and improved confidence, concentration and motivation[263]. Nature kinder programs were also found to help teachers to build stronger relationships and a deeper understanding of the children in their care. Some of the evaluations reported broader community benefits too, with a greater awareness of the value of nature play areas for children and a sense that children being seen out in the community, engaged in real life, was positive.

No doubt English author, Tim Gill, would concur. He writes extensively on the importance of free play for children and describes the sighting of children playing outside as being the key marker of a healthy suburb. Gill refers to these children as being 'sentinel' children[264]. It's heart-warming to see a 'sentinel' child or two in a suburban park, as it means their parents feel comfortable with them navigating the neighbourhood and exploring their home ground rather than having them cooped up inside with a screen.

An Australian leader in the field of early childhood education is Doug Fargher, or 'Bushkinder Doug', as he is known on social media. Doug was involved in Australia's first bush kinder—Westgarth Bush Kinder—which was founded in 2011. This program involves children participating in a three-hour session in the Darebin Parklands as one of their 15 hours of kinder over the course of a week. As with many great innovations, it was born of necessity. Following a government directive that all four-year-old children had to attend 15 hours per week of early learning, the staff at Westgarth had to create additional sessions. They simply didn't have the space to accommodate such a change without extending out into the nearby parklands, and so the Bush Kinder was born.

In the bushland, the children only use what's in the natural environment, no books or other equipment is brought into the park. This provides an opportunity for more creative, open-ended play and exploration. The Westgarth Bush Kinder is a great example of a successful partnership between a kindergarten and a bushland. Balancing the needs of the children with the protection of the natural environment required a spirit of collaboration between the parks and education staff. As a new program, it provided an opportunity for teachers and parents to compare children's behaviour in bush kinder to the regular, indoor 'home kinder'. The program at Westgarth was evaluated in 2012 and the findings were that it 'exceeded all expectations'[263].

The evaluation document beautifully outlines the benefits for the children, teachers and parents involved and describes the ways this type of nature-based program differs from regular, indoor kinder. For example, the types of play in the bushland included 'more imaginative play and periods of sitting, reflecting and philosophical discussion with others, both peers and teachers.' Group dynamics were described as calmer and more level, with a 'softening of the louder, bigger voices and the lifting or empowering of the quieter voices for some children'. The teachers also describe play as having less gender stereotyping and being more inclusive with 'all children [were] welcomed in play'.

Teachers involved in the evaluation described personal professional development benefits, including the growth of investigative skills with mobile technology and the 'increased depth of their observations and interpretations of children's play promoted by the Bush Kinder setting'. Through their involvement in this pilot, the teachers also cultivated relationships beyond the kinder itself, with park rangers, colleagues, researchers, community members and the media. They describe deeper, more diverse and trusting relationships with the parents, perhaps relating to the heightened awareness of risk and the newness of the program. A lovely quote from one teacher which highlights the positives from trying this model is: 'It's all about relationships, belonging and community...the difference is there's no stuff, so the relationships are intensified, your role as a teacher is freed and you become stronger without clutter, it is really quite empowering'.

Broader community benefits were noted, including the desire of children to take their friends and family into the bushland they had come to know through kinder. This increased the number of people visiting and valuing the parklands.

While Westgarth Bush Kinder took the first steps to develop nature-based kinder programs in Australia, others have quickly followed. The bush kinder philosophy has been incorporated into Aboriginal communities too, as a way of helping the next generation of First Australians connect to Country. The Balee Koolin Bubup Bush Playgroup meets in the bushland of the Royal Botanic Gardens Cranbourne in Melbourne. With the guidance of local Elders, community members and an Indigenous officer from the Gardens, children and their families learn Boon Wurrung (local language) words for Country, important cultural stories and knowledge about local plants and animals[265].

## KITCHEN GARDENS

Another exciting innovation occurring in schools is the kitchen garden phenomenon. When my second son was in Prep, it was fun to be a part of developing the kitchen garden program at our local school. With the support of other parents and teaching staff we would organise weekly gardening or cooking sessions with the children during their first year of primary school. One of the wonderful things was seeing how children who were less focussed in the classroom setting could engage in the hands-on approach of our sessions, especially outdoor gardening. It was also great to see children whose parents spent little time out in the garden learning to relax about getting dirty, or wet, and instead become absorbed in the tasks of planting, watering or digging.

For optimal wellbeing we need to know how to eat well and to develop our literacy about which foods are most nutritious. This begins in childhood when young people are taught where their food comes from and how to prepare simple, healthy meals. This kind of learning is practical and hands-on, an experiential 'learning by doing'. A kitchen garden program enables all children, regardless of their family situation, to develop these important life skills. There is nothing quite like eating something you have grown yourself. It is also terrific to see children try different sorts of foods and to approach mealtimes with a curiosity and interest that is often not seen at home. The power of positive peer pressure cannot be underestimated.

My son is now in his twenties, so this school garden experience when he was five is quite some time ago. In the intervening years, the concept of a kitchen garden program has become extremely popular, in large part due to the success of the Stephanie Alexander Kitchen Garden model. Stephanie Alexander is an icon of the Melbourne restaurant and food scene having spent years establishing wonderful restaurants and then publishing what is regarded by many as a 'go to' cooking reference book, *The Cook's Companion* in 1996. This book has now sold some 500,000 copies and is also an app so has been constantly updated and evolving.

Concerned about the lack of knowledge many children had about where their food came from and how to prepare simple, healthy food, Alexander launched the Kitchen Garden Program. It began as a pilot project at a single school and now has a national reach, involving some 800 schools which is 10% of all Australian primary schools. From little things, big things grow.

This way of teaching kitchen gardening has been evaluated and the overall impact on participating schools is impressive[266]. Benefits include increased understanding of how food can be grown, harvested and prepared with flow-on effects into other curriculum areas like maths and science. Children's teamwork, sharing and other social skills improved too. Positive effects rippled out beyond the school and into the community as parents for whom English was a second language could participate in the cooking and gardening whereas they felt less comfortable assisting with reading and other classroom-based tasks. The program provided these parents with a practical way to engage in their children's education.

Food choices made at home were positively influenced with children requesting dishes cooked at school be included in the home menu. The great thing about this is that these meals always included vegetables. With the majority of Australian children not eating the optimal five serves of veggies per day, an excellent outcome of this program is an increase in the variety and quantity of vegetables eaten by children and their families[267]. Teachers in the evaluation study described a shift towards children bringing healthier food from home for snacks and lunch and most becoming more enthusiastic about trying new foods.

The evaluation report has some lovely descriptions of children and their families experimenting with new foods. For example: 'One parent came in to ask "What are capers? My child wants them on her pasta!" and "I had one child and he wouldn't eat the salad, just wouldn't' touch it. "I'm not eating that, it's leaves" and then he tried them and thought they were actually quite nice. The week after, he came back and he said, "I made that leaf thingy that we made last week and I made it for my mum and she liked it too".'

Broad social benefits included the students teaching younger siblings kitchen skills. Many discovered the joy of sharing a meal with others, around a table and learnt table manners, conversation skills and how to clean up co-operatively.

Positives flowed beyond the students through to older generations as children discovered they could talk to their grandparents about cooking and gardening. Older program volunteers formed friendships with children while cooking or gardening. The interaction between student and volunteer was different to that between student and teacher, and helped expand the types of relationships within the community. Research has found the main predictor of happiness to be the formation of meaningful relationships. So this element of the program, with friendships forming across cultures and generations, is truly special.

The volunteers experienced personal growth too, learning new skills, gaining confidence and making friends. One school planned to develop a community garden within its grounds to be used by those in town who no longer gardened at home because of concerns about water quality and drought. An important nutritional, recreational and social resource was created. Some schools also planned to share cooking and gardening facilities to allow others within their region to access kitchen garden learning. In the current environment of schools competing via NAPLAN results and online scorecards, this shared passion for cooking and gardening with children brings about a counter-cultural revolution of collaboration and resource sharing.

Of course, there are deep environmental learnings too. Within the school garden children learnt about biodiversity, composting, water conservation, worm farming and the importance of insects for pollination and soil health. They took these insights home, helping improve community knowledge on these important science and sustainability topics and deepening the value placed on nature.

The program was of the greatest benefit to students living with the biggest disadvantage. Those with the poorest health, educational and social indicators benefit most from having a cooking and gardening program embedded in their school's curriculum by helping such students learn how growing, harvesting, preparing and then eating plants can provide them with a tool to lift their wellbeing. One of the classroom teachers sums up the potentially life-changing value of this type of experiential learning: "I've got a boy in my class who is academically poor, socially inept and you think when he gets older it's going to be really hard and in the kitchen, he wants to be a chef. That's what he wants to do and I can see him following that through and if we didn't have the [kitchen garden] program here he may have been someone who has gone on and is lost but now he might grow up to be that great chef."

In some of the staff interviews, similar observations were made, for example: "Some of the boys are 'hopeless' in the classroom but very, very good in the garden: interested, intelligent, capable." If we are to address the increasing inequity within our society we need to focus on the foundations of health and education. One way to benefit both these core elements is learning within, about, and from nature. A school-based kitchen garden program is one great way to do this.

## SUSTAINABILITY EDUCATION

Learning about sustainably is now a core part of the Australian curriculum. Sustainability is how to live without damaging our environment and this subject is another way for children to learn about and connect to nature. The topic of sustainability tends to focus on water and energy cycles and waste reduction. But a key element is understanding the natural world and its ecosystems.

Unfortunately, a lot of environmental education for children focuses on large scale, complex problems. These can sometimes be presented in a depressing and overwhelming way. Rather than burden young people with problems created by their forbears, educator David Sobel says, "let us allow them to love the earth before we ask them to save it".[268] Children need to be allowed to find the adventure, fun and fascination in nature and to challenge themselves through exploration. Care is needed not to focus on the devastation of climate change, pollution and the destruction of nature and then turn to children and ask them to come up with solutions.

Inspiring leaders can be a positive force. But only if they create opportunities for young people to first understand and then, empowered by their knowledge, develop solutions to environmental challenges within their sphere of influence. If teaching is tailored to a child's developmental stage, a balance can be found where young people learn about problems after they have meaningfully connected to the world around them.

David Sobel proposes three developmentally appropriate phases of environmental learning. He says, "in early childhood, activities should centre on enhancing the developmental tendency toward empathy with the natural world. In middle childhood, exploration should take precedence. And in early adolescence, social action should assume a more central role."[268] This means children under seven can learn to care about the nature around them through story and imaginative play, responding to what they encounter. This will foster a sense of wonder, which feeds curiosity and learning as was discussed in the section on nature play.

Children from eight to eleven can learn how to explore their world further, from home or school, out into local and then more distant communities. At this age, kids will be able to create their own secret places within nature, like a cubby or tree house. David Sobel calls this a 'developmental geography of childhood'. Teachers and caregivers can help children learn through direct experience by going out into nearby nature to explore. In this way children of middle childhood are mapping their home ground and connecting with 'their place'. In his book *How to Raise a Wild Child*, American author Scott D. Sampson, describes this as 'place-based learning'[269] and expands on how experience based school programming can cover the entire curriculum. He says, "Far from being parochial, place-based learning uses direct experiences in local landscapes to inform larger-scale explorations. Much better to understand and intimately experience one's local oak or fir forest before diving into books and videos about the disappearing Amazon rainforest".

As well as learning about their local landscape, the creation of secret places like cubbies or dens provides children with a private place of their own. In their hidden spot, children can nurture their imagination and tend to their inner world. English author, Jay Griffiths, explores this need for privacy and space in her expansive discussion of childhood[237]. She says, "Wanting their secret places, children make dens from the age of about six, building forts and constructing treehouses in a worldwide habit of childhood. You no more have to teach a child to make a den than give a mouse training in burrowing."

Today's children have very little privacy. Monitored from within the womb via ultrasound, in their cots with video baby monitoring and then at childcare and school. Not to mention countless videos and photos uploaded onto their parents' social media pages. Perhaps a quiet, private space of their own outside is just what they need. "Children often don't want anyone to see them entering their dens and they go there sometimes just to sit alone, sometimes to read, to be secluded, often in silence, to hide treasure and keep secrets. The imagination wants its solitudes, its hideaways of intimacy for self-invention, self-discovery and self-making, so a den, dug on the borders of adult notice, is not a matter of ownership but of self-ownership," says Griffiths[236]. As well as backyards in private homes, school grounds and local parks can support this need by providing space for this kind of play, even though to an adult eye it might look unkempt. Alongside 'sentinal children', markers of child-friendly suburbs have playgrounds with areas for nature play and cubby building. The diversity of the cubbies is heart-warming.

Older children, from the age of 12, can move into social action as they are at a developmental stage where it is naturally sought. This may take the form of being environment leaders at school, lobbying for action on protecting natural places or threatened species. If this has followed on from the initial phase of empathy and exploration, it means children feel empowered to make positive change in a place or about an issue that's meaningful to them.

The Australian curriculum has Sustainability as one of three cross-curriculum priorities. The other two are Aboriginal and Torres Strait Islander Histories and Cultures, and Asia and Australia's engagement with Asia. This has reinforced the value of what has already been taking place at forward thinking schools in sustainability education. One exciting example is the Victorian school, Bentleigh Secondary College, where decades of focus on sustainability teaching has led to not only water and energy savings, but also an enormous increase in the amount of biodiversity on campus[270]. A green transformation of the school has seen the creation of a wetland area and urban forest. The forest is habitat restoration back to the landscape prior to white settlement. Young people learn about the Aboriginal history and culture of the site as well as about its biodiversity values.

This approach shows young people they can be positive agents for change by physically making the world a better place and taking direct action against global problems like climate change, biodiversity loss and water pollution. All this is taking place in their school with their peers and contributing, no doubt, to their self-esteem and sense of purpose. The school's environmental projects are deliberately designed to include the students within scheduled class time in a variety of different subjects. They are learning in the real world, about the real world, literally 'being the change' they want to see. It's inspiring stuff.

## Kids Teaching Kids

Another innovative Australian program is Kids Teaching Kids, developed by father and son team, Arron and Richard Wood. With this approach, teachers are supported to help children develop presentations on environmental issues that are important to them locally. The understanding behind it is that children learn best by teaching others. A focus on local issues makes the content interesting and relevant. The annual conference is a program highlight where children share their work with one other. Their creativity and sense of fun is infectious, with presentations including poetry, rap and dance.

Kids Teaching Kids started in 1999 with the first Young People's River Health Conference in Mildura in rural Victoria. This has grown to become the annual Kids Teaching Kids Conference, a national event attended by some 13,000 students from 500 schools. Supporting young people to create positive change by restoring their local natural environment empowers them and energises their learning. This also grows problem solving and resilience, which are key for optimising the emotional health of young people. The Kids Teaching Kids approach has been developed into a program that teachers and schools can incorporate into their curriculum in a way that works best for them. Its flexible ethos seeks to bring about "a cultural shift in the way we perceive and use our natural environment" by promoting the idea that "because the environment is an issue that is accessible and vital to us all, it can be used as the common building block to unite communities and perhaps even the global community."[271] Arron and Richard Wood have written their story and what is essentially a guidebook[272] and the entire model is being shared internationally through the United Nations' UN Works Programme.

The Kids Teaching Kids story, with the father and son relationship of Richard and Arron at its core, highlights the value of children having an adult to mentor them as they develop a relationship with nature. As Rachel Carson said, "it is more important to pave the way for the child to want to know than to put [them] on a diet of facts [they are] not ready to assimilate".[225] As the founder of the modern environmental movement, Rachel Carson was switched on to the importance of children developing a deep connection to nature in their early years as a way of fostering creativity, curiosity and a love of learning about the world.

In his autobiography, *Billabong Boy*[271], Arron Woods describes growing up beside a billabong deeply immersed in nature. He attributes his determination to restore our environment to this beginning. Studies have shown that children growing up with a sense of connection to nature, facilitated by key adult mentors, are likely to pursue a path of environmental activism or have positive attitudes towards protecting our natural environment[273]. Globally, we are facing an enormous number of complex environmental challenges. Providing meaningful nature time from a young age in kindergartens, schools and communities not only optimally supports the health and development of children, it also nurtures the strength and will they need to become the nature leaders – the Rachel Carsons and Arron Woods of the future.

## OUTDOOR ADVENTURE

Having been a mother of three teenage boys, I am deeply aware of the importance of allowing young people to develop their independence, challenge themselves physically and mentally, and take some risks. I have witnessed the growth of self-agency as well as pure happiness, that comes through prolonged time spent out in nature.

For many years, our family undertook a long journey to the far eastern corner of Victoria to spend a week camping in Croajingalong National Park. Spanning some 88,355 hectares including 100 kilometres of wilderness coastline, the park is classified as a World Biosphere Reserve, one of only 12 in Australia. Thurra River campground sits alongside the river, nestled behind sand dunes with the Southern Ocean pounding the adjacent beach. Each campsite is surrounded by tea tree and banksia forest, has white sand underfoot and is visited throughout the day by enormous monitor lizards and families of fairy wrens. At night, the sky is a mass of stars and the background music the melodic pinging of tiny bats. From our campsite, we can cycle to the river, several ocean beaches or the lighthouse.

It was a family ritual to visit Thurra River and we all became strongly connected to this special place even though we only experienced it once a year. We would return from our week away, having been out of range and Wi-Fi-free, restored and ready to take on another year of work or study. This wild camping allowed us to shrug off the stresses of life in the suburbs, to slow down and engage in nature play. Adults and children alike.

One quintessential Croajingalong experience is the 'Raiders of the Lost Ark' adventure that is the dune walk. It begins with a bushwalk through coastal woodland to the edge of an enormous dune field. Then starts an exhausting trek across several vast sand dunes. At the pinnacle of the dunes the snaking Thurra River comes into view. Here, a choice must be made about whether to run down to the river or to ride your boogie board down (that is, if you've made the extra sacrifice of carrying it all the way there with you!) With an almost 45-degree incline the half-jog, half-run down to the water is part terrifying and part hilarious.

Teenagers, or foolhardy adults, pelt down the dune face on boogie boards and plunge into the river. For those of us trying to be more careful at the bottom of the dune, shoes are quickly shucked off and we dive into the cool, fresh water of the river.

After a rejuvenating swim the next phase involves a race to dry off before the March flies bite. Then begins an arduous walk across the base of the dune in the gutter where it abuts the river's floodplain. Each step into the soft, hot sand is hard work and the half an hour or so to reach the river is exhausting. Once in the shallows of the lower river the going gets easier and it's quite a pleasant walk through the water back downstream to camp. If the river's high we need to float our belongings on the boogie boards as the water rises to our chests but it's nice knowing we are on the home stretch. After an hour or so of this we are back to the campground for a much-deserved cool drink and a rest.

This dune walk is a real adventure for us. We feel a huge sense of achievement at having navigated a course through the dune field, to the river, and back. The risk of injury, or getting lost, is always there. But the feeling of achievement, the problem solving, and teamwork are great. This is the type of team building exercise corporations pay thousands of dollars for their executives to experience. It is also like the outdoor programs many schools are adding to their curriculum for teenagers in the middle years of high school. Unfortunately, this is often not available to all children due to cost and logistics despite its inherent value. These sorts of camps are also usually phased out for the final few years of school, so that children and teachers can focus on what's perceived as being of more benefit to achieving high final grades – indoor curriculum.

Young people, at all stages of schooling, benefit from regular adventurous outdoor experiences. The benefits to their wellbeing and emotional growth far outweigh any risk of injury, and programs can be tailored to the developmental stage of the young people involved. For primary school-aged children, initial experiences can include bushwalking, camping and kayaking with appropriate adult support and encouragement. In adolescence, there can be opportunities for multi-day adventures like hiking and canoeing or higher risk activities like abseiling and caving. In these later years of school much of the activity can be done without direct adult supervision. Groups of several peers can go on forays into the wilderness together and some solo time is also important.

During their teenage years, young people experience an increased rate of mood and behavioural issues. This relates to the mismatch between their intellectual maturity in the mid to late teens and their psychosocial maturity between 22-25 years. They need to learn how to manage risk and solve problems without direct adult input. Outdoor experiences can provide a much safer way for this to occur than may otherwise be provided by society. Far better for a teenager to test their body out by participating in an overnight hike or rafting down a rapid, than by train surfing or experimenting with drugs. As Sobel says, "the task in adolescence is to bond with the self, and nature provides the setting and opportunity for challenging rites of passage."[274]

The part of the brain concerned with planning, consequences and creative problem solving, or 'higher functioning', is the frontal lobe. This area undergoes enormous change during adolescence and early adulthood. The frontal lobe tends to shut down when we are stressed, so decisions made at these times can be poor. As discussed earlier, David Strayer's study of participants on a multi-day hike found improved higher functioning after a prolonged time spent in nature. He called this the "three-day effect". During this study, researchers tested people on-site after they had been immersed in the wilderness for several days. Tests were completed to check creativity and problem-solving. The results were compared to a control group who were tested before leaving for the walk. The group tested after extended time outdoors performed 50% better. The researchers thought this was due to "an increase in exposure to natural stimuli that are both emotionally positive and low-arousing and a corresponding decrease in exposure to attention demanding technology, which regularly requires that we attend to sudden events, switch amongst tasks, maintain task goals, and inhibit irrelevant actions or cognitions."[200]

Teenagers today are often online, switching between various devices and from one social media or education platform to another. They are expected to spend a lot of time looking at a screen for school, and the enmeshed social networks are also accessed via their device. Alerts pop up interrupting attention, so the brain is constantly switching between tasks. Scientists call this specific focus on external tasks *directed attention*. In contrast, allowing the mind to wander and to reflect on things, like imagining the future, remembering personal memories and social emotions, is called the brain's *default mode*. Certain parts of the brain are active in default mode when observed on a functional MRI scanner, and this activity is relatively suppressed by attention focused on external tasks[275]. It seems this daydreaming is important for brain development and that today's young people may be missing out on this gentle default mode due to the educational and other screen-based demands.

Rather than removing outdoor activities from the high-pressured, final years of school when young minds are stressed, we should be incorporating nature-based activities into the timetable. This way, not only academic outcomes but also mental health will be improved. Surely both schools and parents want young people to be as calm and happy as possible as the long years of schooling draw to a close. The importance of time in nature for our mind, mood and happiness has been explored in greater detail earlier. I mention it here again because for young people, who are often struggling with mental health issues, nature may help them to either prevent, or manage, these difficulties. If time away in beautiful natural places is embedded into their educational timetable, we are increasing their chances of navigating the challenges of adolescence smoothly.

Let's expand our thinking of education beyond the academic curriculum to also encompass outdoor programs which reach out into national parks and green spaces. Maybe there can be partnerships between schools and nearby nature at primary and high school levels. For senior students, the scale can be bigger with the reach out into nature extending into more remote places. To optimise the learning environment for our young people we can have school grounds rich in nature, connections to local parks and bushland for project work and then adventurous forays into the wilderness for personal challenge, adventure and restoration.

As this chapter draws to a close, I hope you can see the value of nature for the development, learning and wellbeing of our young people. Only natural spaces can provide it all: clean air, mental restoration, space for exploration and physical challenge, endless opportunities for wonder and a place for curiosity and creativity to flourish.

## GROWING UP IN NATURE

- ❤ Nature makes school grounds healthier – the more different trees and shrubs, the better
- ❤ A view of trees and other plants helps learning
- ❤ You can bring nature into the classroom
- ❤ Nature stimulates creativity and problem solving
- ❤ You can learn about any subject in, with, and through nature
- ❤ Learning can extend into nearby nature and wilderness
- ❤ Nature time helps children's brains rest and recover
- ❤ Nature provides awesome opportunities for teenagers to challenge themselves and grow their resilience and self-agency

# EPILOGUE

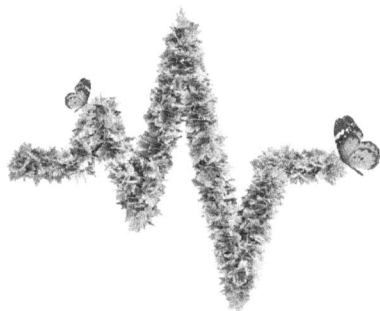

# Harmonising With Nature

*"We cannot win this battle to save species and environments without forging an emotional bond between ourselves and nature as well – for we will not fight to save what we do not love."*

~Stephen Jay Gould.

Our health is intimately connected to Earth's biosphere, to the plants and animals with whom we share this beautiful planet. This web of life is delicate and complex and our relationship to it will determine the future for all. Caring for and connecting to the natural world is necessary for the flourishing of all living things. And for our individual health and wellbeing. We can reject the pervasive ecocidality of contemporary society that has disrupted Earth's climate and triggered mass extinctions. Instead, let's choose to restore the Earth and mend our relationship with nature, to create a new way of being where loving and looking after nature sustains us.

We can learn to live mindfully among the vast tapestry of life by taking our cues from First Nations people for whom this is inherent wisdom. In her book *Braiding Sweetgrass*, First Nations scientist and writer, Robin Wall Kimmerer describes how the Haudenosaunee First Nations people begin their day with the Words That Come Before All Else or the Thanksgiving Address[276]. A ritual of reciting collective thanks to all the elements of the natural world upon which human survival depends, the Thanksgiving Address is an invocation of gratitude. As each part of the living world is honoured and thanked from the birds through to the thunder and winds, it is quite long, much longer than America's Pledge of Allegiance, for example. As Kimmerer writes: "it is also a material, scientific inventory of the natural world. ... As it goes forward, each element of the ecosystem is named in its turn, along with its functions. It is a lesson in Native science."[22]

Here is an excerpt, one of the approximately eighteen sections: "The Plants. Now we turn toward the vast fields of Plant life. As far as the eye can see, the Plants grow, working many wonders. They sustain many life forms. With our minds gathered together, we give thanks and look forward to seeing Plant life for many generations to come. Now our minds are one."[276]

Each section of the address finishes with the words 'now our minds are one', a unifying statement of reflection and intention.

The Thanksgiving Address is spoken at the beginning of each school day for children in Haudenosaunee communities and before all meetings and gatherings. This culture of gratitude runs counter to most modern societies. Wall Kimmerer writes, "In a consumer society, contentment is a radical proposition. Recognising abundance rather than scarcity undermines an economy that thrives by creating unmet desires. Gratitude cultivates an ethic of fullness, but the economy needs emptiness. The Thanksgiving Address reminds you that you already have everything you need".[22]

In Australia, we begin most formal events with an acknowledgment of Traditional Owners and pay our respects to the Aboriginal or Torres Strait Islander Elders of the land. Many also choose to remind those present that sovereignty was never ceded and a Treaty never signed, that the land was stolen. Where I live, in south-eastern Melbourne, the Traditional Custodians are the Wurundjeri Woi-wurrung people of the Eastern Kulin Nation. They mark important events or the arrival of visitors with a Smoking Ceremony. I have been fortunate to participate in several and to have the ritual explained to me. It may be differently performed according to the Elder facilitating but often begins with a fire being lit. This may be comprised of three different types of wood and leaves, representing the children, the Elders and the adults within the community. The Creator spirit Bunjil, the wedge-tailed eagle, is thanked, and visitors are welcomed to the land and invited to walk through the fire's smoke to be cleansed. After this, each newcomer is given a leaf to symbolise they are welcome to take what they need from the land during their visit. This permission comes with the understanding the guest will care for the Country they stay on, ensuring its future health. The giving of a leaf, akin to a passport, reminds the recipient not to take too much and to look after the people, plants and animals they encounter.

Like Australian Aboriginal and Torres Strait Islander people, the Haudenosaunee First Nations people are always mindful that future generations be cared for. They use the term Honourable Harvest to guide the taking of plants and animals for food, shelter and clothing. Kimmerer describes the rules of the Harvest as follows:

*"Know the ways of the ones who take care of you,*
*so that you may take care of them.*
*Introduce yourself. Be accountable as the one who*
*comes asking for life.*
*Ask permission before taking. Abide by the answer.*
*Never take the first. Never take the last.*
*Take only what you need.*
*Take only that which is given.*
*Never take more than half. Leave some for others.*
*Harvest in a way that minimises harm.*
*Use it respectfully. Never waste what you have taken.*
*Share.*
*Give thanks for what you have been given.*
*Give a gift, in reciprocity for what you have taken.*
*Sustain the ones who sustain you and the earth will*
*last forever."*[22]

We can hold the rules of the Honourable Harvest in our hearts when we go to buy our food, remembering the plants and animals whose lives were taken so we could eat. This ecological consciousness makes it difficult to overeat or to waste food or water.

We can begin to address the legacy of ecosystem destruction we have inherited and work with others to repair and restore the lands and seas. In doing so, not only will the soils, waters, plants and animals recover, we will too. Our innate biophilia will be nurtured as we see the land we tend revitalise. The ripples of this cultivation are felt physically, emotionally and spiritually. It is poignant to read how the rehabilitation of Doug Lang's degraded farm has been an integral part of his recovery. Lang's healing through land restoration provides hope and inspiration for us all. He writes, "The tree violet is the true survivor. There are more tree violet bushes on our farm now then there ever was. Tractors, cables, crowbars, gelignite and sprays could not eradicate this plant. It is a plant I have grown to truly admire for its fighting qualities. It is a resilient, shrubby bush that's rough around the edges and I love the way it hangs in there with its fighting 'never give up' spirit. It is a plant that is meant to be in this area. It's a plant where, on a warm spring evening, it comes alive with a mass of insect life, thousands of them, that all play their role in this world of biodiversity. This prickly bush is also a haven for the beautiful blue wrens and finches that enjoy the protective sanctuary it provides –it is a safe playground for these fragile birds."

When Lang describes the return of native birds and animals to his farm following his replanting of lost, once abundant trees and shrubs he relates powerfully to his own healing. "When I witness such things, I can actually feel my mental health and physical health improve. Nature has a way of giving inner peace, nature's tranquiliser. To think we are creating habitat for little creatures is just a wonderful, fulfilling feeling. It is no coincidence that these experiences lift my spirits when I feel lost and totally beaten. It is no coincidence that I have a lot less depressive episodes these days and that I feel calmer more of the time. Nature does this."[137]

Spending time caring for the natural world feeds our soul and calms our mind as well as exercising our bodies. The plants and animals benefit from our tending to them and we receive their gifts in return. It is a relationship of reciprocity exemplified in the simple act of gardening. As Robin Wall Kimmerer says, "In a garden, food arises from partnership. If I don't pick rocks and pull weeds, I'm not fulfilling my end of the bargain. I can do these things with my handy opposable thumb and capacity to use tools, to shovel manure. But I can no more create a tomato or embroider a trellis in beans than I can turn lead into gold. That is the plants' responsibility and their gift: animating the inanimate. Now there is a gift. … A garden is a nursery for nurturing connection, the soil for cultivation of practical reverence. And its power goes far beyond the garden gate – once you develop a relationship with a little patch of earth, it becomes a seed itself. Something essential happens in a vegetable garden. It's a place where if you can't say 'I love you' out loud, you can say it in seeds. And the land will reciprocate, in beans."[22]

We can work to deepen our nature connection in our own way. This might be by planting a vegetable or flower garden on the balcony of our apartment, restoring a degraded area of suburban bushland or rehabilitating a landscape harmed by destructive farming practices. Or perhaps all three. The key is a sense of connection to place and of a care for the land and all the plants and animals who live there with us. To truly feel this deeply requires us to be quiet at times, and to pay attention to what the other living things are telling us. Of course, they can't speak to us; they let us know if their needs are being met by how they look and behave. It's hard not to notice the thirst of a wilting plant or panting bird on a hot summer's day. Simply switching off your phone, removing your headphones and stopping to look carefully at what's around can help turn your nature radar on. Once again, First Nations people have something to tell us about how to best connect to nature. To really listen to the land.

Dadirri (da-did-ee) is a word from the Ngan'gikurunggurr and Ngen'giwumirri languages of the peoples of the Daly River region in northern Australia. It means 'deep water sounds' and describes their way of being on Country. It is focused on quiet, still awareness; inner, deep listening and feeling nature. This way of being contrasts with the way we non-Indigenous people are often quickly moving through the world, either walking, running or driving. We also tend to talk more and ask lots of questions.

Elder, Miriam-Rose Ungunmerr-Baumann, in her reflection on dadirri writes, "in our Aboriginal way, we learnt to listen from our earliest days. We could not live good and useful lives unless we listened. This was the normal way for us to learn – not by asking questions. We learnt by watching and listening, waiting and then acting. Our people have passed on this way of listening for over 40,000 years. ... My people are not threatened by silence. They are completely at home in it. They have lived for thousands of years with Nature's quietness." She goes on to explain the quiet stillness and waiting part of dadirri. "Our Aboriginal culture has taught us to be still and to wait. We do not try to hurry things up. We let them follow their natural course, like the seasons. ... To be still brings peace – and it brings understanding. When we are really still in the bush, we concentrate. We are aware of the anthills and the turtles and the water lillies. Our culture is different. We are asking our fellow Australians to take time to know us; to be still and listen to us... I believe that the spirit of dadirri that we have to offer will blossom and grow, not just within ourselves, but in our whole nation."[277]

The practice of deep listening to Country is widespread, although the language shifts depending on where you are. Given the new understanding we have of the benefits of mindfulness and meditation, perhaps non-Indigenous Australians are beginning to sense this old way. Maybe we can pause and learn from the First Peoples of our ancient land and celebrate their knowledge of how best to be in this place. A strong step towards conciliation will surely be a willingness to practise our own deep listening to the original inhabitants and an acknowledgement that they have much to teach us about how to best be. Both with ourselves and others and with the land itself.

It is not easy for us to slow down, to develop patience and an ability to really listen to the natural world. But it is essential if we are to restore balance, to live in harmony with the living things upon which we depend. To grow our green heart.

Transforming ourselves so we are more in sync with the rhythms of nature requires a shift in our orientation. We can turn our hearts and minds green by consciously planting nature into our lives. This means making time to mindfully notice and be with other living things. It may be guided by a nature prescription or a personal commitment to have at least one 'green hour' per day. It also involves enriching our living, working, and learning spaces with nature.

Imagine a future where healthcare settings are naturally healthy places to be, with fresh air, plentiful plants and images and sounds of nature. Landscape-based health interventions embedded within our medical system will help restore wellbeing to those suffering. Forest bathing programs will see old-growth and native forests protected and cherished for their health-giving values. And degraded ecosystems will be regenerated by those seeking community, friendship and meaning. All children will have the time and space to play in nature. Bush kinders, kitchen gardens and outdoor learning and adventure will be an integral part of young people's lives. They will be given every opportunity to feel the wonder and awe of nature.

This nature-fuelled revolution, invigorated by a sense of care, will intuitively address the twin problems of climate change and biodiversity loss. Those with a green heart and mind, with the spirit of deep listening, will make the right choices.

# Here are some simple steps to begin your journey...

## 1.
## Connect to your place

❤ Learn the first name of the place where you live and the language and stories of its First Peoples.

❤ Look for indigenous plants and animals, seek out their names in the language of the First Peoples and begin to look after them. Understand their needs and restore their habitat. This might be in your own garden, in nearby nature or by volunteering with the local Friends group or council.

❤ Spend some time just being still and tuning in to the nature around you, you may like to use the suggestions in the Green Mind Chapter to help guide this process.

❤ Practise deep listening to place.

## 2.
## Connect to people in your community

❤ Join with others who are interested in the local nature and culture.

❤ Go along to festivals and events that bring together First Nations knowledge, belief systems and nature.

❤ Listen to local First Nations Elders and communities whenever you can, seek out experiences where you can learn and give the respect of deep listening.

# 3.
# Develop a culture of gratitude to the natural world around you

♥ Begin each day with a practise of consciously thanking the living world that sustains your life and that of your family and friends. Look to the Thanksgiving Address and other cultural practises for inspiration.

♥ Begin important gatherings with a ceremonial practice of gratitude to the Traditional Custodians on whose land you are meeting and to the natural world that sustains us all.

♥ Move through the landscape mindfully because you are stepping through a cultural landscape as well as a natural one.

# 4.
# Use resources mindfully

♥ Adopt the Honourable Harvest mindset to take only what you need without compromising the ongoing health of the natural environment or other people.

♥ Consider the effects of your actions and choices on Earth and on future generations.

# FIND OUT MORE

To grow your knowledge on nature and wellbeing and explore some topics in greater detail I recommend the following resources.

## Books

### Biodiversity and Ecological Damage

*Silent Spring* by Rachel Carson

*The Bush* by Don Watson

*Maralinga's Long Shadow, Yvonne's Story* by Christobel Mattingley

*White Beech* by Germaine Greer

*Half Earth* and other writings by E.O. Wilson

*The Legacy* by David Suzuki

*Finding The Mother Tree* by Suzanne Simard

*The Secret Life of Trees* and other books by Peter Wohlleben

*Call Of The Reed Warbler* by Charles Massey

*Fathoms: The World In The Whale* by Rebecca Giggs

*Sea Sick* by Alanna Mitchell

### Climate Change

*This Changes Everything* and other books by Naomi Klein

*Merchants of Doubt* by Naomi Oreskes

*Climate Code Red* by David Spratt and Phillip Sutton

*We Are the Weather Makers* and other books by Tim Flannery

### First Nations' Knowledges

*Dark Emu* and other books by Bruce Pascoe

*The Greatest Estate on Earth* by Bill Gammage

*Braiding Sweetgrass* and other books by Robin Wall Kimmerer

*Treading Lightly* by Tex Sculthorpe and Karl-Erik Svelby

*Sand Talk* by Tyson Yunkaporta

*Tell Me Why* by Archie Roach

*Welcome to Country: A Travel Guide to Indigenous Australia* by Marcia Langton

## Mindfulness Meditation

*Hardwiring Happiness* and other books by Rick Hansen

*Wherever You Go, There You Are* and other books by Jon Kabat-Zinn

*My Year of Living Mindfully* by Shannon Harvey

*The Happiness Plan* by Elise Bialylew

## Nature and Wellbeing

*Forest Bathing* by Dr Qing Li

*Blue Mind* by Wallace J. Nichols

*The Nature Fix* by Florence Williams

*Phosphoresence* by Julia Baird

*The Space Between The Stars* by Indira Naidoo

*The Comfort Of Water* by Maya Ward

*The Nature of Survival* by Doug Lang

## Children and Nature

*The Last Child in the Woods* and other books by Richard Louv

*The Sense Of Wonder* by Rachel Carson

*How to Raise A Wild Child* by Scott D. Sampson

*Kith* by Jay Griffiths

*Billabong Boy* by Aaron Wood

## On screen

*Back To Nature* an 8-part ABC television series hosted by Aaron Pederson and Holly Ringland https://iview.abc.net.au/show/back-to-nature

*Dadirri Film* found on the Miriam Rose Foundation website https://www.miriamrosefoundation.org.au/dadirri/

*Schools Out: Lessons from a Forest Kindergarten* film directed by Lisa Molomot

*Project Wildthing* film by David Bond- access on thewildnetwork

*My Year of Living Mindfully* and *The Connection* films by Shannon Harvey https://www.shannonharvey.com/collections/films

## Online

The International Children and Nature Network (USA) http://www.childrenandnature.org/

The Climate Council https://www.climatecouncil.org.au/

Doctors for the Environment Australia https://dea.org.au/

The Planetary Health Alliance https://www.planetaryhealthalliance.org/planetary-health

Park Rx America- a nature prescribing hub https://parkrxamerica.org/

Kids In Nature Network https://www.kidsinnaturenetwork.org.au/

NHS Forest (UK) https://nhsforest.org

# Courses and experiences

*Wayapa Wuurrk* – a diploma in earth connection practice based on ancient Indigenous wisdom. Training is through an intensive 7-day experiential learning with storytelling, deep listening and other Indigenous ways. https://wayapa.com/about/

*Forest Therapy Guide Course* by International Nature and Forest Therapy Alliance – a six month mentored training course to become a Forest Therapy Guide. https://infta.net/

*Dadirri Tours* – Miriam Rose Ungunmerr-Baumann has issued an open invitation to all Australians to "come and sit with us on country." To experience dadirri visit the Miriam Rose Foundation's website. https://www.miriamrosefoundation.org.au/

*Mindfulness Based Stress Reduction (MBSR)* an 8-week foundational, evidence-based mindfulness course developed by Jon Kabat-Zinn offered globally through accredited teachers. https://mbsrtraining.com/

In Australia MBSR is offered through Openground. https://www.openground.com.au/

*Nature Play Course* a 2-hour online course for teachers from Cool Australia featuring Dr Dimity Williams. https://learn.coolaustralia.org/course/teach-nature-play-cc011/

# GLOSSARY OF TERMS

*Aboriginal* – the original inhabitants of mainland Australia or Tasmania

*Aboriginal and Torres Strait Islander* – original habitant of all lands now known as Australia

*Biodiversity* – biological diversity, the variety of lifeforms on Earth

*Biome* – a geographical grouping of ecosystems

*Biophilia* – the inherent love of nature

*Climate change* – any change in the climate, lasting for several decades or longer, including changes in temperature, rainfall or wind patterns

*Ecocide* – mass damage or destruction of ecosystems

*Ecosystem* – the network of relationships between living things and their physical environment

*First Peoples* – the collective of individual Nations in Australia including those unsure of which Nation they are from

*Fossil Fuel* – a fuel formed in the geological past from the remains of living things

*indigenous* (all lower case) – belonging naturally to a place i.e. a plant or animal

*Indigenous* (capitalised) – refers to First Peoples in an international context or Aboriginal and Torres Strait Islander peoples

*Nature* – the total ecological system of the material world

*Solastalgia* – a form of emotional or existential distress caused by environmental change

*Terracide* – global ecocide

Terminology for Aboriginal and Torres Strait Islander people based upon Public Health Association of Australia's guide.[278]

# ACKNOWLEDGEMENTS

Writing this book has been like walking a multiday hike. So exciting to envisage and plan for, friends to share the experience with at times but ultimately, a deeply personal adventure with all the ups and downs, pain, frustration and, yes of course, exhilaration of any journey worth taking. Along the way I have had my share of challenge, good and bad luck and serendipity. Always, there has been nature to contemplate and seek comfort and rejuvenation from. Also too, the sense that I am not alone, that many others are trying to share their experience and ideas in the hope that doing so will somehow shape the world, to make it a healthier, happier place. Meeting these fellow travellers has proved an unexpected delight and they have all made my life richer.

In its embryonic stage, when this book was merely an itch to be scratched, several people helped push me forward. Professor Mardie Townsend provided ideas and encouragement at this time. My friend Grant Blashki helped with perspective and introduced me to Helen Sykes who kindly reviewed an early draft. But it was really my incredibly patient and supportive husband Andrew who urged me to "just start writing!". I am so very fortunate to have had him steady me as I journeyed forth.

Listening to community radio one day in this early phase I heard writer and comedian Catherine Deveny interviewed about her Gunna's classes. The die was cast. I was slowly drawn into the wonderful world of 'Queen Dev'! Weekends spent writing, laughing and reflecting with others supported me as I progressed my drafts. Deep thanks to Catherine and all her Gunnas for keeping me sane and motivated. As one path leads to another, through Catherine I met Julie Ponstance, a self-publishing coach extraordinaire. Thanks to Julie for her smiling and urging and for those who joined me in Julie's course. All provided encouragement and feedback at different stages, especially Kate and Suze.

My dear friend and colleague, Associate Professor Marion Carey, kindly provided a meticulous and thoughtful review. And Christine Joy, who has taught me so much about nature play and our beautiful environment, generously read the manuscript during an especially challenging time. I am also grateful to Lorna Hendry who gave me some necessarily firm guidance after reading an early draft and for the editorial expertise of Elena Gomez and Amanda Spedding. And huge thanks to Sophie White for her thoughtful and creative book design.

I am thrilled and so very grateful to Dr Bob Brown for finding time within his busy life to write the forward. The passion, intelligence and love he brings to environmental advocacy is inspiring and energising.

*Nature, Our Medicine* is the fruit of my lifelong relationship with the natural world. My first and favourite playground and safe place. I am so grateful for the nature mentors who laid the foundations – especially my mother. This strong base fortified me as I stepped into the world of medicine and then environmental advocacy and activism. I would like to express my gratitude to the following friends, allies and inspirations:

To Sue Pratt and Anna Mezzetti and our merry band of community climate activists during the Families for a Safe Climate years—Lona Parry, Clare Nolan, Claire Ekins, Digna Nichols, Karin Hammarberg and Astrid Kruse-Thorpe—and our friends, children and partners who donned orange t-shirts, made papier mache dinosaurs and placards and created some ruckus in middle-class Melbourne.

To my friends and colleagues at Doctors for the Environment Australia who take time out of their demanding medical work to lobby for change within the health sector and society more broadly. Especially Marion Carey, Katherine Barraclough, Rosalie Schultz, Jessica Kneebone, Brooke Ah Shay and Kenneth Winkel who are passionate about biodiversity and getting more 'green' into healthcare. And to David Shearman, the late Tony McMichael and other leaders for speaking about the relationship between health and the environment for many decades. I'd like to also acknowledge Eugenie Kayak whose calm leadership guided us through the (successful) battle to prevent the development of a coal plant because of its health harms – the first time a health organisation had taken such a move.

To all those who have tried, and are still trying, to protect the Tarkine/takayna. Particularly the GetUp crew from my trip in 2010, and my son Patrick who spoke passionately at school about the forest and why it should be looked after, not destroyed. Also Bob Brown and his partner Paul Thomas who hosted our group in 2017 as we visited takayna's forest, rivers and coastline. Sitting around the fire sipping tea and feasting on Paul's scones as we learnt about the fight ahead was a powerful experience. Knowing there are people still living in the forest, trying to halt mining is both heart wrenching and strongly motivating. May sanity prevail and they be able to come home soon.

To others working to protect nature in courtrooms, boardrooms and tearooms. And to those who've spoken out, often at great personal cost – Greta Thunberg, Jane Goodall, Tim Flannery, Maya Ward, David Suzuki, and many others. And to all First Nations sovereign people who have been fighting for their lives, family, culture and Country since colonisation began.

To those who have devoted their lives to researching and promoting nature-based health interventions like Qing Li, Melissa Lem and Robert Zarr.

To Doug Lang, whose moving memoir speaks to the healing power of nature, for letting me share his story.

To everyone I encountered through the Centre for Sustainability Leadership who forever changed how I think, especially the incredible Jason Clarke and Kate Nicolazzo. Through CSL I met Cecile van der Burgh and Sanne de Swart – thank goodness! Our journey into the world of nature play expanded my horizons and through the Kids In Nature Network we have helped thousands of children get the time and space to be in nature. The Royal Botanic Gardens Melbourne is special for providing KINN with a home base and the expertise of Christine Joy in our foundational period. The Gardens continues to provide partnership and other support and KINN flourishes with its new board and team. Thanks also to David Strickland, a 'true believer' in a suit who provided bureaucratic backing.

To all those who seek to fill children's lives with nature, whether through advocacy, education or everyday life, people like Claire Wardell, David Bond, Doug Faragher, Mick Roberston, Emily Barrow and Richard Louv.

To the many inspiring First Nations people who have generously shared their culture and shown me how to be in relationship with the natural world. Especially Willie Gordon who took my family out on Country, demonstrating how to truly care for it. June Oscar (AO) guided me and others through the special health centre she designed in Fitzroy Crossing. Lionel Lauch's guided walks through the beautiful bushland of coastal Victoria and didgeridoo sound meditation on the clifftop were moving and enlightening. Listening to Archie Roach (AO) and Ruby Hunter perform songs and tell stories on many occasions and reading Archie's memoir helped me grasp the depth of trauma inflicted on the Stolen Generations and understand the healing power of music and the sacredness of Country. Trevor Gallagher performed several Smoking Ceremonies at the Royal Botanic Gardens for Kids In Nature Network events, I discovered something new every time. Listening to Tyson Yunkaporta speak at the Common Ground meditation conference and reading his book, *Sand Talk*, enriched my understanding of Indigenous thinking. Glenn Romanis, Aunty Delmae Barton and William Barton, through their contributions to Kids In Nature Network events, expanded my conception of art and music. While Claire G. Coleman's books, both fiction and non-fiction, have challenged my preconceptions about many things, especially colonization. Aunty Joy Murphy Wandin (AO)'s contribution to the Nature Play Week launch in 2017 where she talked about her book, *Welcome To Country*, taught me about Wurundjeri Woi-wurrung culture and language. And the Miriam Rose Foundation allowed me to mention dadirri.

To my meditation teachers for helping me slow down and find the inner space and quiet to truly pay attention – Nique Murch, Timothea Goddard and Julia Grieves. And to Dr Elise Bialylew for starting me off on the journey with her innovative Mindful In May campaign.

Finally, thanks to Andrew and our beautiful children Ben, Patrick and Luca. Your encouragement and unwavering support keep me going. May you always feel gently held by Earth.

# ENDNOTES

## Chapter 1 – Earth's Biome

1   Mace G et al. Biodiversity. Millennium Ecosystem Assessment. United Naations. 2005: 4: 79-90.

2   Lambers H & Bradshaw D. Australia's south west: a hotspot for wildlife and plants that deserves World Heritage status. The Conversation. 2016 18.2.16.

3   Soil Society America. Soils Overview. 2019. https://www.soils.org/files/about-soils/soils-overview.pdf.

4   Dept. Regional Industries and Regional Development. Dryland salinity in Western Australia. 2022.https://www.agric.wa.gov.au/soil-salinity/dryland-salinity-western-australia-0

5   Mochan K & Gubana B. Salinity crisis destroying Australia's farmland, but farmers hope to stop it Australia: ABC News; 2018 [updated 3.6.18. https://www.abc.net.au/news/rural/2018-06-02/salinity-crisis-for-australias-farmland-but-farmers-fight-back/9826834.

6   McLeman R et al. What we learned from the Dust Bowl: lessons in science, policy, and adaptation. Population and Environment. 2014;35(4):417-40.

7   Shaw E. Difference between a biome and an ecosystem 2018 [cited 2019. https://sciencing.com/difference-between-biome-ecosystem-6468.html.

8   Irish Famine Curriculum Committee. The Great Irish Famine. New Jersey 1998.

9   Department of the Environment & Energy. Leadbeater's Possum- gymnobelideus leadbeateri: Australian Goverment; 2019 [cited 2019. http://www.environment.gov.au/cgi-bin/sprat/public/publicspecies.pl?taxon_id=273.

10  Phillips J. Marine macroalgal biodiversity hotspots: Why is there high species richness and endemism in southern Australian marine benthic flora? Biodiversity and Conservation. 102001.

11  Keith H, Mackey B & Lindenmayer D. Re-evaluation of forest biomass carbon stocks and lessons from the world's most carbon-dense forests. Proceedings of the National Academy of Sciences of the United States of America. 2009;106(28):11635-11640

12  Ellison D. From Myth to Concept and Beyond- The BioGeoPhysical Revolution and the Forest-Water Paradigm. Background study prepared for the thirteenth session of the United Nations Forum on Forests. 2018.

13  Lamb J et al. Seagrass ecosystems reduce exposure to bacterial pathogens of humans, fishes, and invertebrates. Science. 2017;355:731-3.

## Chapter 2 – Our Relationship To Earth

14  Margulis L. Microcosmos: Four Billion Years of Microbial Evolution. New York: University of California Press; 1986.

15  Mc Kinney D. Prof. Suzanne Simard Talks About 'Mother Trees". UBC Reports. Canada. 2011.

16  Wohlleben P. The Hidden Life of Trees:What they feel, how they communicate, discoveries from a secret world. Vancouver: Greystone Books; 2016.

17  Ketcham C. The Life and Death of Pando. Discover Magazine. 19 October, 2018.

18  Baines R. Botanist's bid to save 'King's Holly', world's oldest living plant', from extinction. ABC News. 2014.

19  Clode D. The Wasp and the Orchid Australia: Picador; 2018.

20  Obituaries. Lyn Margulis. The Telegraph. 2011.

21  Sculthorpe T & Sveiby K. Treading Lightly- The Hidden Wisdom of the World's Oldest People. New South Wales: Allen & Unwin; 2006.

22  Kimmerer RW. Braiding Sweetgrass. Minnesota: Milkweed Editons; 2013.

23  Spencer R. Theophrastus Australia: Plants People Planet; 2019. https://plantspeopleplanet.org.au/c1/c1/.

24  Watson D. The Bush. Australia: Pengin Group; 2014.

25  Pascoe B. Salt. Carlton, Australia: Black Ink; 2019.

26  Roach A. Tell Me Why. Australia: Simon & Shuster; 2019.

## Chapter 3 – Human Health Within Earth's Biome

27  Ranadheera SH, Deborah and Barouei, Javad. Explainer: what is the gut microbiota and how does it affect mind and body? Australia: The Conversation; 2016 [cited 2016. https://theconversation.com/explainer-what-is-the-gut-microbiota-and-how-does-it-affect-mind-and-body-40536.

28  Mueller NT, Bakacs E, Combellick J, Grigoryan Z, Dominguez-Bello MG. The infant microbiome development: mom matters. Trends Mol Med. 2015;21(2):109-17.

29  Strachan D. Hayfever, hygiene and household size. BMJ. 1989;299(6710):1259-60.

30  Rook G, Lowry C & Raison C. Microbial 'Old Friends', immunoregulation and stress resilience'. Evolution, Medicine, & Public Health. 2013;2013(1):46-64.

31  Rook G. Regulation of the immune system by biodiversity from the natural environment: An Ecosystem service essential to health. Proceedings of the National Academy of Sciences of the United States of America. 2013;110(46):18360-7.

32  Klaasen HL et al. Apathogenic, intestinal, segmented, filamentous bacteria stimulate the mucosal immune system of mice. Infect Immunol. 1993;61(1):303-6.

33  Sudo N et al. The requirement of intestinal bacterial flora for the development of an IgE production system fully susceptible to oral tolerance induction. J Immunol. 1997;159:1739-45.

34  Kalliomaki M et al. Distinct patterns of neonatal gut microflora in infants in whom atopy was and was not developing. J Allergy Clin Immunol. 2001;107:129-34.

35  Penders J et al. Gut microbiota composition and development of atopic manifestations in infancy: the KOALA Birth Cohort Study. Gut. 2007;56:661-7.

36  Noval Rias M et al. A microbiota signature associated with experimental food allergy promotes allergic sensitization and anaphylaxis. JACI. 2013;131:201-12.

37  Stancel N et al. Interplay between CRP, Atherogenic LDL, and LOX-1 and Its Potential Role in the Pathogenesis of Atherosclerosis. Clin Chem. 2016;62(2):320-7.

38  McDade TW et al. Early origins of inflammation: microbial exposures in infancy predict lower levels of C-reactive protein in adulthood. Proc Biol Sci. 2010;277(1684):1129-37.

39  Kuiper J et al. Immunomodulation of the inflammatory response in atherosclerosis. Curr Opin Lipidol. 2007;18(5):521-6.

40  Gimeno D et al. Associations of C-reactive protein and interleukin-6 with cognitive symptoms of depression: 12-year follow-up of the Whitehall II study. Psychol Med. 2009;39(3):413-23.

41  Valkanova V, Ebmeier KP, Allan CL. CRP, IL-6 and depression: a systematic review and meta-analysis of longitudinal studies. J Affect Disord. 2013;150(3):736-44.

42  Suzuki D. The Legacy An Elder's Vision for our Sustainable Future. Sydney: Allen & Unwin; 2010.

43  Gao B et al. Cone Snails: A Big Store of Conotoxins for Novel Drug Discovery. Toxins. 2017;9(12).

44  Laupu W. Mangosteen Extract's potential to Treat Schizophrenia: a randomized controlled trial: Lambert Academic Publishing; 2016.

45  Guo Mea. alpha-Mangostin Extraction from the Native Mangosteen (Garcinia mangostana L>) and the Binding Mechanisms of alpha-Mangostin to HSA or TRF. PLoS One. 2016;11(9):e0161566.

46  Peel E et al. Cathelicidins in the Tasmanian devil. Scientific Reports. 2016.

47  Higgins I. Australian bush foods are all around us, but the industry is just 'waking up'. Melbourne. ABC News Online. April 2019.

48  Thurston R et al. Aboriginal uses of seaweeds in temperate Australia: an archival assessment. Journal of Applied Phycology. 2018;30:1821-32.

49  Living Culture Victoria, Australia: Living culture; 2020 [home page for living culture- Lionel Lauch]. https://www.livingculture.org.au.

50  School of Biological Sciences. Aboriginal Plants in the Grounds of Monash University- A Guide. Melbourne, Australia: Monash University; 2010.

## Chapter 4 – Nature's Gifts

51  Tyler M et al. Inhibition of gastric acid secretion in the gastric brooding frog, Rheobatrachus silus. Science. 1983;220(4597):609-10.

52  Guerera D, Bhushan B & Kumar N. Lessons from mosquitoes' painless piercing. Journal of the Mechanical Behavior of Biomedical Materials. 2018;84:178-87.

53  Department of Education. From Gumnuts to Buttons [online pdf of educational course for secondary students]. Tasmania: Tasmanian Government; 2019. https://www.google.com/url?sa=t&rct=j&q=&esrc=s&source=web&cd=11&ved=2ahUKEwj_gYG2osPmAhW07HMBHd56C0o4ChAWMAB6BAgDEAE&url=https%3A%2F%2Fwww.theorb.tas.gov.au%2Fbackend%2Fapi%2Fv1%2Fcms%2Fdocuments%2F238%2FFrom_Gumnuts_to_Buttons_Significant_Places_Y9.pdf&usg=AOvVaw3ZBlPOKazS9-30Lscqs22M.

54  Maslow A. Toward a Psychology of Being. New York: Van Nostrand Reinhold; 1968.

55  Cherry K. Peak Experiences in Psychology: verywellmind; 2019. https://www.verywellmind.com/what-are-peak-experiences-2795268.

56  Ward M. The Comfort of Water. A River Pilgrimage. Yarraville: Transit Lounge; 2011.

## Chapter 5 – Nature And Health Today

57  Thunberg G. No One Is Too Small To Make A Difference. United Kingdom: Penguin; 2019.

58  Flannery T. We are the Weather Makers. Melbourne, Australia: Text Publishing; 2006.

59  Allen M et al. Frequently Asked Questions. IPCC. France. 2018.

60  Environmental Investigation Agency. Blowing it: Illegal Production and Use of Banned CFC-11 in China's Foam Blowing Industry. 2018.

61  Buck S. The first American settlers cut down millions of trees to deliberately engineer climate change. Timeline. 2017.

62  Food and Agriculture Organisation of the United Nations. Impacts of climate change on fisheries and accquaculture. Rome, Italy; 2018.

63  Fitzer S. The world's shellfish are under threat as our oceans become more acidic. The Conversation. 2019.

64  Hughes T et al. Global warming impairs stock-recruitment dynamics of corals. Nature. 2019;568;387-90.

65  WWF. Green Turtles and Climate Change 2019. https://www.wwf.org.au/what-we-do/species/green-turtle/green-turtles-and-climate-change#gs.umcxgw.

66  van Oosterzee P and Duke N. Extreme weather explains 'unprecendented' mangrove deaths in NT: study. The Conversation. 2017 March 14, 2017.

67  Babcock R et al. Severe Continental-Scale Impacts of Climate Change Are Happening Now: Extreme Climate Events Impact Marine Habitat Forming Communities Along 45% of Australia's Coast. Frontiers in Marine Science. 2019.

68  CSIRO BoM. State of the Climate 2018. In: Meteorology Bo, editor. Australia: Australian Government; 2018. p. 2-17.

69  Lister B and Garcia A. Climate-driven declines in arthropod abundance restructure in a rainforest food web. PNAS. 2018;115(44):E10397-E406.

70  Carrington D. Insect collapse: We are destroying our life support systems'. The Guardian. 2019 15 Jan 2019.

71  Nicole H. 'Imminent risk': Climate crisis facing Australian rainforests likened to coral bleaching. The Sydney Morning Herald. 2019 April 30, 2019.

72  Wet Tropics Management Authority. A statement from the Board of the Wet Tropics Management Authority regarding serious climate change impacts on the Wet Tropics of Queensland World Heritage Area. In: Authority WTM, editor. Cairns, Queensland2019.

73  Caldwell F. Climate change sparks fears for flying foxes afer 23,000 deaths. Brisbane Times. 2019 March 17,2019.

74  Bowman D. 2019 Tasmanian Fires: Impacts and Management Lessons Fire Centre Research Hub: University of Tasmania; 2019. https://firecentre.org.au/2019-tasmanian-fires-impacts-and-management-lessons/.

75  Harvey F. 'Tipping ponts' could exacerbate climate crisis, scientists fear. The Guardian 2018.

76  Costello et al. Managing the health effects of climate change: Lancet and University College London Institute for Global Health Commission. Lancet. 2009;373(9676):1693-733.

77  Hitch G. Bushfire Royal Commission hears that Black Summer smoke killed nearly 450 people. ABC [Internet]. 2020. https://www.abc.net.au/news/2020-05-26/bushfire-royal-commission-hearings-smoke-killed-445-people/12286094.

78  Doctors for the Environment Australia. Severe Storms, Floods and Your Health. Australia: Doctors for the Environment Australia; 2017.

79  Robine JM et al. Death toll exceeded 70,000 in Europe during summer of 2003. Comptes Rendus Biologies. 2008;331(2):171-8.

80  Dowling J. Melbourne city centre a death trap as heat-island effect takes its toll. The Age. 2014 January 17, 2014.

81  Doctors for the Environment Australia. Heatwaves and Health in Australia. Australia: Doctors for the Environment Australia; 2016.

82  McDermott BM, Lee EM, Judd M, Gibbon P. Posttraumatic stress disorder and general psychopathology in children and adolescents following a wildfire disaster. Can J Psychiatry. 2005;50(3):137-43.

83  Shocket M RS, and Mordecai E. Temperature explains broad patterns of Ross River virus transmission. eLIFE. 2018;7.

84 Sutton B. Health warning on mosquitoes and Ross River virus. Dept. of Health & Human Services, State Government of Victoria, Australia. 2018.

85 Beggs PJ, Bambrick HJ. Is the global rise of asthma an early impact of anthropogenic climate change? Environ Health Perspect. 2005;113(8):915-9.

86 Albrecht G. The age of solastalgia. The Conversation. August 7, 2012.

87 Miller N. 'These issues are global': new NGV exhibit connects country and climate. The Sydney Morning Herald. November 2, 2021.

88 Flood J. The Moth Hunters: Aboriginal Prehistory of the Australian Alps. Canberra: Australian Institute of Aboriginal Studies; 1980.

89 Gale J. History of and Legends relating to the Federal Capital Territory of the Commonwealth of Australia. Queanbeyan: A.M. Pallick & Sons; 1927.

90 Stephenson B, David, Bl, Freslov, J et al. 2000 Year-old Bogong moth (Agrotis infusa) Aboriginal food remains, Australia. Scientific Reports. 2020.

91 Monash University. Aboriginal populations used Bogong moths as a food source 2,000 years ago, researchers find [press release]. 8 February, 2021.

92 Readfearn G. Decline in Bogong moth numbers leaves mountain pygmy possums starving. The Guardian. 2019.

93 Australian Wildlife Conservancy. Feral Cat and Fox Control 2019. https://www.australianwildlife.org/our-work/feral-cat-and-fox-control/

94 Urban M. Accelerating extinction risk from climate change. Science. 2015;348(6234):571-3.

95 The Royal Womens Hospital. Food and nutrition in pregnancy 2019 [cited 2019. https://www.thewomens.org.au/health-information/pregnancy-and-birth/a-healthy-pregnancy/food-nutrition-in-pregnancy.

96 Carson R. Silent Spring. United States: Houghton Mifflin; 1962.

97 Ravindran J, Pankajashan M & Puthur S. Organochlorine pesticides, their toxic effects on living organisms and their fate in the environment. Interdisciplinary Toxicology. 2016;9:90-100.

98 Hasham N. Industrial chemicals: Turnbull government moves to slash safety testing regulations. The Sydney Morning Herald. 2017.

99 Levine H et al. Temporal trends in sperm count: a systematic review and meta-regression analysis. Human Reproduction Update. 2017;23(6):646-59.

100 Swan S. Countdown: How Our Modern World Is Threatening Sperm Counts, Altering Male and Female Reproductive Development, and Imperiling the Future of the Human Race: Scribner; 2021.

101 Pelloura E and Diamanti-Kandarakis E. Polycystic overy syndrome (PCOS) and endocrine disrupting chemicals (EDCs). Review of Endocrinological Metabolic Disorders. 2015;16:365-71.

102 Katz T et al. Endocrine-disrupting chemicals and uterine fibroids. Fertili Steril. 2016;106:967-77.

103 Stephens V et al. The Potential Relsationship Between Environmental Endocrine Disruptor Exposure and the Development of Endometriosis and Adenomyosis. Frontiers in Physiology. 2022;12.

104 Endocrine Society. Endocrine-Disrupting Chemicals 2019. https://www.endocrine.org/topics/edc/what-edcs-are.

105 Calafat A et al. Urinary Concentrations of Bisphenol A and 4-Nonylphenol in a Human Reference Population. Environmental Health Perspectives. 2005;113:391-5.

106 Sanchez-Bayo F and Wyckhuys K. Worldwide decline of the entomofauna: A review of its drivers. Biological Conservation. 2019;232:8-27.

107 Lister B and Garcia A. Climate-driven declines in arthropod abundance restructure a rainforest food web. Proceedings of the National Academy of Sciences of the United States of America. 2018;115;E10397-E406.

108 Hallman C et al. More than 75 percent deline over 27 years in total flying insect biomass in protected areas. PLoS One. 2017;12:e0185809.

109 The Ocean Clean Up. How much plastic floats in the Great Pacific Garbage Patch? 2019 [cited 2019 9.7.19]. https://theoceancleanup.com/great-pacific-garbage-patch/.

110 National Geographic. Great Pacific Garbage Patch 2019. https://www.nationalgeographic.org/encyclopedia/great-pacific-garbage-patch/.

111 World Wildlife Fund. Living Forests Report: Chapter 5- Saving Forests at Risk. 2015.

112 Finn H and Stephens N. The invisible harm: land clearing is a significant issue of animal welfare. Wildlife Research. 2017;44:377-91.

113 Finn H and Stephens N. Land clearing isn't just about trees- it's an animal welfare issue too. The Conversation. July 5, 2017.

114 NITV Staff Writer. International corporation accused of clearing sacred and significant sites. NITV. 7 June, 2019.

115 Queensland Govt. Land cover change in Queensland. In: Science DoEa, editor. Queensland: Queensland Government; 2018.

116 Laurance B and van Oosterezee P. The next global health pandemic could easily erupt in your backyard. The Converstation. 2020.

117 UNEP. UNEP Frontiers 2016 Report- Emerging Issues of Environmental Concern. United Nations Environment Programme. Nairobi; 2016.

118 Parks Australia. Uluru-Kata Tjuta National Park Fact Sheet-Flora. Australia. Australian Government. 2019.

119 Brain C. Report released as feral camel cull ends. ABC News. 21 November 2013.

120 Jack P. Station owners fear feral camels numbers are on the rise, call for better feral animal management. ABC News. 2019;Sect. Rural.

121 Garrick M. Cane toads decimate Kakadu National Park while Commonwealth 'sits on its hands', says experts. ABC News. 2019.

122 Ward-Fear G et al. Sharper eyes see shyer lizards: Collaboration with indigenous peoples can alter the outcomes of conservation research. Conservation Letters. 2019.

123 State Library of Victoria. Introduced Plants 2019. http://ergo.slv.vic.gov.au/explore-history/land-exploration/environment/introduced-plants.

124 Tasmanian Government. Herbicides for Blackberry Control. In: Department of Primary Industries P, Water and Environment, editor. Tasmania: Tasmanian Government; 2019.

125 Californians for Alternatives to Toxics. Toxicological Profile for Triclopyr California: Californians for Alternative to Toxics; 2019. http://www.alt2tox.org/tox_profile-triclopyr.htm.

126 Ecocide Law. 2019. https://ecocidelaw.com.

127 Gauger A et al. The Ecocide Project- 'Ecocide is the missing 5th Crime Against Peace'. London: Human Rights Consortium; 2012.

128 Albrecht G. Ecocide and Solastalgia Australia: Glenn Albrecht; 2019 [updated 22/4/19. https://glennaalbrecht.com/2019/04/22/ecocide-and-solastalgia/.

# Chapter 6 – Our Toxic Relationship With Nature

42  Suzuki D. The Legacy: An Elder's Vision for our Sustainable Future. Sydney: Allen & Unwin; 2010.

129 Department of the Environment. Threatened Species Listings. Canberra, Australia: Australian Government; 2019.

130 Mattingley C. Maralinga's Long Shadow Yvonne's Story. Australia: Allen & Unwin; 2016.

131 Davidson H and Wahiquist C. Australian dig finds evidence of Aboriginal habitation up to 80,000 years ago. The Guardian. 2017 20.7.2017.

132 Lawrence R & Sweeney D. Unfinished Business: Rehabilitating the Ranger Uranium Mine. Sydney, Australia: University of Sydney; 2019 7 May 2019.

133 Townsend M. Quantifying the health and wellbeing benefits of nature. Valuing Nature: Protected Areas and Ecosystem Services. Perspectives on natural systems. Australia: Australian Committee for IUCN; 2015. p. 34-7.

134 Balmford A, Clegg L, Coulson T, Taylor J. Why conservationists should heed Pokemon. Science. 2002;295(5564):2367.

135 Paull D et al. Koala habitat conservation plan. Australia. WWF; 2019.

136 Wilkinson M. Koala numbers dive on east coast. Four Corners. ABC. 2012.

137 Lang D. The Nature of Survival. Victoria, Australia. Doug Lang. 2016.

138 Clark I and Kostanski L. An Indigenous History of Stonnington- A Report to the City of Stonnington. Victoria, Australia: City of Stonnington; 2006.

139 Beath N and Wilmoth L. Gardiner Family. Papers, 1814-65, 1959. National Library of Australia. 1960.

140 Pascoe B. Dark Emu. Black seeds: agriculture or accident? Broome, Western Australia: Magabala Books; 2014.

141 Sutton P and Walshe K. Farmers of Hunter-gatherers? Melbourne, Australia: Melbourne University Press; 2021.

142 Gammage B. The Biggest Estate on Earth. New South Wales: Allen & Unwin; 2011.

143 Yunkaporta T. Sand Talk. Melbourne: The Text Publishing Company; 2019.

144 Minister for the Environment. Stronger protection for threatened species. Dept. of the environment and Energy. Australian Governement. Canberra. 2019. https://www.environment.gov.au/minister/price/media-releases/mr20190218a.html.

145 Hannam P. 'Slashed': Morrison government delays assessments for threatened species. The Age. 2019.

146 Horstman M. Tassie BioBlitz bags 'monster' crayfish among haul of hundreds of species Melbourne: ABC news; 2018. https://www.abc.net.au/news/science/2018-03-24/bioblitz-bags-giant-freshwater-crayfish/9572546.

147 Haswell M and Shearman D. The implications for human health and wellbeing of expanding gas mining in Australia: Onshore Oil and Gas Policy Background Paper. Doctors for the Environment Australia; 2019.

## Chapter 7 – Today's Health Challenges

148 Taylor, M et al. Full Description of Mount Isa Contaminant Research. 2010. Australia. Macquarie University.

149 Gerrard J. Active Transport: Children and young people. An overview of evidence. Melbourne. Vichealth. 2009.

150 Salmon J and Okely T. Sitting less for children. National Heart Foundation of Australia. 2011. https://www.heartfoundation.org.au/getmedia/221f8585-8b43-4f43-af41-f2eca067e0d2/PA-Sitting-Less-Child.pdf.

151 Kolb B and Gibb R. Brain Plasticity and Behaviour in the Developing Brain. Journal Canadian Academy Child and Adolescent Psychiatry. 2011;20(4):265-76.

152 Australian Institute for Health and Welfare. Childhood overweight and obesity. Canberra. 2014.

153 Parikesit D et al. The impact of obesity towards prostate diseases. Prostate International. 2016;4(1):1-6.

154 Lambrot R, et al. Low paternal dietary folate alters the mouse sperm epigenome and is associated with negative pregnancy outcomes. Nature communications. 2013;4(2889).

155 Food Standards Australia and New Zealand. Folic acid fortification Australia2016. http://www.foodstandards.gov.au/consumer/nutrition/folicmandatory/Pages/default.aspx.

## Chapter 8 – Nature-based Solutions

156 Australian Bureau of Statistics. Vitamin D. Canberra: Australian Bureau of Statistics; 2014.

157 Department of Health. Clinical Practice Guidelines Antenatal Care: Module 1: 8.9. Vitamin D deficiency. Australia. Australian Government. 2013.

158 Cancer Council. The SunSmart UV Alert [cited 2016 6/3/16]. information on sunsmart app from Cancer Council. http://www.cancercouncil.com.au/66659/cancer-prevention/sun-protection/local-government-workplace/sunsmart-uv-alert/.

159 French AN et al. Risk factors for incident myopia in Australian schoolchildren: the Sydney adolescent vascular and eye study. Ophthalmology. 2013;120(10):2100-8.

160 Perraton L, Kumar, S, and Machotka, Z. Exercise parameters in the treatment of clinical depression: a systematic review of randomized controlled trials. Journal Evaluation Clinical Practice. 2010;16(3):597-604.

161 Li Q. Effect of forest bathing trips on human immune function. Environ Health Prev Med. 2010;15(1):9-17.

162 Mao GX et al. Therapeutic effect of forest bathing on human hypertension in the elderly. J Cardiol. 2012;60(6):495-502.

163 Li Q. The Japanese Art and Science of Shinrin-Yoku Forest Bathing. New York: Viking; 2018.

164 Dirksen K. Science of 'forest bathing': fewer maladies, more well-being? Youtube; 2016.

165 Prescription Trails New Mexico2016 [cited 2016. website with prescription trails for New Mexico]. https://prescriptiontrails.org.

166 Zarr R, Cottrell, L and Merrill, C. Park Prescription (DC Park Rx): A New Strategy to Combat Chronic Disease in Children. Journal of Physical Activity and Health. 2017;14(1):1-2.

167 Park Rx America. America 2020. https://parkrxamerica.org/about.php.

168 People and Parks Foundation. GP Green Referrals People and Parks Foundation webpage: People and Parks Foundation. http://www.peopleandparks.org/projects-activities/gp-green-referrals-program.

169 Ulrich RS. View through a window may influence recovery from surgery. Science. 1984;224(4647):420-1.

170 Maller C et al. healthy parks healthy people literature review. Melbourne, Victoria: Deakin University and Parks Victoria; 2008.

171 Mc Sweeney J et al. Indoor nature exposure (INE): a health-promotion framework. Health Promotion International. 2015;30(1):126-39.

172 Lohr V and Person-Mims C. Physical discomfort may be reduced in the presence of interior plants. International Human Issues in Horticulture. 2000;10:53-9.

173 Wood R et al. The Potted-Plant Microcosm Sustantially Reduces Indoor Air VOC Pollution: 1. Office Field-Study. Water, Air, and Soil Pollution. 2006;175:163-80.

174 Burchett M, Torpy F & Irga P. Indoor plants work. Sydney: University of Technology, Sydney, Group UPalEQR; 2014.

## Chapter 9 – Green Mind

175 Porges S. The Polyvagal Perspective. Biological Psychology. 2006;74(2):116-43.

176 Australian Childhood Foundation. Polyvagal Theory and its implications for Traumatised Students. Australia: Australian childhood foundation; 2011.

177 Hanson R. Hardwiring Happiness. United Kingdom: Rider; 2013.

178 Taft M. Downtime for the Stone-age Brain. The Wise Brain Bulletin. 2016;10(2):1-8.

179 International Fragrance Association. About the IFRA Transparency List 2019 [30/10/19]. https://ifrafragrance.org/initiatives/transparency/ifra-transparency-list.

180 Silva-Neto RP, Peres MF, Valenca MM. Odorant substances that trigger headaches in migraine patients. Cephalalgia. 2014;34(1):14-21.

181 Grenville K. The Case Against Fragrance. Melbourne, Australia: Griffin Press; 2017.

182 Australian Psychological Society. Australian Loneliness Report. 2018.

183 Gilbert P & Choden. Mindful Compassion. United Kingdom. Robinson. 2013.

184 Australian Bureau of Statistics. Personal Safety Survey. Canberra with Australian Government; 2016.

185 Bryant W and Bricknell S. Homicide in Australia 2012-13 to 2013-14: National Homicide Monitoring Program report. Canberra: Australian Institute of Criminology; 2017.

186 Vassos E et al. Urban-rural differences in incidence rates of psychiatric disorders in Denmark. Br J Psychiatry. 2016;208(5):435-40.

187 Lederbogen F et al. City living and urban upbringing affect neural social stress processing in humans. Nature. 2011;474(7352):498-501.

188 Hallowell E. Driven to distraction at work. Massachusetts: Harvard Business School; 2015.

189 Chandra M et al. Screen time of infants in Sydney, Australia: a birth cohort study. BMJ Open. 2016;6(10).

190 Hancox RJ, Milne BJ & Poulton R. Association between child and adolescent television viewing and adult health: a longitutidinal birth cohort study. Lancet. 2004;364:257-62.

191 Gadberry S. Effect of restricting first graders' TV-viewing on leisure time use, IQ hanged, and cognitive style. Journal of Applied Developmental Psychology. 1980;1(1):45-57.

192 Evans Schmidt M et al. The Effects of Background Television on the Toy Play Behaviour of Very Young Children. Child Development. 2008;79(4):1137-51.

193 Department of Health. Move and Play Every Day-National Physical Activity Recommendations for Children 0-5 years. Canberra. Australia. Australian Government.

194 Strom M. Sydney Observatory wants Australia's first urban dark sky park. Sydney Morning Herald. 2017.

195 Nichols WJ. Blue Mind. Little, Brown & Company. Boston. 2014.

196 Rogers K. Biophilia hypothesis Encyclopedia Britannica [updated 3/5/1131/10/17]. https://www.britannica.com/science/biophilia-hypothesis.

197 Bratman G et al. Nature experience reduces rumination and subgenual prefrontal cortex activation. PNAS. 2015;112(28):8567-72.

198 Williams F. This is Your Brain on Nature. National Geographic. January 2016.

199 Atchley RA, Strayer DL, Atchley P. Creativity in the Wild: Improving Creative Reasoning through Immersion in Natural Settings. PLOS ONE. 2012;7(12):e51474.

200 Planet Ark. Adding Trees- a prescription for health, happiness and fulfilment. Australia: Planet Ark; 2016.

201 Planet Ark. Needing Trees: The Nature of Happiness. Australia: Planet Ark; 2015.

202 Sebba R. The Landscapes of Childhood. The reflection of childhood's environment in adult memories and in children's attitudes. Environment and Behaviour. 1991;23(4):395-422.

203 OLPRO. Camping improves your sex life [press release]. UK, 26.9.13.

204 Slepian M and Ambady N. Fluid movement and creativity. Journal of Experimental Psychology General 2012;141(4):625-9.

205 Harrison E. Meditation and Health. Perth: Perth Meditation Centre; 2001.

206 Hassed C. Driven to distraction: Why be mindful in thie unmindful world? In: Blashki, G & Sykes, H. (editors) Life surfing life dancing. Melbourne, Australia: Future Leaders; 2013.

207 Benson H. The Relaxation Response. New York: Harper Collins; 1975.

208 Hansen R. Positive Neuroplasticity: The Mindful Cultivation of Durable Inner Resources. Australian Meditation Conference; 2018; Melbourne, Australia.

209 Epel E et al. Can meditation slow rate of cellular aging? Cognitive stress, mindfulness, and telomeres. Ann N Y Acad Sci. 2009;1172:34-53.

## Chapter 10 – A Green Mind Approach To Mental Illness, Stress, And Suffering

210 Roszak T. The Nature of Sanity. Psychology Today. 1996, reviewed last June 2016.

211 Burns GW. Sunsets and Seashores. Nature-Guided Therapy in Positive Couple and Family Work. In: Burns GW, editor. Happiness, healing and enhancement. New Jersey: Wiley; 2010. p. 239-51.

212 Gottman JM, Swanson, C.C, & Swanson, K.R. A general systems theory of marriage; Nonlinear difference equation modelling of marital interaction Personality and Social Psychology Review. 2002;6 (4):326-40.

213 Adventure Works. Therapeutic programs and counselling support Australia 2019. [cited 2019]. https://adventureworks.org.au/services/.

26  Roach A. Tell Me Why. Australia: Simon & Shuster; 2019.

214 Autism Awareness Australia. Surfers Healing Australia 2018 Australia: Autism Awareness Australia; 2017 [cited 2018 12/11/18]. http://www.autismawareness.com.au/news-events/events-campaigns/surfers-healing-australia-2018/.

215 The Wave Project. The Wave Project Torquay- Australia Pilot Evaluation report. 2016.

216 Ocean Mind. Changing lives through surfing 2018 [home page of Open Mind]. https://oceanmind.org.au.

217 Ashfar P et al. Effect of White Noise on Sleep in Patients Admitted to a Coronary Care. Journal of Caring Sciences. 2016;5(2):103-9.

218 Alvarsson J, Wiens S & Nilsson M. Stress Recovery during Exposure to Nature Sound and Environmental Noise. Int J Environ Res Public Health. 2010;7(3):1036-46.

219 Townsend M and Ebden M. Feel Blue, Touch Green. Victoria, Australia: Deakin University; 2006.

137 Lang D. The Nature of Survival. Victoria, Australia. Doug Lang. 2016.

220 Adventure Works. A brief survey of the evidence Australia: Adventure Works Australia Ltd.; 2017. https://adventureworks.org.au/a-brief-survey-of-the-evidence/.

221 Active in Parks. Barwon Medicare Local Case Study 2011. http://activeinparks.org/members/case-studies/youth-ambassadors-program/.

222 Australian Indigenous Psychology Education Project Australia: AIPEP; 2020. http://www.indigenouspsyched.org.au/about#overview.

223 North Coast Primary Health Network. Being on Country Brings Greater Engagement and Sharing in Suicide Prevention Workshops [press release]. New South Wales. 2017.

224 Kenyon G. How an Aboriginal approach to mental health is helping farmers deal with drought. Mosaic. 23 April 2019.

## Chapter 11 – Growing Up In Nature

225 Carson R. The Sense of Wonder. New York. Harper & Rowe Publishers; 1965.

226 Winton T. Island home, a landscape memoir. Australia. Hamish Hamilton. 2015.

227 Molomot L. School's Out. Lessons from a Forest Kindergarten. 2013.

228 Hashmi K and Marshall F. You and Me, Murrawee. Victoria, Australia. Puffin; 1999.

229 Children's Garden 2016. https://www.rbg.vic.gov.au/visit-melbourne/attractions/children-garden.

230 Andrews J. Fox Kids Early Learning Centre follows European outside sleeping model for babies. Leader Community News. 16 June 2016.

231 Mirams S. Situated Among the Gum Trees: the Blackburn Open Air School. Provenance: The Journal of Public Record Office Victoria. 2011(10).

232 Bagot K, Allen, F and Toukhsati, S. Perceived restorativeness of children's school playground environments: Nature, playground features and play period experiences. Journal of Environmental Psychology. 2015;41:1-9.

233 Kaplan S. The restorative benefits of nature: Toward an integrative framework. Journal of Environmental Psychology. 1995;15(3):169-82.

234 Matsuoka R. Student performance and high school landscapes: Examining the links. Landscape and Urban Planning. 2010;97(4):273-82.

235 American Institute for Research. Effects of Outdoor Education Programs for Children in California. 2005.

236 International Association of Nature Pedagogy. https://www.naturepedagogy.com.

237 Griffiths J. Kith: The riddle of the childscape. London: Hamish Hamilton; 2013.

238 Department for Environment. The natural choice: securing the value of nature. United Kingdom. HM Government. 2011.

239 Malone K and Waite S. Student outcomes and Natural Schooling. Plymouth: Plymouth University; 2016.

240 Waite S, Passy, R et al. Natural Connections Demonstration Project, 2012-2016: Final Report. Natural England Commissioned reports; 2016.

241 Plymouth University. Transforming outdoor learning in schools- lessons from the natural connections project. Plymouth: Plymouth University; 2016.

242 University of Copenhagen. TrygFondens Udeskole Research Project 2013-2016 (TEACHOUT). University of Copenhagen; 2016.

243 Bolling M et al. Children & Nature network2017. [cited 2017]. https://www.childrenandnature.org/2017/04/06/growing-the-udeskole-movement-finding-balance-in-school-based-outdoor-learning-2/.

244 Meng NC. Speech by Acting Minister for Education (Schools) Ng Chee Meng. Singapore. 2016.

245 Sir Ken Robinson. Do schools Kill Creativity? TED2006. Accessed Oct. 2022. https://www.ted.com/talks/ken_robinson_says_schools_kill_creativity#t-1135208

246 Tes Magazine. Sir Ken Robinson shares five reasons you should take your class outside. TES; 2016.

247 Outdoor Classroom Day. Outdoor Classroom Day UK & Ireland 2017. https://www.tes.com/news/school-news/breaking-news/watch-sir-ken-robinson-shares-five-reasons-you-should-take-your-class.

248 Council on Epidemiology. Air Pollution and Heart Disease, Stroke. American Heart Association; 2015.

249 Brook RD et al. Particulate matter air pollution and cardiovascular disease: An update to the scientific statement from the American Heart Association. Circulation. 2010;121(21):2331-78.

250 Australian Institute of Health and Welfare. Australian burden of disease study: impact and causes of illness and death in Australia 2011. Canberra. 2016.

251 Howarth D. Lead exposure. Implications for general practice. Australian Family Physician. 2012;41(5):311-5.

252 Davand P et al. Risks and benefits of green spaces for children: a cross-sectional study of associations with sedentary behavior, obesity, asthma, and allergy. Environ Health Perspect. 2014;122(12):1329-35.

253 CSIRO. Projections of days over 35 degrees C to 2100 for all capital cities under a no-mitigation case, data prepared for the Garnaut Climae Change Review Aspendale, Victoria. 2008.

254 Doctors for the Environment Australia. No time for games. Children's health and climate change. 2015.

255 City of Melbourne. Urban Forest Strategy. Making a great city greener. 2012-2032. City of Melbourne; 2012.

256 Barlass T. 5000 trees chopped down at NSW schools after Bridget Wright killed in playground, says Education Department. The Sydney Morning Herald. 28 August 2014.

257 Peeples L. Why these goalies are worried about unknown toxins in artificial turf. The Huffington Post. 31 May 2014.

258 Brown D. Artificial Turf. Environment and Human Health Inc; Connecticut. 2007. https://www.ehhi.org/turf_report07.pdf

259 Zhang J; Han IZ, L and Crain, W. Hazardous chemicals in synthetic turf materials and their bioaccessibility in digestive fluids. Journal of Exposure Science and Environmental Epidemiology. 2008;18:600-7.

260 World Commission on the Ethics of Scientific Knowledge and Technology. The Precautionary Principle. United Nations Educational, Scientific and cultural Organisation; 2005.

261 Gosk S. Feds finally take action on crumb rubber turf. NBC News; 12 February 2016.

262 Federal Research on Recycled Tire Crumbs Used on Playing Fields EPA website: EPA; 2016 [24/6/16]. https://www.epa.gov/chemical-research/federal-research-recycled-tire-crumbs-used-playing-fields.

263 Elliott S and Chancellor B. Westgarth Kindergarten Bush Kinder Evaluation Westgarth Kindergarten and RMIT University; 2012.

264 Gill T. Rethinking Childhood. United Kingdom. 2016. [home page for Tim Gill]. https://rethinkingchildhood.com/no-fear/.

265 Victorian Curriculum and Assessment Authority. Snapshot 2- Balee Koolin Bubup Bush Playgroup. Victoria, Australia. Early Years Exchange- Victorian Early Years Learning and Development Framework. 2014.

266 Block K et al. Evaluation of the Stephanie Alexander Kitchen Garden Program. Mc Caughey Centre; 2009.

267 Nutrition Australia. Australian Dietary Guidelines 2013 [cited 2016 17/8/16]. http://www.nutritionaustralia.org/national/resource/australian-dietary-guidelines-2013.

268 Sobel D. Beyond Ecophobia. Yes! Magazine. November 1998.

269 Sampson SD. How to raise a wild child. New York: Houghton Mifflin Harcourt Publishing Company; 2015.

270 Australian Institute for Teaching and School Leadership. Wetlands at Bentleigh Secondary College. 2014.

271 Wood A and R. Billabong Boy. Australia: New Holland Publishers; 2010.

272 Wood A and R. Inspiring the next young environmental leaders (Kids teaching Kids). Victoria: Firestarter; 2007.

273 Wells N and Lekies K. Nature and the LIfe Course: Pathways from Childhood Nature Experiences to Adult Environmentalism. Children, Youth and Environments. 2006;16(1):1-24.

274 Sobel D. Wild Play: Parenting Adventures in the Great Outdoors. San Francisco, CA.: Sierra Book Club; 2011.

197 Atchley RA, Strayer DL, Atchley P. Creativity in the Wild: Improving Creative Reasoning through Immersion in Natural Settings. PLOS ONE. 2012;7(12):e51474.

275 Immordino-Yang M, Christodoulou, JA and Singh, V. Rest is not idleness: Implications of the Brain's Default Mode for Human Development and Education. Perspectives on Psychological Science. 2012;7(4):352-64.

# Epilogue

276 Haudenosaunee Confederacy. Haudenosaunee Thanksgiving Address Greetings to the Natural World. United States of America: Six Nations Indian Museum and the Tracking Project.

22 Kimmerer RW. Braiding Sweetgrass. Minnesota: Milkweed Editons; 2013.

137 Lang D. The Nature of Survival. Victoria, Doug Lang. Australia. 2016.

277 Ungunmerr M-R. Dadirri- Inner Deep Listening and Quiet Still Awareness. In: Miriam-Rose Foundation. Australia. 1988.

278 Public Health Association Australia. Aboriginal and Torres Strait Islander Guide to terminology. ACT: PHAA; 2020.

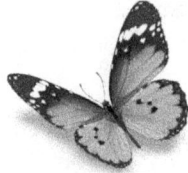

*For more information about Dr Dimity Williams,*

*visit* www.natureourmedicine.com

*email* info@natureourmedicine.com

*or to connect with Dimity*

**f** natureourmedicine

**⊙** natureourmedicine

## DID YOU ENJOY
## READING THIS BOOK?

*If so, it would be wonderful if you could please take a few moments to post a positive review on Amazon.*

*Share your thoughts on what you loved about the book so others can benefit from your experience of Nature, Our Medicine.*

*In turn, they can enjoy it too.*

*Thank you so much!*